Postg

The Canc

Postgraduate Vascular Surgery

The Candidate's Guide to the FRCS

Edited by

Vish Bhattacharya
Queen Elizabeth Hospital

Gerard Stansby
Freeman Hospital

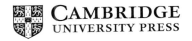
CAMBRIDGE
UNIVERSITY PRESS

CAMBRIDGE UNIVERSITY PRESS
Cambridge, New York, Melbourne, Madrid, Cape Town, Singapore,
São Paulo, Delhi, Dubai, Tokyo, Mexico City

Cambridge University Press
The Edinburgh Building, Cambridge CB2 8RU, UK

Published in the the United States of America by Cambridge University Press, New York

www.cambridge.org
Information on this title: www.cambridge.org/9780521133524

First published 2010

Printed in the United Kingdom at the University Press, Cambridge

A catalogue record for this publication is available from the British Library

Library of Congress Cataloguing in Publication data
Postgraduate vascular surgery : the candidate's guide to the FRCS / [edited by] Vish Bhattacharya,
   Gerard Stansby.
      p. ; cm.
   Includes bibliographical references and index.
   ISBN 978-0-521-13352-4 (pbk.)
   1. Blood-vessels–Surgery–Handbooks, manuals, etc.   I. Bhattacharya, Vish.   II. Stansby,
   Gerard.   III. Title.
   [DNLM: 1. Vascular Surgical Procedures–Handbooks.   2. Vascular Diseases–surgery–
   Handbooks. WG 39]
   RD598.5.P67 2010
   617.4'13–dc22   2010039933

ISBN 978-0-521-13352-4 Paperback

Contents

Contributors

Mohamed Abdelhamid
Department of Vascular Surgery,
University Hospital Birmingham
NHS Foundation Trust, Selly Oak Hospital,
Birmingham, UK

Hassan Badri
Gateshead Health NHS Foundation Trust,
Queen Elizabeth Hospital, Sheriff Hill,
Gateshead, UK

Arun Balakrishnan
The Northern Vascular Centre,
Freeman Hospital, High Heaton,
Newcastle upon Tyne, UK

Vish Bhattacharya
Gateshead Health NHS Foundation Trust,
Queen Elizabeth Hospital,
Sheriff Hill, Gateshead, UK

Paul Blair
Department of Vascular Endovascular
Surgery, Royal Victoria Hospital, Belfast, UK

Julie Brittenden
University Department of Surgery,
Aberdeen Royal Infirmary, Aberdeen,
UK

Rod Chalmers
University Department of Surgery,
Royal Infirmary of Edinburgh,
Edinburgh, UK

Mike Clarke
The Northern Vascular Centre,
Freeman Hospital, High Heaton,
Newcastle upon Tyne, UK

Marcus Cleanthis
The Northern Vascular Centre,
Freeman Hospital, High Heaton,
Newcastle upon Tyne, UK

David M. Cressey
Department of Anaesthesia,
Freeman Hospital, High Heaton,
Newcastle upon Tyne, UK

Chris Davies
Department of Vascular Surgery,
Southampton General Hospital,
Southampton, UK

Robert Davies
University Department of Vascular
Surgery, Heart of England NHS
Foundation Trust, Birmingham, UK

Jeremy French
Transplantation and Hepatobiliary Surgery,
Freeman Hospital, High Heaton,
Newcastle upon Tyne, UK

Dharmendra Garg
Gateshead Health NHS Foundation Trust,
Queen Elizabeth Hospital,
Sheriff Hill, Gateshead, UK

Robbie George
Department of Vascular Endovascular
Surgery, Royal Victoria Hospital, Belfast,
UK

George Hamilton
University Department of Vascular
Surgery, Royal Free Hospital, London,
UK

Mathew Jacob
Transplantation and Hepatobiliary Surgery,
Freeman Hospital, High Heaton,
Newcastle upon Tyne, UK

Mark Kay
Coventry and Warwickshire County
Vascular Unit, University Hospitals
Coventry, UK

David Lambert
The Northern Vascular Centre,
Freeman Hospital, High Heaton,
Newcastle upon Tyne, UK

Tim Lees
The Northern Vascular Centre,
Freeman Hospital, High Heaton,
Newcastle upon Tyne, UK

Asif Mahmood
Department of Surgery, Good
Hope Hospital, Sutton Coldfield,
Birmingham, UK

Derek Manas
Transplantation and Hepatobiliary Surgery,
Freeman Hospital, High Heaton,
Newcastle upon Tyne, UK

Colette Marshall
Coventry and Warwickshire County
Vascular Unit, University Hospitals
Coventry, UK

David C. Mitchell
Department of Vascular Surgery,
Southmead Hospital, Westbury-on-Trym,
Bristol, UK

A. Ross Naylor
Department of Surgery, Leicester Royal
Infirmary, Leicester, UK

William D. Neary
Department of Vascular Surgery,
Southmead Hospital, Westbury-on-Trym,
Bristol, UK

Ian D. Nesbitt
Department of Anaesthesia,
Freeman Hospital, High Heaton,
Newcastle upon Tyne, UK

Colin Nice
Gateshead Health NHS Foundation Trust,
Queen Elizabeth Hospital, Sheriff Hill,
Gateshead, UK

Andrew Platts
Consultant Vascular Interventional
Radiologist, Vascular Unit, Royal Free
Hospital, University College Medical
School, London, UK

Jenny Richards
University of Edinburgh, Royal Infirmary
of Edinburgh, Edinburgh, UK

Mohammed Sharif
Department of Vascular and
Endovascular Surgery, Belfast City
Hospital, Belfast, UK

Cliff Shearman
Department of Vascular Surgery,
Southampton General Hospital,
Southampton, UK

Jonathan Smout
The Northern Vascular Centre,
Freeman Hospital, High Heaton,
Newcastle upon Tyne, UK

Gerard Stansby
The Northern Vascular Centre,
Freeman Hospital, High Heaton,
Newcastle upon Tyne, UK

Rajiv Vohra
Department of Vascular Surgery,
Selly Oak Hospital, Birmingham, UK

Rob Williams
Department of Radiology,
Freeman Hospital, High Heaton,
Newcastle upon Tyne, UK

Alasdair Wilson
Department of Surgery, University of
Aberdeen, Aberdeen Royal Infirmary,
Aberdeen, UK

Preface

Examinations are always challenging although less so for the well prepared. The Intercollegiate Exit Examination in Surgery, in particular, often causes considerable anguish for the candidates. It is expensive to fail the examination, both financially and emotionally. It is a high stake examination and comes at a critical stage in a young surgeon's career when he or she is nearing the end of training.

Over many years, and having discussed the examination with both successful and unsuccessful candidates, we felt that a book was required that would provide a quick, easy read for candidates already under pressure to cover a vast array of subjects. It would need to be pitched at the right level and would complement both clinical experience and aid personal revision.

This book has been divided into two sections. The clinical cases section has been written by two recently successful candidates who have incorporated the views of several trainees to make this section relevant to their needs.

The second section has been written by experts in their respective fields who have provided succinct chapters in a concise format. All the co-authors are surgical trainees, most of whom have passed the examination or are preparing for it. Key points have been mentioned at the beginning of the chapters to aid quick revision before the examinations. References have been deliberately kept to a minimum.

We thank all the contributors for their hard work and timely submission of manuscripts. We are especially grateful to Nick Dunton and Katie James of Cambridge University Press for their continuous support and timely reminders.

Though we appreciate the fact that it takes more than a book to pass the examinations we hope this book serves as a useful tool for candidates to achieve success. Good luck!

Section 1

Final FRCS vascular clinicals

The current format of the Final FRCS clinical examination for vascular candidates consists of both general surgery and vascular clinicals. These examinations have the same layout, and are taken on the same day. Each clinical consists of a series of five short stations taken in rapid succession. For each examination there are two examiners who will take turns in questioning and marking the candidate. The cases are either a patient encounter or interpreting an investigation. With the final examination being directed at ascertaining competence to become a consultant, the questions tend to relate to management issues rather than testing your ability to perform a head-to-toe clinical assessment. However, as senior trainees it is expected that you should know how to examine a patient in an orderly and effective fashion. Failure to demonstrate this in the clinical encounters will ring alarm bells with the examiners.

The short case format of the clinicals should not be viewed as a hurdle, but rather as an opportunity for you to impart your fundamental knowledge on a broad range of topics. The examination process is an efficient way of assessing a wide range of subjects in a limited period of time, in a systematic manner. Candidates who have gone through the clinicals are often left stunned by the number of topics that have been discussed in a blur of 30 minutes. Candidates should therefore see the benefits of this system where a poor performance for one case becomes a small part of the whole marking scheme. It is essential that candidates who feel that they have done badly at one station do not dwell on their misfortune, but compose themselves and get on with the rest of the assessment believing they can still pass.

It is important that as the candidate you listen carefully to the examiner's questions. The instructions will often be extremely focused, and initially seem quite a minor request. The initial 'starter' question will then lead on to more complex issues. The questions are generally not intended to catch you out, so do what you are asked to do. It is essential that you appear comfortable dealing with patients. Although observed examination practice with colleagues is very useful, it can also be helpful to get into a habit of examining patients in outpatient clinics in the same systematic manner as you would use in the examination. Your actions will then become effortless and automatic in the high adrenaline situation of the examination. It is important to get over the 'pass/fail' information and common conditions before moving on to rarities. As the clinical examinations and vivas all depend on verbal interaction to impart your knowledge, it is vitally important to practice viva questioning with colleagues. This will help you formulate a structure to your answers in an orderly fashion, and you should quickly notice an improvement in your performance.

When anticipating cases for your clinical examination, common conditions in mobile patients will appear most frequently. If you have ever been in the situation of organising patients for a clinical examination you realise that the mobile elderly and those with stable chronic disease are easiest to recruit. There will always be a small pool of rarities such as Klippel–Trénaunay syndrome or carotid body tumours that are willing to turn up for examinations. It would be extremely unusual for an acute life-, or limb-threatening problem to turn up to an examination. When performing the clinicals try to smile when introducing yourself to the patients and thank the patients following the encounter (the same applies to thanking the examiners!). The examination day can actually become quite repetitive for the patients and examiners alike. Try hard to make them feel that their participation is valued, and demonstrate that you can put patients at their ease.

Last minute revision can be helpful as topics recently read have a habit of turning up in examinations. Despite this, turning up to the examination sleep deprived will not help your performance; hence a sensible balance must be met. Research has demonstrated that moderate sleep deprivation produces impaired cognitive and motor performance similar to alcohol intoxication. You would not expect to pass an examination whilst intoxicated!

Introduction to the examination and clinical cases

Jonathan Smout and Asif Mahmood

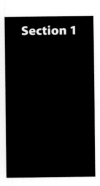

Popliteal aneurysm

The basics

Popliteal aneurysms (PAs) are the commonest peripheral aneurysm (Figure I.1). Approximately half are bilateral and half are associated with an aortic aneurysm. Conversely, 5–10% of patients with an abdominal aortic aneurysm (AAA) have a PA. The majority of PAs present with distal ischaemic complications in either the acute or chronic situation. The prevalence of the PA is thought to be around 1% for those in their eighth decade. When presenting acutely with distal limb ischaemia, limb loss occurs in up to 50% of cases. PAs almost exclusively occur in males. When treatment is indicated PAs are generally treated by surgical exclusion although endovascular management is a newer development in selected cases. Occasionally patients with patent PAs and very diseased run-off may be managed long term with anticoagulation to reduce the risk of aneurysm thrombosis.

The case

Popliteal aneurysms are usually easy to identify as an expansile, or prominent, pulsation in the popliteal fossa. The artery is best palpated against the tibia in the midline of the popliteal fossa, with the knee in the extended position (or with a few degrees of flexion). The artery can also be palpated with the knee flexed to 130°; in this position the popliteal fascia loosens to aid palpation. However, in doing so the manoeuvre deepens the artery from the skin surface. When thrombosed, PAs may be more difficult to diagnose clinically. It is important to assess the distal circulation for evidence of embolisation into the foot or calf vessels. Other posterior knee swellings include a Baker's cyst or a semimembranosus bursa. Remember a PA can exist at any point along the course of the popliteal artery and include the lower SFA as well. In contrast, Baker's cyst originates below the level of the knee joint as it extends beneath the gastrocnemius muscle. A Baker's cyst will often be associated with symptoms and signs suggestive of degenerative arthritis of the knee joint. When present, an enlarged semimembranosus bursa will be located medially under the popliteal edge of the semimembranosus muscle.

Questions

How do PAs present?

In the acute situation PAs usually present with distal ischaemia as a consequence of acute thrombosis or distal embolisation. In the chronic situation they present with intermittent

Postgraduate Vascular Surgery: The Candidate's Guide to the FRCS, eds. Vish Bhattacharya and Gerard Stansby. Published by Cambridge University Press. © Cambridge University Press 2010.

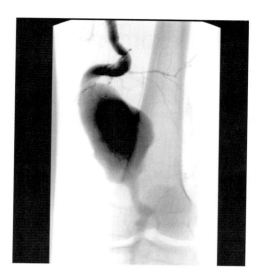

Figure I.1 Angiographic image of a popliteal aneurysm.

claudication as a result of chronic embolisation to the tibial vessels. Asymptomatic PAs are often identified when screening patients with known aortic aneurysms. In contrast to aortic aneurysms, rupture of a PA is a relatively rare occurrence (<5%). Other rarer presentations result from local pressure on surrounding nerves and/or popliteal vein, and they can be the cause of a deep vein thrombosis (DVT).

Tell me about the anatomy of the popliteal artery?

The popliteal artery commences when the femoral artery passes through the adductor hiatus in the thigh. The vessel terminates as it splits into the anterior tibial artery and tibioperoneal trunk at the lower border of popliteus muscle. The popliteal artery gives off genicular branches at several levels to form a large collateral network about the knee joint. The artery is the deepest major structure in the popliteal fossa, and sits beneath the popliteal vein. The tibial nerve lies superficial to the popliteal vein. This organisation is not in the classical vein/artery/nerve configuration.

How would you approach the proximal and distal popliteal artery?

Although the popliteal artery can be approached via posterior or lateral incisions, the most common routes of proximal and distal access are via the medial approach. The supra-geniculate artery is accessed via an incision in the distal third of thigh along the anterior border of the sartorius muscle. This muscle is mobilised posterior and the artery is identified between the medial intramuscular septum anteriorly and semimembranosus muscle posteriorly. The infrageniculate popliteal artery is exposed medially via a longitudinal incision, 1 cm behind the posterior/medial border of the tibia. The long saphenous vein (LSV) is usually located posterior to the incision, and care must me made not to damage it! A tissue plane is bluntly created between the soleus and gastrocnemius muscles. The tendons of sartorius, gracilis and semitendinosus often require division for more proximal access. The popliteal vein must be mobilised as this sits in front of the artery from the medial approach.

What are your indications for elective repair?

In contrast to AAAs, where there is clear consensus on indications for intervention in terms of size, this is not the case for PAs. Most surgeons would treat PAs exceeding 2 cm in diameter although patient factors may influence the decision for intervention. These factors may include patient fitness, the anatomical configuration of the PA, evidence of distal embolisation or the presence of critical ischaemia. Most surgeons would view distal embolisation as a strong indicator for treatment, irrespective of aneurysm size. The presence of mural thrombus on Duplex scanning, and significant distortion of the aneurysm should be viewed as concerning signs. Prevention of aneurysm thrombosis is critical as limb loss is markedly worse in the acute setting than for elective surgery.

When is thrombolysis utilised?

It has been observed that catheter based thrombolysis is associated with higher risks of ischaemic complications when used to manage acute PAs in comparison to treating an acute graft occlusion. During the lysis process a large volume of thromboembolic material is destabilised and inevitably embolised distally. Studies have demonstrated that in at least 10% of patients the limb acutely deteriorates during the lysis process. The main role of thrombolysis is 'on table' to clear thrombus from the run-off vessels during the process of surgical revascularisation. Thrombolysis can sometimes be used where no distal target vessels are seen for surgical bypass on initial angiography and the limb is only in the 'marginally' threatened category.

What major problem faces endovascular treatment of PAs?

It is without doubt that covered endovascular stents can effectively exclude PAs and provide an adequate conduit to supply blood to the lower leg. The main concerns regarding popliteal stent grafts relate to their long-term durability. With the constant flexing of the knee joint, the physical stresses challenge the integrity and positioning of popliteal stent grafts. Endovascular exclusion was first described in 1994, and most of the literature reports come from institutional case series. Endovascular treatment was mainly performed in asymptomatic patients, and initial results were poor. With the development of newer, more flexible devices these results have improved, with 5-year patency rates of >75% being published.

Carotid body tumour

The basics

Carotid body tumours (CBTs) are paragangliomas derived from the neural crest ectoderm. Paragangliomas are a rare neoplasm that can be found in the abdomen, thorax, and head and neck region. They are usually considered benign and complete surgical removal results in cure. The rule of '5%' is often quoted as 5% are bilateral, 5% familial, 5% systemically malignant and 5% locally reoccur. In reality nearer 10% are familial and in these patients one-third have bilateral tumours. In contrast to retroperitoneal paragangliomas, where the majority are hormonally active, <5% of CBTs are hormonally activity. In the neck paragangliomas can also arise from the vagus nerve (glomus vagale), and jugular bulb (glomus jugulare). There are three distinct groups of patients: sporadic (majority); familial; and hyperplastic (associated with chronic hypoxia).

The case

The thought of a CBT in your final examination might overwhelm you with fear, but it shouldn't! With their management being a relatively specialised subject you will not be expected to know a large amount about CBTs or to have treated one. Twenty minutes reading will provide you with all the knowledge you need to impress the examiners. The examination case will take the form of a neck mass, postoperative case and/or a computed tomography (CT)/magenetic resonance (MR) scan to review. The mass will be palpated at the level of (or above) the hyoid bone, along the anterior border of sternocleidomastoid. The CBT is firm in consistency and hence often referred to as a 'potato tumour', the mass is laterally mobile but vertically fixed. The tumour is itself not pulsatile although a transmitted pulsation may be present, or a pulsation may be palpable from an overlying external carotid artery. Differential diagnoses to consider are cervical lymphadenopathy (are there nodes elsewhere?), branchial cyst, carotid artery aneurysm (expansile mass), carotid artery tortuosity or other cervical paragangliomas. Due to the anatomical distortion and intraoperative bleeding, cranial nerve injury is more common when treating CBTs than during carotid endarterectomy (glossopharyngeal, vagus [including laryngeal branches], hypoglossal, accessory).

Questions

How do CBTs usually present?

A CBT usually presents as a painless neck mass (>50%), and can also present with compression of local structures or pain. The most common nerves to be compressed are the glossopharyngeal, vagus and hypoglossal nerves. CBTs rarely present with symptoms of cerebral ischaemia.

What are the typical CT/MR findings?

Due to the location of the CBT they typically splay the carotid bifurcation on angiography (arterial/CT or MR) – Figure I.2. If the tumour does not display this feature it is more likely to be another type of paraganglioma. The tumour derives its blood supply from the external carotid artery. The tumours are usually well defined, and when large can encase the carotid vessels.

What is the preoperative assessment?

All patients should have had a Duplex scan and neurological examination as part of their initial investigations. Further investigations include laryngoscopy (vocal cord assessment), plus selective catecholamine screening in patients experiencing hypertensive episodes or those with other neuroendocrine tumours (and contralateral CBTs on imaging). Magnetic resonance imaging (MRI) scanning is valuable for diagnostic purposes, and to identify the cranial limits of the tumour. Angiography is useful with larger tumours to identify their blood supply.

What classification system is used for CBTs?

The Shamblin classification (I to III) is used to stratify CBTs. Shamblin I tumours are small and easily dissected from the vessel wall, Shamblin II tumours are of medium size and partially encircle the carotid vessels. Shamblin III tumours are large (>4 cm) and more completely encircle the carotid vessels. The Shamblin class III tumours classically require excision and a vascular reconstruction with an interposition graft.

What endovascular interventions can be helpful in managing large tumours?

CBTs have a rich blood supply, and can be associated with significant perioperative blood loss. In addition, operative bleeding can make a safe dissection more difficult. The tumours

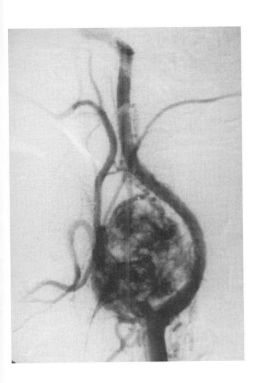

Figure I.2 Intra-arterial angiography of carotid body tumour. Note splaying of the carotid bifurcation and high vascularity of the tumour.

derive their blood supply from external carotid artery branches. Preoperative tumour embolisation, or covered stent placement over the external carotid artery feeding vessels, have both been advocated to reduce bleeding for particularly large tumours. Both of these options remain controversial as they both pose a small risk of cerebral embolisation.

Femoral anastomotic pseudoaneurysms

The basics

Femoral anastomotic pseudoaneurysms (FAPs) often occur as a consequence of previous aortobifemoral bypass surgery (Figure I.3(a) and (b)). The relationship of the anastomosis to a constantly moving hip joint may be a contributory factor in the degeneration of the arterial wall at the site of the anastomosis. Compliance may also be an issue in the pathogenesis of FAPs at the junction between the elastic artery and an inelastic prosthetic material. Their incidence at 5 years is around 5–10%; studies with longer-term follow up naturally demonstrate higher occurrence for FAPs.

Continued smoking and wound infection at the time of the original operation are thought to be risk factors for FAP development. In the case of aortobifemoral surgery the aneurysms are often bilateral.

The case

FAPs are an ideal examination case with their chronic nature and obvious clinical signs. On clinical examination femoral anastomotic pseudoaneurysms are easy to palpate due to

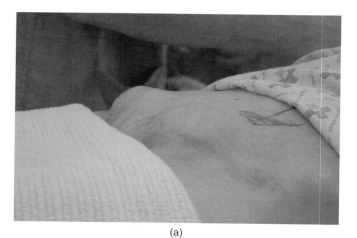

(a)

Figure I.3 Femoral anastomotic pseudoaneurysms. (a) Visible on bilateral groin inspection as late consequence of aortobifemoral surgery. (b) Angiogram of same patient, demonstrating bilateral femoral artery aneurysms. Note full length bilateral superficial femoral artery occlusions.

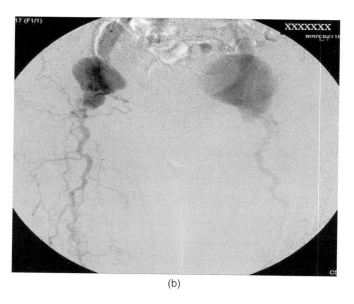

(b)

their superficial location. The leg and abdomen should be inspected for scars from the previous surgery. The main differential diagnoses are of other aneurysm of the femoral artery including atherosclerotic, mycotic, traumatic (including iatrogenic) and aneurysms related to connective tissue disorders.

Questions

How do FAPs present?

FAPs usually present with a visible or palpable pulsatile groin lump. Due to local pressure effects the patient can experience pain from peripheral nerve irritation (mass effect). Patients may also present less frequently with distal embolisation, rupture and aneurysm thrombosis.

What factors predispose to FAP formation?

Factors that may predispose to FAP formation include infection (early and late), poor surgical techniques (i.e. inadequate tissue bites, undue graft tension), concomitant endarterectomy, and the continued processes of arterial degeneration from atherosclerosis (hence promoted by continued smoking).

What are your indications for surgery?

Aneurysms >2–3 cm (debatable) in diameter should be considered for surgery. Patient factors and rate of growth may influence the size for intervention. The presence of distal embolisation should lower the threshold for repair.

What is your approach to surgical repair?

The approach to surgical repair will be influenced by evidence of an infective process in the aneurysm or groin. For chronic FAPs where infection is not suspected the aneurysm can be repaired by placement of an interposition graft between graft and normal native artery. The aneurysm should be controlled proximally and distally and the aneurysm should be opened throughout its length. The anastomosis should be tension free and good bites of healthy arterial wall should be taken. Foggarty occlusion balloons may be useful for controlling back-bleeding side branches, as scarring in the groin may have made the initial dissection difficult. For cases where infection is evident the surgery should include local debridement and removal of infected graft material. The revascularisation should be performed through healthy tissue using an autologous conduit where possible. In all cases tissue should be sent for culture. The laboratory should be made aware that slow growing bacteria such as staphylococcus epidermidis may be implicated. Antibiotic therapy should be discussed with the microbiologists and reflect the likely causative organisms in your local area.

Vascular access
The basics

Dialysis utilising arteriovenous fistulae has been practiced since the 1960s. The classical Cimino-Brescia fistula connects the radial artery to the cephalic vein at the wrist level. For use as a dialysis conduit, flow rates of at least 200 ml min^{-1} are required and there needs to be a suitable length of vein for access. Preoperative Duplex scanning should be performed in the presence of poor peripheral pulses, equivocal veins, failed fistula in the limb, a previous subclavian catheter or signs of proximal venous obstruction.

The case

The autologous arteriovenous (AV) fistula is the preferred method of dialysis in patients with long-term, end-stage renal failure. In the examination you may be presented with an arm to examine in a patient with an AV fistula. On inspection the arm should examined for dilated superficial veins and scars from a current (or previous) fistula. The arm should be inspected for scarring consistent with current needle punctures for dialysis. It is also important to examine the arm for evidence of distal ischaemia, particularly in the digits. On palpation the fistula should have a palpable 'thrill', or if occluded a thrombosed vein may be palpable. The distal pulses should be assessed. On auscultation a machinery murmur will be audible if the flow is sufficient. Proximal to the fistula there should be a sufficient length of vein for two needle dialysis.

Questions

What is the preferred location for a primary AV fistula?

The preferred location for an AV fistula is as distal as possible (artery and veins permitting) in the non-dominant arm. Although many surgeons utilise the radial artery and cephalic vein at the wrist for primary fistulae, some surgeons have demonstrated good results with fistulae made with these vessels in the anatomical snuff box. Distal sites are utilised to allow new fistulae to be created at more proximal locations in the case of fistula failure, plus a lower risk of distal ischaemia. The non-dominant arm is used to allow the recipient to perform activities during the dialysis process. Use of the non-dominant arm also means that if any complications occur as a consequence of the intervention they will have a lesser impact on the patient's function.

What findings on palpation can suggest that a fistula is at risk?

In a fistula functioning for dialysis a thrill will be easily palpable in the majority of cases. The presence of a weak thrill suggests the presence of inflow disease or narrowing at the site of the anastomosis. Pulsatility in the fistula suggests the presence of a stenosis or occlusion in the venous run-off. If a thrill is unclear in the examination you should also listen with a stethoscope.

Why is cardiac failure problematic in patients with AV fistulae?

Most fistulae used for dialysis have a blood flow of 500–1000 ml min^{-1}. In patients with more proximal fistulae, such as those in the antecubital fossa, the flow rates may be even higher than this. These high flow rates can be demanding on patients with existing cardiac failure. High-output cardiac failure can be diagnosed by observing a fall in pulse rate on manual occlusion of the fistula (Branham's sign). Patients with poor cardiac output will also be at risk of fistula occlusion or insufficient flow for effective dialysis from poor flow.

What are the complications of an AV fistula?

- Bleeding – bleeding can occur in the postoperative period from the anastomosis or divided vessels. Early exploration is advocated if there is any concern that the pressure effects from the haematoma could compromise the fistula.
- Thrombosis – early thrombosis can occur due to technical problems with the anastomosis or underlying arterial or venous disease. Re-exploration has been advocated to correct these technical issues unless there is evidence of non-correctible arterial or venous problems at the time of the operation. This view has been challenged by others with the observation that re-explored fistulae often re-thrombosis, hence, the creation of a new fistula at a more proximal location may be a better option.
- Failure to mature – an autologous AV fistula requires time for remodelling and venous dilatation prior to commencement of dialysis. This should be at least 4–6 weeks. In fistulae that remain small and have a poor flow investigations should be performed to look for an underlying reversible cause.
- Steal – steal occurs more commonly in proximal than distal fistulae. Treatment can involve surgical narrowing of the fistula or ligation or ligation of the retrograde blood

flow into the fistula from the distal limb. In some situations the fistula must be ligated. More complex interventions such as the Distal Revascularisation-Interval Ligation (DRIL) procedure have been successfully performed whereby the fistula is ligated at the artery just distal to the anastomosis. A distal bypass is then performed from a more proximal to a more distal arterial location to re-perfuse the distal arm. If there was a case of steal with digital ischemia available to the organisers this would be a good examination case.

- Infection – superficial sepsis usually respond to antibiotics. Severe infection may present with a major haemorrhage requiring fistula ligation.
- Aneurysm formation – although aneurysmal dilatation of the fistula is common it does not usually require surgical intervention.
- Ischaemic neuropathy – monomelic ischaemic neuropathy occurs with steal and usually presents within hours of surgery. This condition will not correct unless the fistula is reversed. If the condition is left untreated permanent neurological damage can occur.

Lymphoedema

The basics

Lymphoedema occurs when the circulation of lymph from the peripheral tissues back to the central system is impaired. The majority of cases are due to obliteration of the lympatics (80%) although proximal obstruction and lymphatic valvular dysfunction are also causes. Lymphoedema is generally classified into primary and secondary causes. Primary causes are sub-classified by the age of onset into 'congenital' (<1 year), 'praecox' (<35 years) and 'tarda' (>35 years).

The case

Lymphoedema of the lower limbs is a regular vascular examination case (lymphoedema of the arm following treatment for breast cancer treatment is also commonly seen in the vascular or general surgical examinations). The clinical findings are of a leg swelling that does not easily pit. The skin and subcutaneous tissues become fibrosed and less compliant with time, hence the ability to 'pit' the skin is lost. The skin can also become thickened and hyperkeratotic in appearance. Typical features of lymphoedema include a tree-trunk appearance of the lower leg (NB step for the trunk at the ankle), 'buffalo' hump on the dorsum of the foot and squared-off toes (in cross section) (Figure I.4). 'Stemmer's' sign occurs when it is no longer possible to pinch the skin on the dorsum of the 2nd toe. Chylous vesicles may appear on the shins. It is important to examine the patient for other causes of leg swelling and evidence of secondary causes of lymphoedema (see below).

Questions

What are the secondary causes of lymphoedema?

Secondary lymphoedema mainly falls into three categories; infective, malignancy and iatrogenic. The commonest cause worldwide is from the parasitic infestation filariasis. In the UK the commonest cause for lymphoedema is malignancy; either due to the

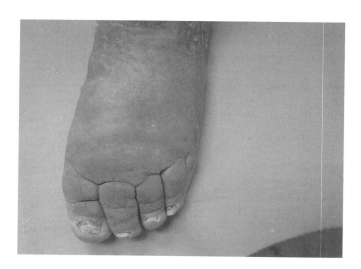

Figure I. 4 Lymphoedema of the foot.

disease process itself or as a consequence of its treatment. Recurrent minor infections can cause lymphoedema by chronic lymphangitis and progressive damage to the lymphatic system.

1. Infective – parasitic (filariasis), bacterial (*Staphylococcus*, *Streptococcus*, TB).
2. Malignancy – infiltration or compression of lymphatic vessels and nodes.
3. Iatrogenic – radiotherapy, surgery (either direct surgery on the lymph nodes, via 'collateral' damage during vascular surgical procedures, or by major surgery obliterating lymphatic routes).

How is lymphangioscintigraphy performed?

The colloid of a radioactive isotope (technetium) is injected bilaterally into the interdigital spaces between the 2nd and 3rd toes. The proximal progression of the isotope is assessed using a high-resolution collimator, which takes images at regular intervals. Bilateral ilioinguinal node visualisation with isotope should occur within 1 hour in the normal individual. The images demonstrate the progression (or hold up) of lymphatic flow. Abnormalities that may be seen include an interruption of lymphatic flow, collateral lymph vessels, dermal backflow, delayed flow, delayed visualisation or non-visualisation of lymph nodes, a reduced number of lymph nodes and dilated lymphatics.

What findings on MRI are suggestive of lymphoedema?

On MRI scanning there is generalised subcutaneous oedema with a honeycomb pattern. The latter is a result of the subcutaneous fibrosis. MRI can also demonstrate anatomical detail of lymphatics and is complementary to scintigraphy.

What surgical procedures are performed to manage lymphoedema?

Surgery is infrequently performed to manage lymphoedema. The mainstay of management is with complex decongestive therapy. Surgery is confined to severe cases where conventional measures have failed. Surgery is divided into debulking procedures and lymphatic bypass surgery. The classic Homan's procedure involves incisions along the affected portion of the limb. The lymphoedematous subcutaneous tissue is excised with preservation of the skin flaps. The skin flaps are cut to size and closed. Several procedures may be necessary to manage severe disease. The Charles' procedure is a slightly more aggressive procedure whereby the affected subcutaneous tissue is resected down to muscle fascia and then covered with a skin graft (Charles never actually performed this procedure on the leg!). Although the results from the operation can be good in selected cases, there is significant morbidity including delayed wound healing, infection and nerve injury.

Diabetic foot

The basics

In around half of diabetic patients who develop foot ulceration, ischaemia is the primary cause of a significant contributing factor. The remaining cases will predominantly be neuropathic in their aetiology. Limb loss is 15 times more frequent in diabetic than non-diabetic patients, and it is commonly preceded by foot ulceration. The diabetic foot is prone to ulceration for a number of key factors, including neuropathy, impaired vascularity at micro- and macro-vascular levels, deformity and immune effects. Diabetes is frequently complicated by renal failure, and this accelerates the development of vascular disease. Diabetic retinopathy also makes wound care all the more difficult.

The case

Patients with chronic diabetic foot disease are in plentiful supply and often more than willing to attend hospital for an examination. No matter where the foot lesion is located the same basic assessment of the foot must be performed. During the examination you must assess the vascularity, look for evidence of neuropathy, assess foot deformity, look for signs of infection and comment on the wound condition. Where bone can be probed at the base of an ulcer the likelihood of osteomyelitis is greatly increased. It is probably easiest to perform a general inspection of the foot and then assess each aspect in turn.

Questions

How does diabetic neuropathy influence foot disease?

To describe the changes it is best to split them up into motor, sensory and autonomic. The motor changes are thought to predominantly affect the small muscles of the foot with preservation of the long flexors and extensors. This leads to clawing of the toes with prominence of the plantar metatarsal heads. Patients are often unaware of their sensory neuropathy, and its presence impedes their ability to avoid injuries and protect healing wounds. Autonomic neuropathy has several effects; first, it reduces sweating and causes dryness and fissuring of the skin. Second, it alters foot microcirculation, causing blood to shunt from the skin circulation.

How is neuropathy tested?

The simplest and most practical method for testing for neuropathy utilises pressure perception with a 10 g nylon monofilament (Figure I.5). Buckling of the monofilament with pressure indicates a skin pressure of 10 g. The skin is tested in a standardised pattern at several

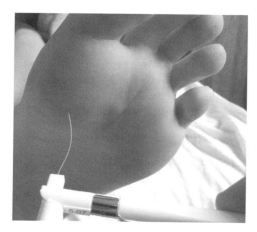

Figure I.5 Testing neuropathy with a 10 g monofilament.

points on the foot. Impaired sensation demonstrated by this method has been shown to correlate with the risk of ulceration. The presence of neuropathy can also be assessed using a biothesiometer (vibration sensation), or by nerve conduction studies.

What are the principles in managing acute diabetic foot disease?

- Vascular assessment and revascularisation where necessary.
- Treating infection – draining sepsis, antibiotics.
- Wound care – debridement, wound dressings, and 'off loading' of wound.

Following wound healing, prevention is of paramount importance.

What is 'Charcot's foot'?

Charcot's neuroarthropathy is a complex condition whereby bony destruction and joint deformity occurs. The changes result from neuropathy, and diabetes is the commonest cause of neuropathy in the Western world. Presentation is often delayed due to the impaired sensation of pain. In the early phase the foot is often warm and swollen, and these changes are often mistaken for cellulitis. As the condition progresses the foot becomes structurally deformed with collapse of the medial arch. There is a rocker bottom deformity to the foot with bony prominences. The skin temperature is often several degrees higher in the affected foot. Bony changes will usually be obvious on plain X-rays, although in the initial phase the imaging may be normal. Once the diagnosis is suspected the foot must be immobilised until the deformity has stabilised.

What imaging aids the diagnosis of osteomyelitis?

Osteomyelitis is often difficult to diagnose in the diabetic foot. The presence of neuropathy and adjacent ulceration can complicate the situation. In around 70% of cases there will be plain radiographic evidence of bony destruction. Serial plain radiographs in suspected cases are valuable in looking for changes in the bony integrity; the serial radiographs should be taken at 2-week intervals. Three phase bone scans and isotope white cell scans can also be used in combination with plain radiographs to improve accuracy. In combination with plain radiographs, these modalities are sensitive for osteomyelitis in over 90% of cases. MRI scanning is now becoming established as the investigation of choice in diagnosing osteo-myelitis and deep infections in the diabetic foot. MRI findings of osteomyelitis include a decreased bone marrow T1 signal, increased T2 signal, and post-gadolinium enhancement. MRI can also identify associated abnormalities such as cellulitis, abscess formation, sinus tracts, and cortical bone destruction.

Complications of carotid endarterectomy

The basics

The main complications of carotid endarterectomy (CEA) include stroke, nerve injury, haemorrhage, cardiac ischaemia and death. Carotid patch infection is fortunately a rela-tively infrequent complication (<1%), and you are unlikely to see one in the examination.

The case

In previous examinations candidates have been introduced to a patient with a visible scar from a CEA. The candidates have been asked about the patient's likely intervention, and then questioned about various aspects of carotid surgery. Pre- or postoperative carotid patients are a common examination case.

Questions

Which cranial nerves are at risk during carotid endarterectomy?

The cranial nerves most commonly injured during carotid surgery include the hypoglossal, vagus and laryngeal nerves.

- The hypoglossal nerve is the most commonly injured major nerve during CEA. The hypoglossal nerve crosses the internal carotid artery and external carotid artery near the upper limit of internal carotid artery dissection. Due to its location it runs the risk of division, diathermy or traction during surgery. Hypoglossal nerve injury classically presents with tongue deviation towards the side of nerve injury. Injury during CEA occurs in 5–10% of cases and is usually a transient phenomenon. It is more common if the nerve has been mobilised.
- The vagus nerve is usually located posteriorly in the carotid sheath. This posterior location makes it vulnerable to clamp injuries if the arterial clamp is carelessly placed beyond the artery.
- The superior laryngeal nerve is susceptible to injury where it descends behind the internal carotid artery and then passes posteriorly close to the superior thyroid artery. Injury to the superior laryngeal nerve probably goes unnoticed most of the time.
- The non-recurrent laryngeal nerve, when present, is at particular risk during carotid endarterectomy. Non-recurrent nerves occur in 0.5–1% of people and are commonest on the right-hand side. In its non-recurrent course, the nerve passes transversely from under the carotid sheath and will be at right-angles to the normal position.
- The glossopharyngeal nerve is rarely damaged during a straightforward CEA. The glossopharyngeal nerve is susceptible to injury when a more extensive cranial dissection is performed. The nerve is deep too and courses in a similar direction to the posterior belly of the digastric muscle.

- The spinal accessory nerve exits the skull in posterior direction just deep to the styloid process. The nerve is susceptible to injury during 'high' carotid dissections or during the retrojugular approach to the carotid artery. The spinal accessory nerve provides motor innervation to the trapezius and sternocleidomastoid.

Would you use local or general anesthesia?

The general anaesthetic versus local anaesthetic for carotid surgery (GALA) trial showed no advantage for either. It remains a choice between the patient and surgeon concerned. You should have a view on what you should do in your practice and be prepared to justify it.

Does patching reduce the risk of perioperative stroke?

The Cochrane Stroke Review Group has published a meta-analysis comparing carotid patching to primary closure. The analysis demonstrated a reduction in the ipsilateral stroke rate and restenosis with patching. Most surgeons use a Dacron patch although some may use vein patches or material such as bovine pericardium. The best current practice is to use a patch on virtually all patients.

What should be performed prior to bilateral carotid surgery?

The vocal cords should be checked for evidence of recurrent laryngeal nerve injury from the first procedure. Bilateral nerve injury can cause significant difficulties with voice, swallowing and obstruction of the upper airway – the neutral position of the cords is in the midline.

What is the risk of disabling stroke or death?

The risk of death or disabling stroke in both the European and North American carotid endarterectomy trials (NASCET and ECST) was approximately 3%. The combined rate of death and all strokes is virtually double this figure. Data from the European and North American asymptomatic carotid endarterectomy trials (ACST and ACAS) 30-day any stroke or death rates are near 2.5%, suggesting that the asymptomatic patients and/or the surgery is lower risk. Vascular units should strive to audit their own results and present their own complication rates when consenting patients.

What is the frequency of haematoma formation?

Data from randomised trials often identify much higher rates of complication than self-reported case series. In the GALA trial haematoma rates were close to 10% and just over one third of these cases required re-exploration for bleeding. Haematoma in the neck can result in airway obstruction and should be considered a serious problem as per thyroid surgery. The mechanism of airway obstruction is through a combination of laryngeal oedema plus direct compression. Re-intubation should be considered sooner rather than later where airway compromise is suspected.

When would you use a carotid shunt?

Unless conclusive trial evidence becomes available controversy will reign over approaches to carotid shunting. Policies include shunting all patients, selective shunting and not-shunting. You should decide on your policy and be able to justify it in the examination. An appropriate policy is to shunt all CEAs under general anaesthetic and selectively shunt those under local anaesthesia.

How is cerebral perfusion monitored during CEA?

Although sophisticated methods exist to measure cerebral perfusion such as xenon washout, infra-red spectroscopy and electrophysiological studies, none are ideal for everyday carotid practice. Commonly used methods include awake testing (local anaesthetic procedures), measurement of stump pressures, and Transcranial Doppler (TCD). In cerebral monitoring you want a device that is simple and cheap to use, is able to identify ipsilateral cerebral blood flow, can identify embolic events and looks at neurological function. Unfortunately, none of the methods available can satisfy all of the requirements fully. Awake testing may seem the most ideal, but it will not necessarily warn you of embolisation; once cerebral compromise is apparent inserting the shunt may be more difficult due to patient agitation. TCD can assess reduction in cerebral blood flow (>50% reduction in middle cerebral artery flow) and provide evidence of embolic events before and during shunt insertion; however, it does not demonstrate whether the patient's neurology has been affected. Stump pressure measurement is cheap and readily available, stump pressure <50 mmHg are taken to indicate the need for a shunt. Stump 'pressures' are taken as a proxy measurement of cerebral blood 'flow', and will not identify changes during the shunting period, unless repeatedly measured.

How would you manage a postoperative cerebrovascular event (CVE) following recent carotid endarterectomy?

The management of a postoperative CVE will be contentious and dependent on the timing and facilities available as well as when the event occurs. Whatever investigations and treatments are instituted, all patients should have their cerebral perfusion and oxygenation optimised and this will usually require admission to an area such as a high dependency unit (HDU) or an intensive therapy unit (ITU). Intubation and ventilation may be needed if the conscious level is impaired or the patient is confused. The intention with these patients is to identify those with carotid artery thrombosis, prevent further events (correct technical problems, antiplatelet therapy, mange hypertension and hypotension) and to identify patients with haemorrhagic strokes.

When the CVE is apparent on waking, or occurs in the recovery room, the patient is in the ideal location to return to theatre to correct carotid artery thrombosis or technical problems. Ideally a Duplex scan should be performed immediately to see if the endarterectomised vessel is patent or if there are technical problems with the endarterectomy. If the scan is normal and the surgeon was 'happy' with the operation the benefits of re-operation will be questionable, and perhaps the best course of action is to exclude other causes of embolisation and optimise antithrombotic therapy. These patients should have a cerebral CT scan as soon as possible to exclude a haemorrhage, particularly where enhanced antithrombotic therapy is being considered. The scan should also include angiography, this is particularly important if the aortic arch and intracranial vessels have not been previously imaged.

In patients where the blood pressure has been labile and there have been periods of significant hypertension a haemorrhagic stroke should be more strongly considered. In these patients a cerebral CT should be performed immediately to exclude a haemorrhage. It should be remembered that cerebral haemorrhage occurs in the minority of patients, and a case review has suggested that this represents about 10% of postoperative strokes. CVAs that occur after the immediate postoperative period are less likely to derive the same benefit from re-exploration, and should be urgently imaged with carotid Duplex (if available), CT and CT angiography (CTA).

Buerger's disease

The basics

Buerger's disease (thromboangiitis obliterans) is an inflammatory arteriopathy that predominantly affects small- and medium-sized arteries. The changes are pathologically distinct from atherosclerosis. The lower extremity is predominantly affected although this is not exclusive. The disorder classically affects young male smokers; however, the pattern of disease is changing. Leo Buerger first described the condition in pathological specimens in 1908, and termed the disease thromboangiitis obliterans. In contrast to the common clinical presentation of atherosclerosis with intermittent claudication, patients with Buerger's disease tend to present with rest pain and tissue loss. Near to half of patients diagnosed with Buerger's disease who continue to smoke end up requiring an amputation of some sort. The exact pathogenic mechanism linking Buerger's disease to tobacco is unknown.

The case

Consider the diagnosis in any young patient with symptoms or signs of critical ischaemia. Patients with Buerger's disease are young and mobile enough to attend examinations, and they have good clinical signs. In the clinical encounter the level of vascular disease should be established and other alternative diagnosis considered. Do not make this diagnosis too glibly but suspect it in young male smokers with significant ischemia and preserved proximal pulses.

Questions

What are the pathological and radiological features of Buerger's disease?

- The pathological features at a microscopic level involve an acute hypercellular thrombosis causing arterial occlusion. There is a striking perivascular inflammation that can also affects veins. Despite the intravascular thrombosis patients with Buerger's disease have not been demonstrated to be hypercoagulable.
- The radiological features are of relatively normal arteries to the knee level with abrupt occlusions of the tibial vessels with 'corkscrew' collateral feeding of the distal vessels at the ankle (Figure I.6).

How is the diagnosis made?

There are several diagnostic criteria described (Tel Aviv, Oregon) for Buerger's disease. The consistent factors in these schemes are:

- exclusion other causes;
- tobacco use;
- distal extremity disease (femoral pulses nearly always preserved);
- young age of onset (< 45);
- The presence of upper limb disease, phlebitis migrans or Raynaud's phenomena, and radiological signs strengthen the diagnosis.

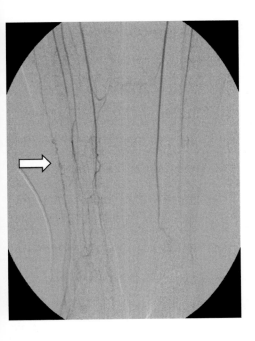

Figure I.6 Peripheral angiogram of tibial vessels in Buerger's disease. Arrow indicating corkscrew collaterals.

What other forms of vasculitis are relevant to the vascular surgeon?

- Takayasu's arteritis – this affects larger elastic arteries such as the aorta and its branches. The majority of patients are female and present in their 2nd and 3rd decade. Two phases exist of acute pre-pulseless and chronic pulseless.
- Giant cell arteritis (temporal arteritis) – this is a granulomatous vasculitis affecting large- and medium-sized arteries, with the cranial vessels most commonly affected. This can present with cranial ischaemia (visual loss, jaw ischaemia, headaches) or with chronic constitutional symptoms.
- Polyarteritis nodosa – this is a necrotising vasculitis affecting small- and medium-sized arteries. The disease is more common in males and usually presents in middle age. Renal and gastrointestinal involvement is common.
- Drug induced – penicillins, sulphonamides, NSAIDs, cocaine, etc.

Connective tissue disorders should be considered in patients with digital ulceration, without typical findings of atherosclerosis. Other rarer vascular disorders are also considered in the popliteal entrapment scenario.

How is Buerger's disease managed?

The absolute goal for managing Buerger's disease is establishing permanent abstinence from smoking. Aspirin should be prescribed for its antiplatelet effects, and analgesics for pain control. Prostaglandin infusions may help with symptom control, although it is uncertain if they alter the progression of tissue loss. Distal ischaemic lesions will often auto-amputate or may require surgical amputation. Awaiting demarcation is helpful even if surgery is planned. Antibiotics may be needed intermittently for any infective episodes. A lumbar chemical sympathectomy is helpful in selected cases for chronic pain control.

Vascular malformations

The basics

Vascular anomalies fall into two main categories, haemangiomas and vascular malformations. Haemangiomas will be evident at birth, and have a distinct natural history (proliferation, plateau and involution). Most will disappear during the first decade of life. Previous terminology utilised the term 'haemangioma' for both lesions appearing around birth and those appearing later in life. More recent terminology has defined the self-involuting tumours as haemangiomas (hence the port wine stain is no longer considered a haemangioma). Vascular malformations grow during childhood, and may enlarge following hormonal change, trauma and sepsis. Most vascular malformations are sporadic although some can be part of a specific syndrome, such as Klippel–Trénaunay. Vascular malformations are derived from aberrations in vasculogenesis, and generally do not undergo spontaneous involution. Although several classifications exist, they are most simply considered in two main clinically relevant categories: fast- and slow-flowing lesions.

- Fast-flow: arterial malformation, arteriovenous malformations and arteriovenous fistulae.
- Slow-flow: venous malformations, lymphatic malformations, capillary malformations.

First-line investigations include Duplex and MRI scanning. Duplex scanning demonstrates flow dynamics and morphology of the lesion. MRI scanning provides more detailed information on structure and relationship to other soft tissues. MRI is also able to differentiate between slow- and fast-flow malformations. Invasive investigations such as arteriography and venography are still performed second line, and can provide valuable additional information when planning treatment.

The case

Due to the diversity of lesions we will run through the more common groups of malformation for this scenario.

Capillary malformations

Capillary malformations are intra-dermal vascular anomalies. The malformations appear as pink/red areas of discolouration, and can occur throughout the body. The lesions can cause hypertrophy of the surrounding soft tissues. Capillary malformations may be spontaneous or part of a syndrome such as Klippel–Trénaunay or Sturge-Weber. Imaging will often be performed to look for associated abnormalities. Pulsed dye laser is an established treatment for these lesions.

Venous malformations

Venous malformations are the most prevalent vascular malformation and tend to occur in the head and neck. Because of their slow flow they often take considerable time to enlarge. The lesions have previously been referred to as 'cavernous haemangiomas'. On examination they will be deep blue in colour and easily compressible. The lesions can calcify, and local thrombosis can cause pain. Limb hypertrophy is seen with some extremity lesions. Treatment is conservative with compression where possible. Sclerosant therapy is usually the first-line intervention, and repeat treatments are often needed. Surgical excision can be performed for severe symptoms with or without preoperative sclerotherapy.

Arteriovenous malformations

Arteriovenous malformations are fast-flowing connections that bypass the capillary bed. The lesions are usually apparent at birth, and enlarge in size as their blood flow increases. The lesions are usually warm and pink/blue in colour. Arteriography is often required to establish the anatomy of their arterial supply. Small lesions can be excised (including the feeding vessel). Larger lesions often require a combination of embolisation and surgical excision. Ligation of the feeding vessel alone can cause collateralisation, making further treatment more complex. When these lesions enlarge they can become destructive and lead to cardiac failure.

Lymphatic malformations

Lymphatic malformations have historically included lymphangiomas and cystic hygromas. These lesions are slow flow and usually occur in the cervical region. The majority will be apparent within the first years of life. These lesions can be associated with both soft tissue and skeletal overgrowth.

- Cystic hygroma: this consists of a collection of lymphatic sacs that have failed to connect properly with the normal channels. The lesion are often found in the posterior triangle at the base of the neck. They can rapidly fill up in response to an infection or trauma, and can become very large. On palpation the lesion will be smooth and transilluminate spectacularly.
- Lymphangioma circumscriptum: this is at the other spectrum where small localised lymphatic vesicles are present that do not connect to the normal lymphatic system. They are usually found around the shoulder, axilla, groin and buttocks. If these lesions contain old blood they may turn brown in colour.

MRI scanning is useful in defining the anatomy of the larger lesions. The main sources of symptoms for these lesions are infection and intra-lesional bleeding. Sclerotherapy has been performed with a variety of agents with acceptable results. Surgery is reserved for severe symptoms and recurrence is high. The aim of surgery is complete excision of the lesion to minimise the risk of recurrence. Surgery can be complex and involve multiple procedures. Lymphangioma circumscriptum requires wide local excision if treatment is required.

Vascular malformations (specific syndromes): Klippel–Trénaunay syndrome

The basics

Klippel–Trénaunay syndrome (KTS) was first described by the French physicians Maurice Klippel and Paul Trénaunay in 1900. Most cases are sporadic although there have been reports that the condition has occurred in an autosomal dominant pattern. KTS is a complex and variable syndrome; hence treatment is planned on a case-by-case basis. The venous component of the disease tends to be the most problematic. The physical signs will become evident early in life and there is no gender predominance.

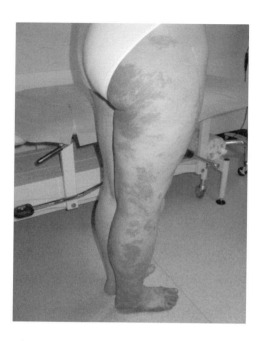

Figure 7 Port-wine' staining and varicose veins in Klippel–Trénaunay syndrome. There is a scar over the hip from a leg shortening procedure.

The case

KTS is an excellent vascular case with its various manifestations and physical signs (Figure I. 7). The clinic findings are discussed below.

Questions

What are the pathological components of KTS?

- Venous abnormalities (varicosities).
- Bony and soft tissues hypertrophy.
- Cutaneous angiomata ('port wine' stains).

Each component of the syndrome may be present to a varying degree. The limb hypertrophy can be secondary to increased bony length and/or increased soft tissue girth. Abnormally developed lymphatics have also been associated with this syndrome.

What is the distribution of varicosities in KTS?

Unlike the typical distribution of greater or lesser saphenous varicosities, the varicosities seen in KTS tend to be located on the lateral side of the thigh and lower leg. The 'port wine' stains from cutaneous angiomata tend to be located in similar lateral distribution to the varicosities. The 'port wine' stain has a distinct, linear border, and the lesion possesses neither a proliferative nor a regressing phase.

What concerns would you have over performing superficial venous surgery in KTS?

In KTS the deep venous system can be abnormally developed. The superficial veins may provide an important role in venous function; hence, they should be left intact unless adequate venous drainage has been demonstrated.

What surgical options are available to treat KTS?

The surgical options for KTS have mainly included de-bulking procedures and venous surgery. The de-bulking procedures are only really considered for severe cases where conservative options have failed. Venous surgery in KTS is associated with a higher rate of recurrence than with conventional venous anatomy.

What non surgical options are available?

Compression therapy is an important treatment modality in the management of limb swelling. Maintaining good compression therapy can reduce pain, swelling and inflammation. The potential side effects of compression therapy include displacement of fluid into other locations, and the compression therapy itself may impede circulation through the limb. As with lymphoedema management, massage therapy can provide an improvement in symptoms. Liquid or foam sclerotherapy offer a less invasive option to treat the varicosities than conventional surgery.

Vascular malformations (specific syndromes): Parkes-Weber syndrome?

Parkes-Weber syndrome was first described by Frederick Parkes-Weber, an English dermatologist and physician to Queen Victoria. Parkes-Weber syndrome is similar in many of its features to KTS; however, in KTS the cutaneous malformations are slow-flowing, whereas in Parkes-Weber syndrome the vascular malformations are fast-flowing arteriovenous abnormalities, with associated limb hypertrophy (haemangiectatic hypertrophy). So, in essence, Parkes-Weber syndrome is a fast-flow arteriovenous malformation in association with the other abnormalities found in KTS such as cutaneous capillary malformation and skeletal or soft tissue hypertrophy.

Vascular malformations (specific syndromes): Proteus syndrome

Proteus syndrome is an extremely rare congenital condition and unlikely to be seen in a clinical examination. The condition is highly variable in appearance, and is named after the Greek sea-god Proteus, who could change his shape at will. The condition consists of cutaneous abnormalities (nevi), vascular abnormalities (capillary, venous, or combined), plus skeletal and soft-tissue abnormalities such as hemihypertrophy. Proteus syndrome is extremely disfiguring as a result of an overgrowth of skin, bones, muscles, fatty tissues, and blood and lymphatic vessels. The changes often only occur over half of the body. The condition was publicised in the 1980s film *The Elephant Man*, about the life of Joseph Merrick, a Proteus sufferer.

Vascular malformations (specific syndromes): popliteal entrapment syndrome and cystic adventitial disease

The basics

Popliteal entrapment usually presents with calf claudication in young athletic individuals. The symptoms may commence following a period of strenuous activity. Foot pulses will be normal at rest unless a complication of the disease process has occurred. Sudden onset claudication in a young person may indicate a vessel occlusion. Popliteal entrapment syndrome can be classified into its anatomical and functional varieties. Long-term complications include localised fibrosis and stenosis, aneurysmal dilatation, and embolisation from the diseased segment of artery.

Making a diagnosis of this condition is particularly problematic for the functional group, as at least 10% of the asymptomatic population demonstrate compression of the popliteal artery with active dorsal or plantar flexion of the ankle joint. The diagnosis of popliteal entrapment is usually made in younger individuals with symptoms of claudication and evidence of vascular compromise on active ankle flexion. Primary atherosclerosis, other arterial disorders, and alternative causes of leg pain must be excluded. Anatomical entrapment should be corrected by removal of the entrapment mechanism (usually release of the medial head of gastrocnemius) with or without resection of the involved segment of artery. This prevents further damage to the artery and distal vasculature.

The case

The patient should have a lower limb vascular examination. Attention should be made to assessing the quality of the ankle pulses in the plantar- and dorsi-flexed positions. The patient should be inspected for venous skin changes, vasculitic lesions and examined for sources of embolisation. The candidate should also indicate to the examiner that they would perform a musculoskeletal examination of the lower limb.

Questions

What two important embryological factors are pertinent in the development of anatomical popliteal entrapment?

Two important embryological factors that can be implicated in the development of popliteal entrapment involve the differing embryonic origins of the mid portion and the distal popliteal artery, and secondly, the migration of the medial head of gastrocnemius.

- In the definitive human anatomy the mid portion of the popliteal artery is a remnant part of the primitive axial artery and definitive distal vessel (original axial vessel lying beneath the popliteus muscle) from a more superficially placed vascular plexus. This process of vascular development occurs between the 8th and 12th week of embryology.
- The medial head of gastrocnemius migrates from a lateral location during embryonic development. This process occurs around a similar time to the changes in the popliteal artery.

What are the common configurations causing popliteal artery compression?

- The popliteal artery can be located medially to the medial head of the gastrocnemius. This abnormal position can occur to a varying degree depending on the final location of the gastrocnemius muscle.
- The popliteal artery may be located within the medial head of the gastrocnemius muscle.
- The popliteal artery may exist deep to the popliteus muscle.
- In functional cases it is thought that muscle hypertrophy from exercise plus a 'vulnerable' location of the artery between the gastrocnemius heads predisposes to the condition.

What other structures can be involved in the compression syndrome?

Popliteal vein and the tibial nerves can also be compressed.

Do you know any classification schemes for popliteal entrapment?

A classification scheme for popliteal entrapment has been suggested by Levien and Veller [1]. Types I to III involve misplacement of the artery in relation to all, or part of, the medial head of gastrocnemius. In Type IV the popliteal artery is developed main in an anomalous way beneath the popliteus muscle. This layout is therefore unrelated to the positioning of the gastrocnemius muscle. Type V was subsequently suggested as an addition to include cases where the popliteal vein is involved. Functional entrapment, where there is compression of the vessel in stressed positions without any apparent anatomic abnormality, is termed Type VI.

What other rare vascular disorders can causes arterial claudication in the younger patient?

- Fibromuscular dysplasia (FMD) – FMD is the commonest cause of 'renal' hypertension in children. Most FMD affects the media of the arterial wall. The renal and carotid vessels are most commonly affected, although the external iliac artery (EIA) is the most commonly involved vessel in the lower limb vasculature. Disease of the EIA usually presents with claudication, although it can be complicated by embolisation, aneurysm or thrombosis. The classic appearance on arterial imaging is of a 'string of beads', angioplasty has been successfully used to treat this disease.
- Persistent sciatic artery – the sciatic artery is the embryonic axial limb artery. In the normal individual the majority of the vessel obliterates, apart from the the segments becoming the internal iliac artery, part of the popliteal artery and the peroneal artery. The condition may present with a pulsatile mass in the buttock. Aneurysmal degeneration of the anomalous artery can occur due to trauma in the sciatic foramen. The patent sciatic artery is associated with hypoplasia of the iliofemoral vessels. The blood supply through these abnormal vessels may be inadequate during exercise, and the diseased sciatic artery may acutely thrombose.
- Cystic adventitial disease (CAD) – CAD of the popliteal artery is thought to exist due to inclusion, or extension, of mucin-secreting structures between the media and adventitia of the popliteal artery. The condition usually presents with claudication in the fourth and fifth decades. On clinical examination, flexing the knee joint may cause the distal pulses to disappear. The typical appearance on angiography is of an 'hourglass' narrowing of the popliteal artery with normal distal vessels.
- Endofibrosis – arterial endofibrosis is a recently discovered condition that can affect highly trained athletes, with cyclists predominantly at risk. Repetitive movement of the hip joint and the cycling posture are thought to lead to chronic arterial injury, resulting in progressive intimal thickening. The endofibrosis most often affects the external iliac arteries. The presence of an arterial pressure drop is useful sign as peripheral pulses and ankle brachial pressure index (ABPI) will usually be normal at rest. The condition has been treated with resection and revascularisation using autologous vein. Prosthetic materials should be avoided due to compliance issues.
- Premature atherosclerosis – lipid disorders and hyperhomocystinaemia should be considered.
- Dissection – aortic dissection can be complicated by acute limb ischaemia. Claudication may be a longer-term consequence of the event. Young patients with

acute dissection usually have significant hypertension or a collagen disorder such as Marfan's. Isolated spontaneous dissections have been described in the peripheral vasculature.

- Embolisation – as with dissection, embolisation should present with a well-defined acute event. Claudication may be an ongoing consequence if the presentation is delayed or embolus is left untreated. Proximal sources of embolisation should be sought.
- Drug induced arteriopathies – cocaine, amphetamines, ergot, etc.
- Pseudoxanthoma elasticum (PXE) – PXE is a rare genetic disorder that produces progressive calcification and fragmentation of elastic fibres in the skin, cardiovascular system and retina. Extensive arteriosclerosis often occurs in the third or fourth decade of life. The disease tends to spare the aorta, but involves lower limb arteries, producing intermittent claudication. Patients with PXE often have coronary and valvular heart diseases.
- Vasculitis.

Venous disease: varicose veins

The basics

Varicose veins are a common clinical condition and an extremely common examination case. Although many patients may seek treatment for cosmetic reasons, a broad range of symptoms such as heaviness, itching, aching, mild swelling, cramps can be attributed to varicose veins. Symptoms tend to be worse towards the end of the day, and after prolonged episodes of standing. In females the symptoms are often worse around the time of menstruation. Varicose veins frequently present as uncomplicated entities, but can also be associated with changes of chronic venous insufficiency (CVI). The main patterns of venous incompetence involve the long (greater) and short (lesser) saphenous veins. With the advent of Duplex scanning a Giacomini vein is often mentioned in reports. This is a thigh extension from the short saphenous vein that joins with the long saphenous vein first described by Giacomini.

The case

Varicose veins should initially be examined in the standing position.

- Inspection – comment on the extent of varicosities and their distribution in relation to the superficial venous systems. The lower abdominal wall and perineal areas should also be inspected for venous collaterals. Inspect for associated skin changes or areas of ulceration suggestive of CVI. Look for a bluish tinge to the skin in the groin suggestive of a saphena varix. Later in the examination you will want to examine the patient in the supine position to ensure that the varicosities disappear on leg elevation (venous occlusion, tricuspid disease).
- Palpation – the skin should be examined for oedema, thickening, and the veins compressed to establish their patency. The saphenofemoral and saphenopopliteal junctions should be palpated for the presence of a varix. The lower limb pulses should be examined for co-existing arterial disease (+/- ABPI). Where abdominal wall venous collaterals are seen Harvey's test can be performed to determine the direction of the flow of the veins. The test is performed by placing two fingers on a segment of vein

several centimetres apart. By sliding one finger along the vein to empty it and then releasing one finger (repeated in both directions) the direction of venous filling can be determined.

- Percussion and auscultation – the 'Tap' test is best performed where a long segment of LSV is palpable. Normally when a column of blood is present in the LSV, transmission of a percussion wave should only occur in an antegrade direction. Where the valves in the system are incompetent is a percussion wave can also travel in a retrograde direction. Auscultation may be useful when looking for evidence of an arteriovenous shunt ('machinery' murmur).
- Tourniquet test – it is worth understanding (and being able to perform) the tourniquet test, although it is infrequently performed in modern clinical practice.
- Hand Held Doppler (HHD) examination for junction reflux. The HHD can be used to identify reflux at the saphenofemoral junction, popliteal fossa and also in the long saphenous vein itself, whilst the patient is in the standing position. When listening for reflux, care must be taken to only apply light pressure to the area of interest, as veins can easily be compressed, hence abolishing audible venous flow. Significant reflux (bidirectional venous blood flow) is taken as >0.5 s in duration. The saphenofemoral junction is located medial to the femoral artery, 2 cm below the level of the pubic tubercle. Reflux can be augmented by compression of the calf muscle or during a Valsalva manoeuvre. The saphenopopliteal junction is much more variable in location, hence HHD examination is less reliable. Reflux in the popliteal fossa is detected by identifying the arterial signal close to the midline, and then moving the probe laterally. The calf muscle is again squeezed to augment reflux. Popliteal fossa reflux will either relate to short saphenous, gastrocnemius or popliteal venous incompetence. Examining the LSV at knee level with HHD is useful where junction reflux is not present, but the varicosities appear distributed in the LSV territory.

Following the peripheral examination you would then wish to examine the abdomen, and rectum, vagina and testes where appropriate for evidence of malignancy or pelvic mass. Prior to intervention, or where varicosities have newly developed, a pregnancy test should be performed (pregnancy causes pelvic venous compression, and increased progesterone levels cause smooth muscle relaxation and alterations in the structure of collagen).

Venous disease: chronic venous insufficiency (CVI) and ulceration

The basics

The prevalence of venous ulceration increases with age, with a rate of 20 per 1000 in subjects over 80 years of age. Healing of venous ulcers is a major cost burden to society with the best healing rates in specialist centres of 70% at 3 months. Venous ulcers are often recurrent and usually have a history of venous disease. The skin at the site of the ulcer is often tender, painful and inflamed prior to the development of the ulcer, and the ulcer formation can often be triggered by minor trauma or scratching of the skin. Around half of patients with venous ulcers have superficial venous incompetence without deep incompetence or obstruction. Chronic leg

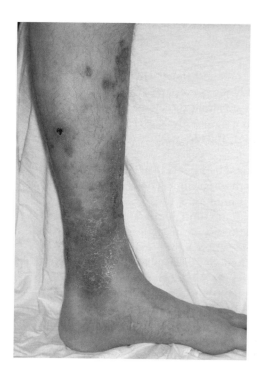

Figure I.8 Image of lower limb venous skin changes – lipodermatosclerosis and pigmentation. .

ulcers are attributable to venous disease in 60–80% of cases; in around 20% of these cases there is underlying arterial insufficiency. Venous ulcers are also often associated with diabetes. Pure venous ulcers are usually relatively painless; if pain is a significant feature you should consider an inflammatory or arterial condition as a cause. Patients with chronic ulcers often develop limited mobility at the ankle joint, this process further compromises function of the calf muscle pump mechanism.

CVI is a complex condition whereby venous hypertension causes inflammation, thickening and fibrin deposition within the skin and subcutaneous tissues. Clinical features of CVI include swelling, ulceration, pain, skin changes (sclerosis, pigmentation, eczema) – Figure I.8. Hypothesis for the formation of CVI skin changes include the white cell trapping, perivascular fibrin cuff formation, tissue pressure effect, and macromolecule leakage theories.

The case

Venous ulceration classically occurs in the gaiter area, usually in the medial location. Ulceration occurring primarily in the foot is unlikely to have a venous cause. The venous ulcer is usually shallow with gentle sloping edges. The surrounding skin will often have skin changes of chronic venous insufficiency. Although the ulcer base may contain some slough, once removed there should be pink epithelium where healing is taking place. There may be areas of white fibrous tissue scarring in the ulcer from the healing process. Where there have been previous venous ulcers there may be pale scars visible ('atrophie blanche'). The absence of visible varicosities does not exclude a venous cause to an ulcer.

Questions

What are the secondary causes of varicose veins?

- Venous obstruction.
- Extrinsic compression – pelvic mass (including pregnancy), increased abdominal pressure, and retroperitoneal fibrosis.
- Intrinsic obstruction – post deep vein thrombosis (DVT), May–Thurner syndrome (DVT as a consequence of compression of the left common iliac vein by the overlying right common iliac artery).
- Valve destruction – post phlebitic limb.
- High flow – arteriovenous fistula.

How does the calf muscle pump function?

The calf muscle pump is an integral part of the process for re-circulating blood from peripheral veins back into the centre venous system. The soleal muscles contain large valveless venous sinusoids with a total capacity of over 100 ml in the adult. At rest the sinusoids fill, and during muscular activity blood is expelled from these veins. Valves in the deep and perforating veins direct blood from the superficial system, and then through the deep system, in a retrograde direction. In the standing subject at rest there is a standing column of blood that exerts a hydrostatic pressure down to the foot level of around 90 mmHg (equivalent to its vertical weight from the point of measurement to the right auricle of the heart). Following repeated calf muscle contraction the hydrostatic venous pressure in the foot falls until it reaches a lower plateau level of 20–30 mmHg (ambulatory venous pressure). If the patient stands still the pressure returns back to a resting pressure of around 90 mmHg. Where deep venous obstruction or incompetence occurs (following a DVT) the pressure produced by the calf muscle pump forces blood into the superficial system causing superficial venous hypertension.

What are the physiological mechanisms of venous hypertension?

- Superficial venous reflux.
- Deep venous reflux.
- Perforator incompetence.
- Deep venous obstruction.
- Calf pump failure.

Any of the above may exist in isolation or combination.

How does venous claudication differ from arterial claudication?

Exercise in the presence of venous insufficiency causes an increase in blood flow to the limb with a compromise to normal venous return. The process can cause distension and a 'bursting' type discomfort to the leg. Unlike the rapidly resolving pain of intermittent claudication (IC), relief in venous claudication takes much longer to occur, and often requires sustained elevation to the limb.

How do you manage venous ulcers?

- Debridement – slough and debris should be regularly cleaned from the surface of an ulcer. Soaking the limb in a bowl of tap water often helps local dressing removal and the debridement of slough.

- Emollients – surrounding areas of dry skin should be kept moist with emollients. (Topical steroids are occasionally used to treat surrounding venous eczema; if there are persistent problems with eczema always consider an allergy to the dressings.)
- Dressing – ulcers can be dressed with non-adherent, hydrocolloid and foam dressings. The benefits of each depend on the current state of the wound. An important factor in dressing performance is that it does not stick to the wound, hence removing valuable granulation tissue on dressing change.
- Graduated compression – the mainstay in managing venous ulcers is with graduated compression therapy. It is useful to try to minimise pre-existing swelling of the limb with rest and elevation prior to commencing therapy. Compression therapy should produce maximum pressure at the ankle, gradually reducing towards the knee level. Compression bandaging is multilayer, with a variety of layers for dressing support, padding, elastic compression and an outer cover. The layers vary between compression systems.
- Antibiotics – antibiotics are only prescribed for ulcers where there is evidence of active infection (i.e. progressing cellulitis) rather than just colonisation. Topical antibiotics are generally not given to treat infections, although metronidazole gel is sometimes used for malodorous wounds.

What is the role of superficial venous surgery in managing venous ulcers?

The recent long term results of compression therapy alone versus compression plus surgery in chronic venous ulceration (ESCHAR) trial has addressed the question of correction of superficial venous reflux in addition to standard compression therapy [2]. The study assessed 500 legs managed in specialist nurse-led leg ulcer clinics (three centres). The investigators demonstrated that surgical correction of superficial venous reflux in addition to compression bandaging did not improve ulcer healing. However, superficial venous surgery did reduce ulcer recurrence at 4 years and also resulted in patients having a greater proportion of ulcer-free time.

What factors influence sub-bandage pressure?

Sub-bandage pressure is proportional to TN/CW. Where T is the bandage tension, C is the circumference of the limb, W is the width of the bandage and N is the number of layers.

From analysing the formula it is clear that a bandage applied with a constant tension will automatically produce a graduated fall in sub-bandage pressure from the narrow ankle to the wider calf. The ankle, being the lowest diameter, will have the highest area of pressure, providing the bandage tension remains the same throughout the dressing. Hence there is an inverse relationship between leg circumference and pressure applied. Bandages are generally applied with a 50% overlap. Care must be taken when applying bandaging around bony prominences (malleoli and tibial crest) not to form areas of localised pressure. Ankle sub-bandage pressures of 40 mmHg are often utilised in treating venous ulcers.

How is compression hosiery classified?

Compression hosiery has commonly been prescribed by the 'Class' system. This system often leads to confusion due to the differing British standard (BS 6612:1985) and European standard (SS-ENV 12718) categories. Whereas the British system is divided into three

Table I.1 Classification of compression hosiery

Class	British (mmHg)	European (mmHg)
I	14–17	18–21
II	18–24	25–32
III	25–35	36–46
IV	NA	Over 59

classes the European has four classes according to the level of ankle compression. The pressure levels in the European 'classes' are higher than those in the British systems (see Table I.1). In clinical practice the best way to prescribe compression hosiery is by the level of compression in mmHg, hence 18–24 mmHg compression hosiery should be requested rather than simply 'class II'.

Aortic aneurysm suitability for endovascular aneurysm repair (EVAR)

The basics

EVAR is now established based upon the UK EVAR trials but techniques, suitability and assessment methods are continually evolving. Assessment of suitability requires a computed tomography (CT) angiogram with a minimum slice thickness of 3 mm. Axial images produced by CT should be assessed to gain a general picture of the aneurysm, patency of visceral arteries and anatomy of the thoracic aorta and arch. Multi-planar reconstructions are then performed on CT work stations to allow measurements of diameters perpendicular to the axis of the aorta and length measurements. Diameters that must be measured are the neck of the aneurysm, the distal landing zone (usually common iliac arteries) and the aortic bifurcation. Important length measurements are length of aortic neck, distal sealing zone, distance from lowest renal artery to aortic bifurcation and distance from aortic bifurcation to intended landing zone (iliac bifurcation). Three-dimensional volume rendering modes using automated techniques to plot the centre-line give the described lengths.

The case

You are shown an abdominal CT scan with an AAA. These will be axial scans but may contain reconstructed images.

Questions

What CT features of an AAA would you consider in assessing it for a conventional stent graft?

Adverse anatomical factors vary for different types of stent but in general these can be classified as shown below. The limitations for EVAR are becoming less. In the EVAR trials 50% of AAAs were suitable for stenting whereas currently using a variety of different devices, approximately 80% can be treated using EVAR. Although no single anatomical problem should prevent one from performing EVAR, several anatomical constraints may prevent sealing and fixation, thereby increasing the risk of endoleak and migration.

Graft introduction

Factors making insertion of the stent difficult include iliac artery tortuosity especially in combination with circumferential calcification preventing straightening of the vessels. Stenotic or occlusive disease of the iliac arteries may prevent access although minor degrees can be overcome by angioplasty, use of 'peel-back' sheaths or even dilating within a sheath for more severe cases. Ultimately a uni-iliac device may be used if one-sided access is impossible with a femoro-femoral cross-over graft used to perfuse the limb with the diseased iliac arteries.

Proximal sealing and fixation

A non-favourable neck may have angulation of more than 60° (although newer devices may allow greater degrees of angulation), conical neck (more than 3 mm increase in diameter distally for 1 cm length of neck for sealing), thrombus or calcification. The length of the neck should be at least 10–15 mm for an adequate proximal seal. Stent grafts come in various diameters and there will be a few AAAs that have a neck diameter that is too large (normally 32 mm diameter of neck, which requires 20% oversizing).

Distal sealing zone

Similar principles apply to the distal sealing zone as they do to the neck. Ideally this should be close to the iliac bifurcation with a sealing length of 10–15 mm. With modern devices iliac diameters as large as 25 mm can be treated. If the landing zone involves the external iliac artery and coverage of the internal iliac artery, there may be a risk of buttock claudication or ischaemic colitis if done bilaterally. Coverage would in addition require embolisation of the internal iliac artery to prevent a Type II endoleak. The internal iliac artery may be preserved by using customised 'iliac-branched grafts'.

Length from renal arteries to aortic bifurcation

The length of the aneurysm from the renal arteries has to be appropriate to allow the short stump of the contralateral limb to fully open. Similarly any 'waisting' at the aortic bifurcation may not allow this to be possible, hence the importance of measuring the diameter of the aortic bifurcation.

How do you classify endoleaks and how are they managed?

Endoleaks are classified as four different types. Types I, III and IV endoleak require intervention whereas most Type II leaks are benign and can be monitored conservatively unless there is continued sac expansion. Table I.2 summarises classification, pathogenesis and management.

Consent for an AAA repair

The basics

The discussion about consent will depend on whether the patient is to undergo open or enodovascular repair and also the ability to obtain consent. The General Medical Council (GMC) has published guidelines for good practice in obtaining consent.

Table I.2 Classification of endoleaks

Type	Pathogenesis	Management
I (proximal)	Poor seal or fixation at neck	Balloon moulding (at first procedure) Palmaz stent Banding of aortic neck
I (distal)	Poor seal or fixation at distal landing zone	Balloon moulding (at first procedure) Upsizing distal limb with extension
II	Feeding IMA or iliolumbar vessels	Conservative treatment if AAA not expanding. If it expands, then CT or selective catheter angiography to diagnose the cause. These may be embolised, IMA may be ligated surgically (open or laparoscopic) or translumbar injection of thrombotic material directly into AAA
III	Modular disconnection or tears in stent graft	Intraoperatively junctional zones can be ballooned. Postoperatively, bridging stent required
IV	Porosity of stent graft or undetected endoleak	Intraoperative porosity or 'sweating' is benign. Endotension resulting in continued sac growth requires relining with new stent graft or explantation

Notes: IMA, inferior mesenteric artery; AAA, abdominal aortic aneurysm; CT, computed tomography.

The case

There will usually be a patient who most likely is about to or has undergone the procedure. Communication is the key. You must assess how much the patient knows about the procedure and then go on to describe the procedure, its benefits and risks. The risks as stated on the consent form should be those that are frequent or serious and in addition should take into account the patient's personal circumstances. These can be divided into general and specific and furthermore early and late.

The benefits of surgery depend on the presentation. For asymptomatic AAAs, the reason for intervention is to prevent rupture. In cases of distal embolisation the aim is limb salvage and in acute cases of rupture or bleeding from fistulation, the aim is to save life. Rarely, large aneurysms may cause obstruction of the duodenum.

The risks of open AAA repair

Early complications

1. These are related to aortic cross clamping and the systemic inflammatory response. Although cardiac complications were the main causes of early mortality, more modern series suggest that multi-organ failure (MOF) is an equal cause of death in elective repair including both primary MOF and MOF secondary to visceral ischaemia and pneumonia.
2. Isolated respiratory failure is the other prominent cause of mortality. With improvements in optimization of cardiac function, patient selection, advancements in anaesthetic and postoperative critical care, early mortality rates have been reduced to 5%.

3. Other complications to mention include distal embolisation leading to limb loss, ischaemic colitis requiring a colostomy, renal failure and impotence. The frequency of these complications will depend on the complexity of the aneurysm including suprarenal clamping, thrombus adjacent to the renal artery origins and patency of visceral and internal iliac arteries.

Late complications

1. Poor coverage of the graft by either the sac of the aneurysm or by an omental flap may lead to graft-to enteric fistulae and graft infection.
2. False aneuryms particularly with anastamoses onto the femoral artery.

The risks of EVAR

Early complications

1. General complications are related to vascular surgical (groin seroma, haematoma and false aneurysm) and radiological procedures involving contrast agents (direct effects of contrast related to volume including renal failure and idiosynchratic reactions).
2. Specific complications are classified as those relating to the stent and those relating to the surgery. Stent related complications include endoleak and rupture. Coverage of both internal iliac arteries in the presence of diseased visceral vessels may lead to ischaemic colitis. Coverage of one internal iliac artery may lead to buttock claudication. Inadvertent coverage of renal arteries may necessitate stenting the renal artery to 'open' the ostium covered by the stent graft. Bilateral occlusion normally necessitates open conversion with renal revascularisation. Balloon moulding has a small risk of rupture in addition, which may be treated by a covered stent graft or open conversion. The 30-day mortality for EVAR is 2%.

Late complications

1. Continued expansion and rupture (1% annual risk) can occur because of either endoleak or endotension alone or in combination with stent migration.
2. Limbs of the stents may also occlude from kinking as a result of changes in conformation of the stent due to sac shrinkage.
3. Although the risk of graft infections is lower than open repair, procedures utilising uni-iliac stents, which need a femoro-femoral cross-over graft, may have a higher risk.

References

1. Levieri LS, Veller MG. Popliteal enfragment synchrome: more common than previously recognized. *J Vcox Surg* 1999; **30**: 587–98.
2. Gohel et al. Long term results of compression therapy alone versus compression therapy alone versus compression plus surgery m chronic venous ulceration (eschar): randamized controlled trial. *BMG* 2007; **335**: 83–87.

Section 2

Final FRCS vascular topics

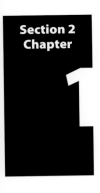

Vascular risk factors and their management

Alasdair Wilson and Julie Brittenden

Key points

- Peripheral arterial disease (PAD) is an under-diagnosed and under-treated condition
- Patients with PAD have a cardiovascular risk profile equivalent to or worse than those with coronary or cerebrovascular disease
- PAD patients with concomitant symptomatic cardiac or cerebrovascular disease, diabetes or a low ankle pressure index are at even higher risk of sustaining a vascular event
- Patients with PAD should receive the same risk factor management as patients with other cardiovascular diseases
- Patient awareness of the need for cardiovascular secondary prevention therapy in PAD is low

The need for cardiovascular risk factor management in patients with peripheral arterial disease

PAD is a condition that is frequently under diagnosed and often the subject of suboptimal care. The first line treatment for patients with PAD is cardiovascular risk factor management with the aim of improving patient survival. This is because patients with PAD have a two- to threefold increased risk of cardiovascular mortality compared to an age- and sex-matched control population. The risk of a patient with PAD dying from a heart attack is believed to be equivalent to those patients who have already survived their first myocardial infarction.

The global Reduction of Atherothrombosis for Continued Health (REACH) registry has recently been established to determine atherothrombotic risk in more than 68 000 at-risk patients [1]. To date it has shown that, compared to patients with coronary heart disease or cerebrovascular disease, those with PAD had the highest rates of cardiovascular death, myocardial infarction, stroke, or hospitalisation for atherothrombotic events at 1-year follow up (Figure 1.1). It also showed that the number of events increased with the number of clinically involved vascular beds. Thus patients with PAD and symptomatic cardiac or cerebrovascular disease have increased risk compared to those with PAD alone (Figure 1.1).

The risk of developing cardiovascular events in patients with PAD is also known to increase with the severity of disease, such that patients with rest pain or tissue loss have a worse prognosis than patients with intermittent claudication (Figure 1.2) [2]. However,

Postgraduate Vascular Surgery: The Candidate's Guide to the FRCS, eds. Vish Bhattacharya and Gerard Stansby. Published by Cambridge University Press. © Cambridge University Press 2010.

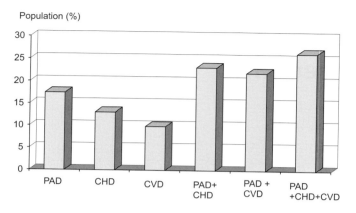

Figure 1.1 One-year cardiovascular event rates in outpatients with atherothrombosis. Data for graph obtained from: Steg PH, Bhatt D, Wilson PWF, D'Iagostino R, Ohman EM, Rother J et al. *JAMA* 2007; **297**: 1197–206. Reproduced with permission. PAD, peripheral arterial disease; CHD, coronary heart disease; CVD, cerebrovascular disease.

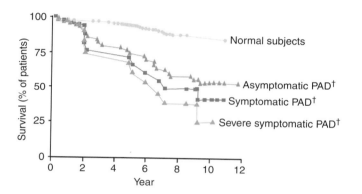

Figure 1.2 Kaplan–Meier survival curves based on mortality from all causes in patients with large vessel disease. Criqui MH, Langer RD, Fronek A, Feigelson HF, Klauber MR, McCann TJ et al. Mortality over a period of 10 years in patients with peripheral arterial disease. *N Engl J Med* 1992; **326**: 381–6. Reproduced with permission. PAD, peripheral arterial disease.

patients who are asymptomatic but have PAD as defined by an ankle brachial pressure index (ABPI) less than 0.9 have also been shown to have a reduced survival compared to a sex- and age-matched control population. In one study, patients who had PAD involving the large vessels were found to have a 6.6-fold (95% confidence interval 2.9–14.9) increased risk of death from coronary heart disease at 10-year follow up compared to patients with no PAD. Overall, less than one-quarter of patients with severe symptomatic large vessel PAD survived 10 years (Figure 1.2) [2].

The ABPI has also been shown to predict overall survival, independently of the metabolic syndrome and other conventional cardiovascular risk factors. The hazard ratio for mortality has been shown to increase consistently with decreasing ABPI for both males and females (Figure 1.3)[3].

Why do we as vascular surgeons need to treat risk factors?

Despite the increased cardiovascular risk in patients with PAD, risk factor management in these patients has been shown to be inadequate in both primary and secondary care settings. In particular, when compared to patients with coronary heart disease (CHD), patients with PAD (despite comparable risk) received less intensive treatment for lipid disorders and hypertension and were prescribed antiplatelet therapy less frequently than were patients with CHD.

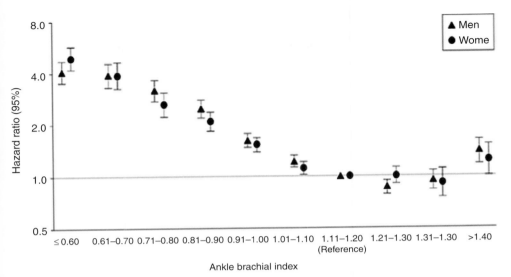

Figure 1.3 Hazard ratios for total mortality in men and women by ankle brachial pressure index (ABI) for all studies in the ABI collaboration. Ankle Brachial Index Collaboration. Ankle Brachial Index combined with Framingham risk score to predict cardiovascular events and mortality. A meta-analysis. *JAMA* 2008; **300**: 197–208. Reproduced with permission.

In addition to being under-treated, PAD is often under-diagnosed and public awareness of the condition has been shown to be poor throughout Europe and the USA. Patients are also unaware of the need for secondary prevention therapy. Thus it is the responsibility of the vascular surgeon to initiate risk factor management if this has not already been commenced in primary care and also to educate the patient on the need for this treatment.

Risk factors

The major risk factors for PAD are the same as for CHD. They can be considered as either 'modifiable' or 'non-modifiable' and those that are modifiable may be treated by 'lifestyle changes' or drug treatments. Of all the modifiable risk factors smoking is the most important but others include management of dyslipidaemia, hypertension, diabetes, and the use of antiplatelet therapy. Evidence-based medicine has shown that reducing cardiovascular risk in patients with symptomatic PAD improves survival. The rationale and targets for treating these risks factors have been addressed in a number of national and international guidelines. The Scottish Intercollegiate Guidelines Network (SIGN) guidelines [4] on the management of peripheral arterial disease and the Transatlantic Society (TASC) guidelines have both been recently updated [5]. All vascular surgeons should check that their PAD patients have stopped smoking, check that they are on an antiplatelet and a statin unless contraindicated, check that their hypertension is adequately treated, exclude diabetes and give lifestyle advice. The management of these risk factors is further summarised below.

Smoking

Smoking cessation is the most important component of secondary prevention in patients with PAD. Cigarette smoking doubles the risk of a patient developing PAD and for those who

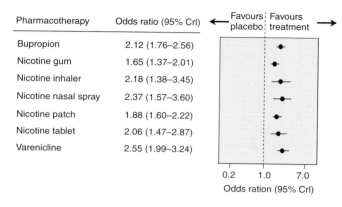

Pharmacotherapy	Odds ratio (95% Crl)
Bupropion	2.12 (1.76–2.56)
Nicotine gum	1.65 (1.37–2.01)
Nicotine inhaler	2.18 (1.38–3.45)
Nicotine nasal spray	2.37 (1.57–3.60)
Nicotine patch	1.88 (1.60–2.22)
Nicotine tablet	2.06 (1.47–2.87)
Varenicline	2.55 (1.99–3.24)

Figure 1.4 Pharmacotherapy for smoking cessation: a meta-analysis of randomized controlled trials. Permission for use requested. Eisenberg MJ, Filion KB, Belisle P et al. Pharmacotherapies for smoking cessation: a meta-analysis of randomized controlled trials *CMAJ* 2008; **179**: 135–44. Reproduced with permission.

continue to smoke the chance of disease progression is also increased by twofold. Cessation of smoking may not improving walking capacity in patients with PAD but can prevent the onset of critical limb ischemia and reduces the risk of bypass graft occlusion by threefold. However, most importantly, smoking cessation is associated with a reduction in all major cardiovascular events. A recent Cochrane review of smoking cessation for the secondary prevention of coronary heart disease has shown that smoking cessation is associated with a 36% reduction in all- cause mortality [6].

The vascular surgeon has an important role in promoting smoking cessation and should 'strongly and repeatedly advise patients to stop smoking' (Figure 1.4) [5, 7], and arrange referral to a smoking cessation program. Encouraging patients to stop smoking through smoking cessation support programs has been shown to double the smoking cessation rate. Nicotine replacement therapy also increases the quit rate by approximately twofold. The combination of these two methods has been associated with a 22% cessation rate at 5 years. Antidepressants such as bupropion have also been found to be useful in achieving smoking cessation and have a synergistic effect when used with nicotine replacement therapy. More recently interest has focused on the role of the nicotine receptor partial agonist varenicline in smoking cessation. This may reduce dependence by mimicking the actions of nicotine on neuronal nicotinic receptors in the brain, thus maintaining some dopamine levels and reducing withdrawal symptoms that are associated with reduced dopamine release. In addition to this action, varenicline may also competitively inhibit binding of cigarette nicotine to these receptors. A recent randomised controlled trial has shown that varenicline results in four times greater odds of stopping smoking compared to a placebo and two times greater odds than bupropion. Although effective, these drugs may have side effects (bupropion can cause seizures, varenicline can cause depression and suicidal ideation). Pharmacotherapy treatments are usually provided within a smoking cessation program that involves counselling and usually uses nicotine replacement as first-line treatment (Figure 1.5).

Smoking: current recommendations

- Patients with PAD who smoke should be advised to quit.
- Vascular surgeons should take the opportunity to advise all patients who smoke with PAD to quit when they attend for a consultation.
- Patients with PAD who smoke should be referred to an intensive support service.
- Patients with PAD who are planning to stop smoking should be offered nicotine replacement therapy (NRT) or varenicline or bupropion.

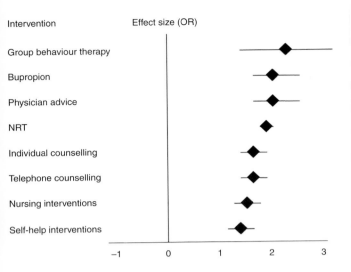

Figure 1.5 Effectiveness of smoking cessation interventions. Eisenberg MJ, Filion KB, Belisle P et al. Effectiveness of smoking cessation interventions among adults: a systemic review of reviews. *Cancer Prevention* 2008; **17**: 535–44. Reproduced with permission.

Dyslipidemia

Epidemiological, post mortem and angiographic studies have consistently shown a strong positive correlation between plasma total cholesterol and the incidence of CHD. In Western populations the increased risk of future cardiovascular events is observed with serum cholesterol levels that were considered to be in the normal range and increase progressively in a linear manner with rising cholesterol concentrations. In patients with PAD, elevated levels of total cholesterol, low density lipoprotein cholesterol, triglycerides and lipoprotein A are independent risk factors for adverse vascular events. In contrast, increased levels of high-density lipoprotein are protective.

Statins competitively inhibit the enzyme 3-hydroxyl-3-methylglutaryl coenzyme A (HMG-CoA), which catalyzes the conversion of HMG-CoA to mevalonate, an early step in the biosynthesis of cholesterol. This leads to a reduction in hepatocyte cholesterol concentration and increased expression of low-density lipoprotein (LDL) receptors, which are involved in the clearance of LDLs and LDL precursors from the circulation. Statin therapy to lower LDL cholesterol is recommended in all patients with PAD, even in those patients whose cholesterol levels are within what is considered the normal range. This guidance is based on the results of the Medical Research Council (MRC) Heart Protection study, which showed that treatment with simvastatin 40 mg daily resulted in a 22% (95% confidence interval: 15–29) relative risk reduction in the rates of myocardial infarction, stroke and of revascularisation in patients with PAD who had a cholesterol level greater than 3.5 mmol l^{-1} [8]. There was also a significant reduction in all-cause mortality and in particular that due to cardiac causes in patients with PAD allocated to simvastatin therapy compared to placebo (Figure 1.6).

These benefits were observed irrespective of the baseline level of cholesterol and occurred in patients with and without clinical disease in other arterial beds. In addition to starting a patient with PAD on a statin it is also important to monitor the reduction in cholesterol levels achieved. The reduction in cardiovascular risk achieved by statin therapy has been shown to be proportional to the achieved reduction in LDL cholesterol reduction (Figure 1.7) [9]. Overall statins reduce the 5-year incidence of major coronary events, coronary

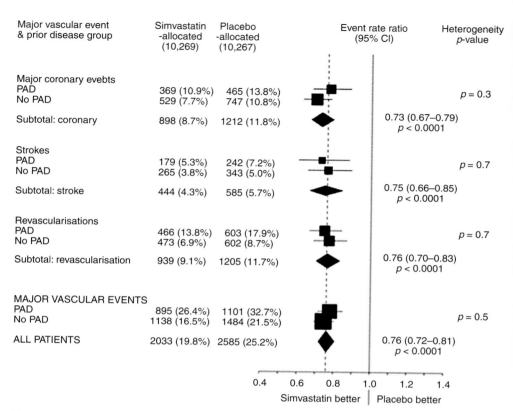

Major vascular event & prior disease group	Simvastatin -allocated (10,269)	Placebo -allocated (10,267)	Event rate ratio (95% CI)	Heterogeneity p-value
Major coronary evebts				
PAD	369 (10.9%)	465 (13.8%)		$p = 0.3$
No PAD	529 (7.7%)	747 (10.8%)		
Subtotal: coronary	898 (8.7%)	1212 (11.8%)	0.73 (0.67–0.79) $p < 0.0001$	
Strokes				
PAD	179 (5.3%)	242 (7.2%)		$p = 0.7$
No PAD	265 (3.8%)	343 (5.0%)		
Subtotal: stroke	444 (4.3%)	585 (5.7%)	0.75 (0.66–0.85) $p < 0.0001$	
Revascularisations				
PAD	466 (13.8%)	603 (17.9%)		$p = 0.7$
No PAD	473 (6.9%)	602 (8.7%)		
Subtotal: revascularisation	939 (9.1%)	1205 (11.7%)	0.76 (0.70–0.83) $p < 0.0001$	
MAJOR VASCULAR EVENTS				
PAD	895 (26.4%)	1101 (32.7%)		$p = 0.5$
No PAD	1138 (16.5%)	1484 (21.5%)		
ALL PATIENTS	2033 (19.8%)	2585 (25.2%)	0.76 (0.72–0.81) $p < 0.0001$	

0.4 0.6 0.8 1.0 1.2 1.4
Simvastatin better | Placebo better

Figure 1.6 Heart Protection Study. Randomized trial of the effects of cholesterol-lowering with simvastatin on peripheral vascular and other major vascular outcomes in 20 536 people with peripheral arterial disease and other high-risk conditions. Heart Protection Study Collaborative Group. *J Vasc Surg* 2007; **45**: 645–54. PAD, peripheral arterial disease.

revascularisation and stroke by one-fifth per mmol l-1 reduction in LDL-cholesterol, irrespective of the patient's baseline lipid profile. Furthermore, recent trials involving patients with acute coronary syndromes and stable coronary disease have shown a greater reduction in cardiac events in patients receiving high-dose compared to conventional dose statin therapy [8] This is likely to be the case for patients with PAD and as such the TASC guidelines recommend more aggressive lowering of cholesterol in those patients with PAD most at risk such as those with concurrent disease in other vascular beds. This should also be considered for those with diabetes or a low ABPI. In addition to statin therapy, dietary measures are also recommended but when used alone have been shown to result in only a 10% reduction in LDL-cholesterol and long-term compliance is known to be low. The main limitations to using statins are side effects, principally muscle aches and rarely rhabdomyolysis.

For blood sampling and other lipids, non-fasting samples are satisfactory for assessing LDL-cholesterol levels. Triglycerides would need to be measured in fasting samples but are not routinely directly targeted in patients with PAD. High-density lipid (HDL)-cholesterol levels are known to be protective and a number of new pharmacological agents are currently under investigation to increase HDL-cholesterol.

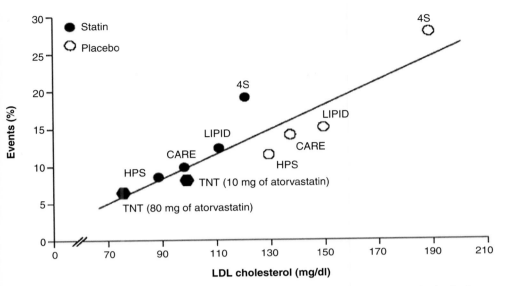

Figure 1.7 Relationship between level of cholesterol reduction achieved with statin therapy and reduction in events. La Rosa JC, Grundy SM, Waters DD. Intensive lipid lowering with atorvastatin in patients with stable coronary disease. *N Engl J Med* 2005; **352**: 1425–1435. Reproduced with permission. *Note*: 100 mg dl^{-1}=2.6 mmol.

Dyslipidaemia: current recommendations

- Patients with PAD with a total cholesterol >3.5 mmol l^{-1} should be commenced on statin therapy (this will be the vast majority of patients and you do not need to wait for lipid levels to come back before starting therapy).
- The aim is to lower the LDL cholesterol to less than 2.0 mmol l^{-1}.
- Patients with PAD and known disease in other vascular beds should be considered for more aggressive treatment with the aim of achieving LDL-cholesterol levels below 1.8 mmol l^{-1}.

Statins and inflammatory response

This is still a controversial area but statins appear to do more than just lower cholesterol. LDL-cholesterol is oxidized by free radicals and may cause direct oxidative damage. A reduction in the levels of LDL cholesterol by the use of statin therapy will result in reduced superoxide production. While many of the anti-inflammatory effects may be due to the reduction in LDL-cholesterol, the reduction in vascular events achieved by statin therapy is greater and occurs earlier than would be predicted from the lipid lowering effects alone. The non-lipid lowering effects of statins have been attributed to their ability to inhibit the generation of proteins called isoprenoids. Mevalonate is the precursor of these compounds and inhibited by statins. The isoprenoids bind to a number of signalling proteins (Rho and Ras) on the cell membrane, which are involved in the inflammatory response. Through these mechanisms statins have widespread effects on the endothelium, coagulation pathways, and platelet function, all of which are implicated in the pathogenesis of acute ischaemic events and have been shown to be activated in patients with PAD.

Vascular surgery has been shown to result in endothelial activation and a pro-thrombotic state, as indeed has lower limb angioplasty. Statin therapy has been shown to decrease the incidence of perioperative cardiac events in patients undergoing vascular surgery. Statin therapy leads to plaque stabilisation and may also have beneficial effects on walking distances. One study has shown that patients with PAD on statin therapy have a lower annual decline in lower extremity performance compared to those who are not on statins. A further study has suggested that statins may increase walking distances in claudicants.

Hypertension

Elevated blood pressure is an independent risk factor for cardiovascular and cerebrovascular morbidity and mortality (SIGN) [4]. In the Framingham trial the age-adjusted risk ratio for intermittent claudication in hypertensive patients compared to controls was increased two and half to fourfold [3]. In the UK, treatment of hypertension in patients with PAD should follow the recommendations of the British Hypertension Society Guidelines [10]. The current targets are a level of less than 140/90 mmHg or 130/80 mmHg for patients with diabetes or chronic renal disease. It can be seen from Figure 1.8 that the recommended first-line drug treatment varies depending on the age and race of the patient. ACE inhibitors are first-line drugs for the treatment of hypertension in patients with PAD but should be commenced with careful monitoring due to the possibility of co-existing renal artery stenosis. The prevalence of this is difficult to ascertain but one study, involving a selective group of patients with PAD who were undergoing angiography, found renal artery stenosis

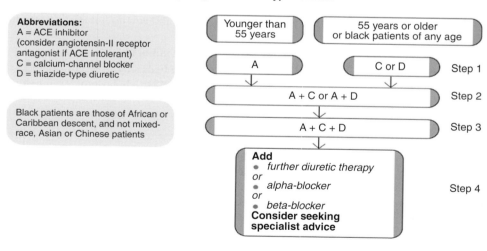

Choosing drugs for patients newly diagnosed with hypertension

Abbreviations:
A = ACE inhibitor
(consider angiotensin-II receptor antagonist if ACE intolerant)
C = calcium-channel blocker
D = thiazide-type diuretic

Black patients are those of African or Caribbean descent, and not mixed-race, Asian or Chinese patients

Younger than 55 years | 55 years or older or black patients of any age

A | C or D — Step 1

A + C or A + D — Step 2

A + C + D — Step 3

Add
• *further diuretic therapy*
or
• *alpha-blocker*
or
• *beta-blocker*
Consider seeking specialist advice — Step 4

BHS

NHS
National Institute for Health and Clinical Excellence

Figure 1.8 Current British Hypertensive Society and National Institute for Health and Clinical Excellence (NICE) guidelines for treatment of newly diagnosed hypertension.

in a quarter of patients. Since the publication of the Heart Outcomes Prevention Evaluation (HOPE) study there has been a move towards recommending the use of ACE inhibitors in patients with PAD even in the absence of hypertension [11]. ACE inhibitors have been shown to have various pleiotropic effects beyond their blood pressure lowering capacity. While there appears to be a promising reduction in cardiovascular mortality, morbidity, and stroke associated with ACE inhibitors, the TASC and SIGN guidelines do not recommend their use in patients with PAD other than for their blood pressure lowering effects. Only 30% of patients in the HOPE study were on statin therapy, and thus the pleiotropic effects of ACE inhibitors, in addition to standard medical therapy in patients with PAD who do not have hypertension, requires to be evaluated further. However, some recent evidence suggests that the ACE inhibitor ramipril may improve pain-free and maximum walking time in patients with PAD.

Beta-adrenergic blocking agents (β-blockers), in particular those with vasoconstrictor properties, were previously not recommended in patients with PAD. However, a meta-analysis of 11 randomised controlled trials has shown that they do not worsen the symptoms of claudication and can be used safely in patients with PAD. Furthermore, β-blockers may offer additional cardio-protection to patients with symptomatic PAD and cardiovascular disease. A number of studies have shown that perioperative use of β-blockers may reduce the postoperative cardiovascular events in PAD patients undergoing major vascular surgery. Their use is therefore recommended in the TASC guidelines. However, this is still a controversial area and a more recent study (POISE study) has shown that they may actually increase mortality [12]. Current advice would be to continue β-blockers if the patient is already on them but not to use them first line for blood pressure control or general risk reduction.

Hypertension: current recommendations

- Patients with PAD and hypertension should be treated to reduce their blood pressure to <140/90 mmHg.
- Patients with PAD, hypertension and either diabetes or renal impairment should be treated to reduce their blood pressure to <130/80 mmHg.
- Beta-adrenergic blocking drugs are not contraindicated in patients with PAD.

Antiplatelet therapy

Antiplatelet therapy is recommended in all patients with PAD. The Antithrombotic Trialists' Collaboration found that antiplatelet therapy (aspirin, ticlopidine or dipyridamole) was associated with a 23% reduction in non-fatal myocardial infarction, non-fatal stroke and vascular death in patients with PAD. Low dose aspirin (75–150 mg) is recommended as it has been shown to be equally as effective as high doses and is associated with a lower rate of gastrointestinal side effects [9].

Clopidogrel, a thienopyridine, has been shown to be of benefit in the treatment of PAD. The use of clopidogrel versus aspirin in patients at high risk of ischaemic events trial (CAPRIE) showed that clopidogrel reduced the relative risk of major vascular events by 8.7% (95% confidence interval 0.3–16.5%) compared to aspirin. In a subgroup analysis, clopidogrel reduced the relative risk of major vascular events by 23.8% (95% confidence interval 8.9–36.2%) compared to aspirin in patients with PAD. A subsequent economic analysis by the National Institute of Health and Clinical Excellence (NICE) has shown that the use of clopidogrel as first-line antiplatelet therapy is cost-effective for 2 years but not beyond this time period [13]. It remains to be determined if clopidogrel is cost effective in the 'higher risk' PAD groups. If used, clopidogrel should be prescribed as monotherapy. A combination antiplatelet therapy of aspirin and clopidogrel has not been shown to be of benefit to patients with PAD, and is not recommended due to the increased risk of bleeding complications.

Platelet activation, despite the use of antiplatelet therapy, has been shown to be increased in patients with PAD compared to healthy controls. Studies have shown 'aspirin resistance' occurs in 11% to 40% of patients with PAD. Similarly, a large variation in response to clopidogrel has also been shown to occur in patients with intermittent claudication, with 10% of patients showing no reduction in platelet activation after a loading dose.

Antiplatelet therapy: current guidelines

- Patients with PAD should be prescribed antiplatelet therapy.
- If aspirin is prescribed it should be used at low dose (75–150 mg).
- If clopidogrel is prescribed it should be used as monotherapy.
- There is currently no evidence for the use of dual antiplatelet therapy in PAD.

Diabetes

Diabetes and its poor control have long been recognised as a major risk factor for peripheral arterial disease. Diabetes increases the risk of PAD by two- to threefold. Approximately 20% of patients with PAD will have diabetes, but undiagnosed diabetes is common and may occur in 12% or more of new patients referred to a vascular clinic. Thus patients attending vascular clinics should be screened for the presence of possible diabetes. Tight diabetic control has been shown to reduce the risk of developing microvascular and macrovascular complications. The UK diabetes prospective study showed that each 1% rise in haemoglobin A1c (HbA1c) was associated with a 28% increased incidence of PAD and a 28% increased risk of death [14]. Furthermore, each 1% reduction in HbA1c achieved by treatment was found to correlate with a 14% reduction in myocardial infarction and a 43% decrease in amputation or death from PAD (Figure 1.9).

The current National Diabetic Guidelines recommend a HbA1c of less than 7% [15]. Thus in vascular clinics the opportunity to measure the HbA1c level should be taken. The current National Guidelines recommend that patients with a HbA1c level of greater than 6.5% should be started on a medical therapy after a trial of lifestyle measures [15]. All too often patients have been maintained on 'lifestyle measures' alone despite persistently elevated HbA1c levels. Furthermore, the presence of PAD and diabetes means that the patient falls into a high-risk category and should have aggressive cardiovascular risk factor management and appropriate foot care. In patients with type II diabetes and PAD, intensive blood pressure control has been shown to significantly reduce the risk of cardiovascular events, as has intensive treatment of dyslipidemia.

Diabetes: current recommendations

- Patients with diabetes and PAD should have aggressive control of blood glucose with the aim of obtaining a HbA1c level of <7%.
- Patients with PAD should be screened for the presence of diabetes.

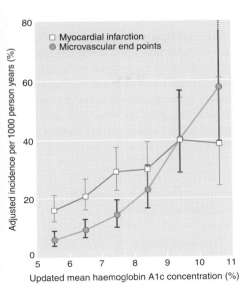

Figure 1.9 Diabetes, haemoglobin A1c and macrovascular events. Stratton IM, Adler AI, Neil HAW, Mathews DR, Manley SE, Cull CA, et al. Association of macrovascular and microvascular complications of type 2 diabetes (UKPDS:35): prospective observational study. *BMJ* 2000; **321**: 405–12. Reproduced with permission.

Lifestyle: weight reduction, diet and exercise

Obesity, in particular a BMI greater than 30 kg m^{-2} is associated with increased cardiovascular risk (SIGN). Thus obese patients with PAD should be offered help with weight reduction in terms of diet and exercise [4]. Patients with intermittent claudication who are physically active have been shown to have improved survival compared to patients who are sedentary [16].

There is abundant evidence to show that exercise can improve walking distance in claudicants if it is provided as a supervised exercise programme. However, there is little evidence that simple advice to exercise more is effective on its own. Where they are available patients with claudication should be referred to a local exercise programme. There are no studies looking at long-term risk reduction benefits of exercise in PAD specifically, however, they are proven to be effective in coronary disease and heart failure patients and prevent both future events and need for hospitalisation.

Weight reduction: current recommendations
- Patients with PAD who are obese should be treated to reduce their weight.

Exercise: current recommendations
- Patients with PAD should be encouraged to exercise and when available referred to a supervised exercise programme.

Homocysteine

This is currently a controversial risk factor for vascular disease. High plasma levels of the non-essential sulphur-containing amino acid homocysteine appear to be an independent risk factor for all types of atherosclerosis including PAD. Vitamins B6, B12 and folate are involved in its metabolism. Hyperhomocysteinemia is common, present in up to 60% of patients with PAD, and may be treated by folic acid and vitamin B6 supplements. However, currently there is no evidence from randomised trials that treatment in patients with PAD will alter the natural history of the disease and indeed evidence from one study in patients with cardiovascular disease suggests that treatment may have the potential of causing harm. There is still debate about whether homocysteine itself, or cofactors such as folic acid, are the causative agents. Thus the TASC guidelines currently recommend that patients with PAD should not be given folate supplements routinely. Homocysteine should probably only be measured in patients who develop PAD at a young age in the absence of traditional risk factors.

Homocysteine: current recommendations

- Patients with PAD should not routinely have homocysteine levels measured.
- Patients with PAD should not routinely be given folate supplements.

References

1. Steg PH, Bhatt D, Wilson PWF et al. One-year cardiovascular event rates in outpatients with atherothrombosis. *JAMA* 2007; **297**: 1197–206.
2. Criqui MH, Langer RD, Fronek A et al. Mortality over a period of 10 years in patients with peripheral arterial disease. *N Engl J Med* 1992; **326**: 381–6.
3. Ankle Brachial Index Collaboration. Ankle Brachial Index combined with Framingham Risk Score to predict cardiovascular events and mortality. *JAMA* 2008; **300**: 197–208.
4. Scottish Intercollegiate Guidelines Network (SIGN). *Diagnosis & Management of Peripheral Arterial Disease* 2006; Guideline no. 89.
5. TASC II guidelines at http://www.tasc-2-pad.org
6. Eisenberg MJ, Filion KB, Belisle P et al. Effectiveness of smoking cessation interventions among adults: a systemic review of reviews. *Cancer Prevention* 2008; **17**: 535–44.
7. LaRosa JC, Grundy SM, Walters DD et al. Intensive lipid lowering with atorvastatin in patients with stable coronary heart disease. *N Engl J Med* 2005; **352**: 1425–35.
8. Antithrombotic Trialists' Collaboration. Collaborative meta-analysis of randomised trials of antiplatelet therapy for the prevention of death, myocardial infarction and stroke in high risk patients. *BMJ* 2002; **324**: 71–86.
9. Heart Protection Study Collaborative Group. MRC/BHF Heart Protection Study of cholesterol lowering with Simvastatin I 20, 536 high risk individuals: a randomised placebo controlled trial. *Lancet* 2002; **360**: 7–22.
10. Stratton IM, Adler AI, Neil HAW et al. Association of macrovascular and microvascular complications of type 2 diabetes (UKPDS:35): prospective observational study. *BMJ* 2000; **321**: 405–12.

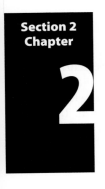

Management of acute limb ischaemia

Arun Balakrishnan and David Lambert

Key points

- Acute limb ischaemia (ALI) is associated with significant mortality and morbidity
- Clinical assessment is paramount for planning management
- All cases of ALI should be assessed by a vascular specialist
- All cases should be started on intravenous heparin as soon as possible to prevention extension of thrombus
- Surgery is preferred with severe ALI as time is of the essence
- Thrombolysis is associated with a lower mortality rate but higher failure rates
- Surgery is more durable but is associated with a higher mortality rate
- If compartment syndrome likely or suspected a fasciotomy is required

Definition

Acute limb ischaemia (ALI) can be defined as a sudden compromise of the blood supply to a limb, threatening its viability. Symptoms are usually of less than 2 weeks in duration. The lower limbs are more commonly affected than the upper limbs.

Background

Patients with ALI present depending on the severity of their symptoms. In patients with acute arterial occlusions and no collaterals symptom onset is immediate and severe. This scenario is seen in patients with embolic occlusions, trauma, thrombosed aneurysms and occluded grafts. If the acute event occurs with a background of an artery or a graft narrowing/occluding over a period of time then usually there are developed collaterals. In these patients the symptoms are often not as severe.

After 3–6 hours of severe ischaemia muscle and nerve undergo irreversible changes. Ischaemia of the limb for greater than 6 hours usually results in functional impairment or limb loss. Time is therefore of the essence – the less the time interval between the event and treatment the better the outcome. Acute limb ischaemia is a genuine surgical emergency with a high incidence of mortality and morbidity. These patients are best managed by a dedicated vascular service [1].

Aetiology

Acute limb ischaemia can be caused by occlusion of a native vessel or a graft. Arteries are mainly occluded by thrombus or emboli (Table 2.1). Emboli tend to lodge in the bifurcation

Postgraduate Vascular Surgery: The Candidate's Guide to the FRCS, eds. Vish Bhattacharya and Gerard Stansby. Published by Cambridge University Press. © Cambridge University Press 2010.

Table 2.1 Causes of arterial occlusion

Embolic

- Mural thrombus following myocardial infarction
- The atrium in patients with atrial fibrillation [2]
- The atrium in patients with rheumatic heart disease
- Valvular vegetations in patients with endocarditis
- Atrial myxoma
- Aneurysms and atherosclerotic lesions proximal to the ischaemic limb
- Paradoxical emboli from the venous system in patients with atrial septal defects

Thrombotic

- Thrombosis of an artery due to atheroma
- Thrombosed aneurysm with peripheral embolisation
- Thrombosis of a reconstructed artery or bypass graft
- Arterial dissection
- External compression
- Popliteal entrapment
- Cystic adventitial disease
- Blunt trauma resulting in disruption of the intima
- Penetrating trauma resulting in division of the artery
- Compartment syndrome
- Low flow states in the limb
  - Hypotension
  - Low cardiac output
  - Vasoconstrictor drugs
  - Severe venous thrombosis

of an artery. The usual sites in the limbs are at the bifurcation of the common femoral artery, iliac artery, popliteal artery, aorta and brachial artery. Almost all emboli are part of a thrombus although foreign body or tumour emboli can occur. Emboli lodging at the aortic bifurcation are termed saddle emboli.

Assessment of the acutely ischaemic limb

The limb is cool, pale with decreased sensation and muscle weakness. The clinical features of an acutely ischaemic limb are often described as the '6 P's':

Pain	Sudden onset, constant and severe
Pallor	The limb is pale
Pulselessness	Unilateral loss of pulses
Paralysis	Inability to move limb
Paresthesia	Altered sensation
Perishingly cold leg	Cool or cold skin

Table 2.2 Classification of acute limb ischaemia

Category	Description	Capillary return	Muscle paralysis	Sensory loss	Arterial Doppler signals	Venous Doppler signals
I Viable	Not immediately threatened	Intact	None	None	Audible	Audible
IIa Threatened	Salvageable if promptly treated	Intact/slow	None	Partial	Inaudible	Audible
IIb Threatened	Salvageable if immediately treated	Slow/absent	Partial	Partial/complete	Inaudible	Audible
III Irreversible	Primary amputation	Absent Staining	Complete Tense compartment	Complete	Inaudible	Inaudible

Rutherford RB. Suggested standards for reports dealing with lower extremity ischemia. *J Vasc Surg* 1986; **4**: 80–94. Reproduced with permission.

However, this is a rather simplistic approach best suited to medical students rather than a vascular specialist. Patients rarely complain of any of these specifically, except pain. Most commonly they describe the sudden onset of pain, inability to stand or walk on the leg and then the onset of numbness in the foot.

An acutely ischaemic limb must be carefully assessed to determine the severity of ischaemia. The main questions to answer are the following:

- Is the ischaemia reversible?
- Is the leg viable?
- Is the limb immediately threatened?

The severity of ischaemia influences management and decision making. A viable limb has minor or no sensory or motor impairment. The presence of rest pain, decreased sensation and weak muscles indicate a threatened limb. Limbs with severe pain in the presence of fixed mottling and tender muscles are irreversibly ischaemic. A viable limb allows time for investigation to decide on appropriate intervention (Table 2.2). When the cause for limb ischaemia is thrombosis in situ the symptoms/signs may be less pronounced. This is because occlusion occurs in an artery/graft that has narrowed over a period of time, permitting collaterals to develop.

Management

The severity of ischaemia influences management, urgency and decision making (Figure 2.1). When a diagnosis of severe ALI is made the patient should be adequately resuscitated. The following measures in particular should be instituted:

1. Oxygen should be administered.
2. Intravenous (IV) access and fluids to achieve adequate hydration.

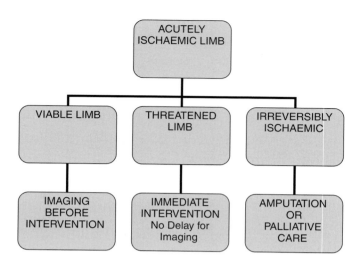

Figure 2.1 Flow chart showing initial decision-making pathway.

3. Heparin therapy: a bolus of 5000 units IV followed by the infusion of heparin at a rate of 1000 units per hour. The APTR is monitored and heparin infusion adjusted accordingly to maintain adequate anticoagulation.
4. Adequate analgesia.
5. Urine output should be monitored – usually a catheter is inserted.

Heparin is used to prevent propagation and extension of thrombus. It also reduces the incidence of cardiovascular events and improves prognosis [3].

Investigation

All patients should have the following baseline tests, although treatment should not be delayed for the results.
1. Full blood count.
2. Urea and electrolytes.
3. Blood glucose.
4. Clotting if already on anticoagulant therapy.
5. Electrocardiogram (ECG).
6. Group and save serum.

Vascular imaging is only indicated to guide treatment if the limb is viable. If the limb is threatened then imaging will not usually change the planned procedure and will delay revascularisation. Imaging will define arterial anatomy and help decide if surgery or endovascular therapy is appropriate. If required on-table angiography may be preferred to avoid delays. If the limb is not immediately threatened then standard imaging modalities including Duplex and computed tomography angiography (CTA) or magnetic resonance angiography (MRA) may be appropriate.

Treatment strategies for acute limb ischaemia

The various available treatment options are:

1. Surgical revascularisation.
2. Surgery in the form of amputation.
3. Endovascular including thrombolysis.
4. Palliative care.

If the limb is immediately threatened then immediate intervention is indicated.

Surgical revascularisation

Embolectomy

Femoral embolectomy can be performed under a local or general anesthetic depending upon the fitness of the patient. If performed under a local anesthetic then an anaesthetist should be present in theatre and the patient adequately monitored. The patient is appropriately prepared and draped. In the absence of a femoral pulse both groins are exposed. The limbs should be visible throughout the procedure and the feet should be placed in transparent bags. The femoral vessels on the affected side should be accessed through a vertical incision centred on the mid inguinal point. The common femoral, superficial femoral and profunda femoris arteries should be dissected free and controlled with slings. A transverse arteriotomy should be fashioned proximal to the bifurcation of the common femoral artery into the superficial femoral and profunda femoris arteries in order to permit selective catheterisation of both arteries. The embolus usually lodges in the femoral bifurcation, iliac bifurcation or the aortic bifurcation. If there is an embolus at the femoral bifurcation this is removed using forceps or suction. This manoeuvre will establish a good flow of blood down the common femoral artery if there are no other proximal lesions. A Fogarty catheter is passed down the superficial femoral and profunda arteries in an attempt to remove any thrombus that may have dropped down these arteries. An intraoperative angiogram can be performed to check if the arteries have been adequately cleared. If the embolus is proximal to the femoral artery then a Fogarty catheter will need to be passed cranially. If flow cannot be established down one side then the patient should have a femoral to femoral artery bypass if there is a normal pulse on the other side. If this is not the case then the patient should have an ipsilateral axillary to femoral artery bypass.

Some patients with an ischaemic limb have a good femoral pulse with an embolus at the popliteal bifurcation. If this diagnosis is suspected then the below-knee popliteal artery should be exposed through an incision behind the medial border of the tibia. The below-knee popliteal, anterior tibial, peroneal and the posterior tibial arteries should be dissected free and controlled with sloops. An incision should be made proximal to the bifurcation of the popliteal artery. Each of the above arteries can now be cleared by selectively catheterising them with a Fogarty balloon catheter. An angiogram can be performed to check clearance of the vessels. The arteriotomy is usually closed with a vein patch to avoid narrowing of the vessel.

If a saddle embolus is suspected at the aortic bifurcation then the femoral arteries are dissected free and controlled in both groins. A Fogarty catheter is passed in a cranial direction on both sides and the clot removed.

In the case of upper limb ischaemia the brachial artery and its bifurcation into the radial and ulnar arteries should be accessed through a lazy S shaped incision in the ante cubital fossa. The arteries are dissected free and controlled with sloops. A transverse arteriotomy is made just proximal to the brachial bifurcation. Clot at the bifurcation can be removed with forceps or by suction. A Fogarty catheter is then passed cranially and into the distal branches to clear any possible embolic material. When good flow has been established the arteriotomy is closed with prolene.

If an angiogram reveals the presence of residual clot in the vessels then intraoperative thrombolysis can be used to dissolve the clot. An infusion of 100 000 units of streptokinase or t-Pa 15 mg in 100 ml of normal saline can be used into the distal vessels over 30 min [4]. An angiogram is repeated to check adequacy of clearance.

Thrombosed arteries, thrombosed aneurysms and grafts can also present with threatened limbs. In these scenarios the surgical approach is different. If there is an absent femoral pulse and inflow cannot be established by embolectomy because of iliac atherosclerosis the patient should have a femoral to femoral or axillary to femoral artery bypass.

The superficial femoral artery cannot be cleared sometimes due to atherosclerotic disease. The patient should have an on table angiogram. Attempts should be made to clear residual thrombus with intra arterial thrombolysis. If there is endovascularly treatable disease this should be treated by an angioplasty. Lesions not amenable to angioplasty may require distal bypass.

Bypass grafts may occlude in the immediate postoperative period or further down the line. Grafts that thrombose in the immediate postoperative period should be explored as this is usually due to technical reasons. Late graft occlusions are usually due to lesions proximal to, in the graft, or distal to the graft due to vein valve site stenosis, neo intimal hyperplasia or progression of disease. These are better first approached by thrombolysis. These patients are sometimes primarily operated on due to the severity of their ischaemia. Late graft occlusions are unlikely to be resurrected. They should have an on table angiogram. If a distal vessel is identified then they should have a bypass procedure as long as good inflow is established.

Thrombosed popliteal artery aneurysms require urgent intervention. An on table angiogram will identify patent vessels if any are distal to the aneurysm. Embolic material in the runoff should be cleared by thrombolysis. A bypass procedure should be performed and the aneurysm excluded by ligation.

In the immediate postoperative period all patients should be anticoagulated with heparin. They should be then anticoagulated with warfarin for a period of 3–6 months.

Surgery in the form of emergency amputation

A proportion of patients will present with irreversible ischaemia. They tend to have severe rest pain, fixed staining and mottling, paralysis and profound sensory loss and usually undergo above-knee amputation. No attempts should be made to revascularise these limbs as the reperfusion injury is likely to prove fatal to the patient. About 10% of patients present with an already nonviable limb and the 30-day amputation rate following ALI is 25–30% [5].

Endovascular treaments

Thrombolysis

Catheter directed thrombolysis is indicated in limbs that fall into categories I and IIa. [5]. As the limb is not severely ischaemic, time is available to pursue thrombolysis.

Table 2.3 Contraindications to thrombolysis

- Active bleeding
- Cerebrovascular accident within 2 months
- Recent gastrointestinal (GI) bleeding
- Pregnancy
- Neurosurgical procedure within 2 months
- Vascular surgical procedure within 2 weeks
- Abdominal surgery within 2 weeks
- Bleeding disorder
- Extensive trauma

The advantages of thrombolysis are decreased risk of trauma to the endothelium, dissolution of clot in vessels that cannot be accessed by means of an embolectomy catheter and low pressure reperfusion of the limb. They may reveal stenotic lesions that are amenable to angioplasty. This will improve long-term patency rates if these lesions are angioplastied.

Complications associated with thrombolysis include the following:

1. Myocardial infarction.
2. Cerebrovascular accidents.
3. Bleeding from puncture site.
4. Embolisation.

If persistent bleeding is an issue then the effect of the lytic agent can be reversed by administering aprotinin. Fresh frozen plasma may be required and other clotting products may need to be replaced.

The use of thrombolysis will depend upon availability, patient's clinical condition and local expertise. There is evidence from randomised clinical trials that at similar time intervals the limb salvage rates with thrombolysis are comparable to surgery but with a lower mortality rate [6–8]. Contraindications to thrombolysis are given in Table 2.3.

Other endovascular treatment options are percutaneous aspiration thrombectomy and percutaneous mechanical thrombectomy.

- Aspiration thrombectomy involves the use of a large bore end hole catheter to aspirate thrombus.
- Mechanical thrombectomy involves the use of devices that agitate, disperse and aspirate thrombus.

The above procedures can be used along with thrombolysis to optimise results.

Palliative care

A proportion of patients will present with acute limb ischaemia while being very unwell. The likely outcome for these patients is death. Attempts should not be made to intervene as this will not change the outcome of their illness.

The aim of treatment should be to alleviate their symptoms. The local palliative care team should be involved and the care of the dying pathway should be instituted.

Complications of acute limb ischaemia

Compartment syndrome

This is due to reperfusion of ischaemic tissue. Typically immediately after surgery the treated limb is noted to be perfused but the patient complains of pain in the calf and inability to dorsiflex the foot.

Reperfusion of an ischaemic muscle results in oedema of the muscle. Swelling is due to failure of cellular membrane function and leaking of capillaries. As muscles are enclosed in a bony fascial compartment this increases the volume and ultimately pressure within the compartment. As the pressure within the compartment increases, muscle perfusion decreases resulting in further ischaemic injury. This in turn increases muscle edema. Thus a vicious circle is established resulting in obstruction of veins, arteries, capillaries, nerve dysfunction and infarction of the muscle. The anterior compartment is the most vulnerable.

If compartment syndrome is clinically suspected or with compartment pressures of more than 20 mm Hg a fasciotomy is indicated. There are several techniques but usually a four compartment fasciotomy should be performed.

Partially closed fasciotomy

The leg is cleaned and draped. The skin over the proximal part of the compartment is incised. The deep fascia that is exposed through this incision is then incised. The remainder of the deep fascia is then divided using scissors that are passed subcutaneously. This technique is used in cases of chronic compartment syndrome. The anterior compartment is most commonly affected. In an acute situation this technique should not be used and an open, full length fasciotomy should be performed.

Open fasciotomy

The leg is cleaned and draped. A four compartment fasciotomy is performed to decompress the four compartments in the leg adequately. An anterolateral incision is made along the fibula from below the knee down to the ankle. Through this incision the fascia overlying the anterior compartment and peroneal compartment is incised. A posteriomedial incision is made along the length of the leg. The underlying fascia is divided and the gastronemius muscle in the superficial posterior compartment is exposed. The attachment of the soleus muscle to the tibia is divided to decompress the deep posterior compartment. The fibula can be excised through an anterolateral incision to achieve adequate decompression of all compartments. The lateral ends of all the fascial envelopes are attached to the fibula. Excision of the fibula therefore decompresses all compartments.

The open wounds should be dressed with non adherent dressing material such as bactigras and a loose bandage. The wounds are allowed to heal by secondary intention or split skin grafts can be used.

Rhabdomyolysis

Muscle breakdown as a result of ischaemic injury can release myoglobin into the blood stream. This can cause acute tubular necrosis leading to renal failure. Patients have dark urine, elevated levels of serum creatine kinase and myoglobin in the urine. Treatment is hydration, alkanising the urine and removing the source of myoglobin. Patients may require haemofiltration or dialysis.

References

1. Clason AE, Stonebridge PA, Duncan AJ et al. Acute ischaemia of the lower limb: the effect of centralising vascular surgical services on morbidity and mortality. *Br J Surg* 1989; **76**: 592–3.

2. Earnshaw JJ. Demography and aetiology of acute leg ischaemia. *Semin Vasc Surg* 2001; **14**: 86–92.

3. Blasidell FW, Steele M, Allen RE. Management of lower extremity arterial ischaemia due to embolism and thrombosis. *Surgery* 1978; **84**: 822–34.

4. Earnshaw JJ, Gaines PA, Beard JD. Management of acute lower limb ischaemia. In: Beard JD, Gaines PA, eds. *Vascular and Endovascular Surgery*. Elsevier, 2006; 169.

5. Norgren L, Hiatt WR et al. Acute limb ischaemia. In: TASC II Inter-Society Consensus on Peripheral Arterial Disease. *Eur J Vasc Endovasc Surg* 2007; **33**: Supplement 1.

6. Critchley JA, Capewell S. Smoking cessation for the secondary prevention of coronary heart disease. *Cochrane Database of Systematic Reviews* 2005; Issue 1. Art. No.: CD003041. DOI: 10.1002/14651858. CD003641.pub2.

7. Results of a prospective randomized trial evaluating surgery versus thrombolysis for ischaemia of the lower extremity. The STILE trial. *Ann Surg* 1994; **220**: 251–66.

8. Ouriel K, Shortell C, Deweese J et al. A comparison of thrombolytic therapy with operative revascularisation in the initial treatment of acute peripheral arterial ischaemia. *J Vasc Surg* 1994; **19**: 1021–30.

9. Ouriel K, Veith F, Sasahara A. A comparison of recombinant urokinase with vascular surgery as initial treatment for acute arterial occlusion of the legs. Thrombolysis or Peripheral Arterial Surgery (TOPAS) Investigators. *N Engl J Med* 1998; **338**: 1105–11.

10. Williams B, Paulter NR, Brown MJ et al. The BMS Guidelines Working Party guidelines for management of hypertension: report of the Fourth Working Party of the British Hypertension Society. *J Hum Hypertens* 2004; **18**: 139–85.

11. Heart Outcomes Prevention Evaluation Study Investigators. Effects of angiotensin-converting enzyme inhibitor, ramipril, on cardiovascular events in high risk patients. *NEJM* 2000; **342**: 145–53.

12. POISE Study Group, Deveraux PJ, Yang H et al. Effects of extended-release metoprolol succinate in patients undergoing non-cardiac surgery (POISE Trial): a randomised controlled trial. *Lancet* 2008; **371**(9627): 1839–97.

13. Karnon J, Brennan A, Pandor A et al. Modelling the long term cost effectiveness of clopidogrel for the secondary prevention of occlusive vascular events in the UK. *Curr Res Med Opin* 2005; **21**(1): 101–12.

14. Heart Protection Study Collaborative Group. MRC/BHF Heart Protection Study of cholesterol lowering with Simvastatin I 20, 536 high risk individuals: a randomised placebo controlled trail. *Lancet* 2002; **360**: 7–22.

15. National Collaborating Centre for Chronic Conditions. *Type 2 Diabetes: National Clinical Guideline for Management in Primary and Secondary Care (Update)*. London: Royal College of Physicians, 2009.

16. Gardner AW, Montgomery PS, Parker DE. Physical activity is a predictor of all cause mortality in patients with intermittent claudication. *J Vasc Surg* 2008; **47**: 117–22.

Final FRCS vascular topics

Chronic lower limb ischaemia, critical ischaemia and the diabetic foot

Chris Davies and Cliff Shearman

Key points

- Peripheral arterial disease (PAD) affects approximately 30% of the adult population
- PAD is a powerful marker of cardiovascular risk and the risk is related to the severity of the PAD
- Risk factor management has been proven to reduce cardiovascular risk but many patients do not receive adequate treatment
- The optimum treatment to improve walking in patients with intermittent claudication is best medical treatment, supervised exercise and angioplasty
- Angioplasty and surgery appear to be equivalent in treating critical limb ischaemia (CLI). However, angioplasty is cheaper due to reduced length of hospital stay
- Diabetic foot complications are a common cause of hospital admission and often precede amputation. The majority of amputations in the UK are carried out in patients with diabetes
- Patients with diabetes should be screened annually for neuropathy and PAD
- Multi-professional team approach to the management of diabetic foot complications can reduce amputation rates

Epidemiology

Atherosclerotic arterial disease affecting the legs, peripheral arterial disease (PAD), is very common. In many patients it is asymptomatic but commonly the first manifestation of PAD is pain in the leg on walking, intermittent claudication. In some patients the blood supply to the leg becomes further reduced to a level when pain is experienced at rest and ulceration and gangrene occur (critical limb ischaemia, CLI). In the Edinburgh Artery study it was found that 4.5% of men and women over 55 years of age had intermittent claudication but a further 25% had evidence of asymptomatic disease. In one-third of the asymptomatic group evidence of a major vessel occlusion was found. At 5-year follow up those that had subsequently developed claudication were found to have come from the asymptomatic group, suggesting there may be a window of opportunity to prevent disease progression. Further evidence of this high prevalence comes from the PAD Awareness Risk & Treatment: New Resources for Survival (PARTNERS) study, which screened 6979 subjects over 70 years of age or over 50–69 with a risk factor for vascular disease in 320 primary care practices in the

Postgraduate Vascular Surgery: The Candidate's Guide to the FRCS, eds. Vish Bhattacharya and Gerard Stansby. Published by Cambridge University Press. © Cambridge University Press 2010.

USA. The study found 5.5% had symptomatic PAD and in total 29% of subjects had PAD. Further, it is estimated that the prevalence of limb threatening or CLI is 220 per million of the population [1].

A number of studies have identified that the majority of patients with PAD do not significantly deteriorate from the point of view of their legs. In the Edinburgh Artery study the annual risk of limb loss was less than 1–2%. However, 5–10% of subjects suffered a cardiovascular event per year, commonly a myocardial infarction or stroke. This is an extraordinarily high cardiovascular risk and patients with PAD are six times more likely to die from cardiovascular disease over 10 years than non-PAD subjects.

The severity of PAD is a prognostic indicator of cardiovascular risk, those with the most severe symptoms faring worse. In patients with CLI the cardiovascular death rate is even worse and one in five will be dead within one year of diagnosis. Although less marked even the asymptomatic group have an increased cardiovascular risk.

Over the past decade this observation has often led to the main focus of treatment shifting to address cardiovascular risk in patients with PAD by attempting to modify their risk factors. However, it is important to remember that many patients with intermittent claudication are extremely handicapped by their symptoms and these may need addressing in their own right. Although it might seem appealing to screen the adult population for PAD there is currently no strong evidence that this approach would reduce cardiovascular risk or be cost effective.

Intermittent claudication

History

Tight, cramp like pain in the muscles of the calf, thigh or buttock is characteristic. Calf claudication is the most common symptom, simply because the most common site for of PAD is in the superficial femoral or popliteal arteries. More proximal disease is required for buttock or thigh claudication. Occasionally buttock claudication can occur from isolated internal iliac artery blocks – usually bilateral – but this is rare. Typically the pain of claudication comes on only after walking for a pain free distance, is usually worse on hills, and is relieved by resting in the standing position. Most other causes of hip or leg pain, such as arthritis, may be exacerbated by walking but will also cause some pain at rest or in certain positions or postures. If the pain only subsides when the patient sits down this suggests the symptoms may be related to their back rather than arterial disease. Spinal canal claudication typically produces numbness, weakness or heaviness in the leg rather than pain localised to a specific muscle group. Spinal canal claudication, due to a narrow spinal canal, may actually be easier going uphill as leaning forward opens the spinal canal up.

It is usual, when taking a history of claudication, to ask the patient to quantify their walking distance – but this is notoriously inaccurate as it will vary with speed and terrain. Additionally patients are often extremely poor at estimating distances. For research purposes walking distances are usually assessed by walking on a treadmill at a set speed and degree of slope. Usually the 'initial claudication distance', which is the distance at which the pain first starts and the 'absolute claudication distance', which is the distance at which the patient stops, are recorded.

Examination

A full cardiovascular examination is important to detect other manifestations of cardiovascular disease. Upper limb peripheral pulses should be palpated and the cardiac rhythm checked. Measurement of blood pressure, cardiac auscultation and abdominal examination for the presence of an abdominal aortic aneurysm should be performed. An abdominal aortic aneurysm cannot be fully excluded by clinical examination and any suspicion should prompt an ultrasound scan.

Examination of the peripheral circulation should include inspection for clinical signs such as ulceration and gangrene. Other, less definitive signs of ischaemia such as cracked skin, hair loss and nail damage should be recorded but are not very useful in their own right. Capillary return is notoriously unreliable unless particularly prolonged, but it should probably also be assessed. In a patient with diabetes it is important to look for signs of abnormal foot shape and callus formation. Skin colour and temperature should also be recorded. The most important aspect of the peripheral examination is peripheral pulse palpation. The femoral, popliteal, posterior tibial and anterior tibial/dorsalis pedis pulses should be identified. In a small number of normal subjects (10–15%) the dorsalis pedis may be absent and in some individuals it is possible to palpate the anterior communicating branch of the peroneal artery on the lateral side of the ankle.

Usually it is sufficient to judge whether a pulse is present or absent. Lower limb pulses can be difficult to feel and trying to judge whether a pulse is strong or weak is rarely of great use. In some patients a hard calcified vessel may be palpated, which is important to identify as it may have implications for treatment. A rough rule is that in patients with calf claudication the disease will be predominantly in the superficial femoral artery and so the popliteal pulse will be absent. For thigh and buttock claudication the disease is predominantly in the aorto-iliac segment and the femoral pulse will be weak or absent. Although this is not infallible, it is a useful concept to bear in mind when examining the peripheral circulation.

Thigh and buttock claudication may be associated with male impotence (Leriche syndrome). It may therefore also be appropriate to enquire about the ability for a male to attain an erection. A small number of patients will have isolated disease of their internal iliac arteries causing their claudication and so will have palpable femoral pulses. This may also be seen in patients who have had therapeutic occlusion of their internal iliac arteries to allow endovascular repair of an aorto-iliac aneurysm.

Auscultation over the femoral artery may detect the presence of a bruit. We believe this is of limited significance as it simply implies turbulent flow proximally. However, in patients with a good history of claudication but palpable pulses a bruit may signify proximal disease, which is only haemodynamically significant during exercise.

Ankle brachial pressure index (ABPI) measurement

Measurement of the ABPI is the third part of the diagnostic triad. The ankle pressure is expressed as a ratio compared to the brachial pressure. An ABPI of 0.9 or less is usually taken to be abnormal. In some patients, especially those with diabetes, the peripheral arteries may be stiff or calcified, which can give an artificially high ankle pressure. This is usually obvious but if doubt remains further investigation may be required. In symptomatic patients with an ABPI of <0.9 there is a 95% sensitivity of diagnosing PAD. To measure the ABPI you need a hand held Doppler with an 8 MHz probe, sphygmomanometer and cuff. Make sure the patient is lying flat, ideally for 10 min before starting. The test is invalid if the patient's legs are not at the same level as the heart. Secure the cuff around the arm as if taking a blood pressure reading in the normal manner. Apply gel over the brachial pulse and apply the Doppler probe over the brachial pulse, at an angle of 60° to the skin. Repeat on the other arm and use the higher of the two readings to calculate the ABPI. When measuring pressures in the dorsalis pedis and posterior tibial arteries make sure the cuff is placed on the lower calf.

Toe pressures/pole test

Patients with diabetes, renal failure and other conditions causing vascular calcification can develop incompressible tibial arteries, causing falsely high systolic pressures when measuring the ABPI. Measurement of toe pressures provides an accurate alternative measurement. The toe pressure is normally about 30 mmHg less than the ankle pressure and an abnormal toe brachial index (TBI) is defined as <0.70. Usually this is not done using a hand held Doppler but by using a system of automatically inflating cuffs on the great toes (sometimes other toes as well) and by recording the pulse using a plethysmographic technique or laser Doppler.

To measure ABI using the pole test the leg is slowly elevated from the horizontal position until the Doppler signal disappears. The height above the left ventricle is measured using a calibrated pole (i.e. a ruler) to record the hydrostatic pressure in equivalents to mmHg. For example 70 cm is equivalent to 50 mmHg.

Differential diagnosis

In the majority of patients the diagnosis of intermittent claudication due to PAD can be confidently confirmed by the simple measures outlined above. Other conditions that should be considered in the differential diagnosis are nerve root irritation due to degenerative lumbar spine disease in which the pain often takes longer to wear off and may only be relieved by sitting. True spinal canal stenosis is relatively uncommon and again the pain is characteristically relieved by sitting or flexing the lumbar spine. Other muscular skeletal conditions such as osteoarthritis are usually possible to identify due to their associated symptoms of nocturnal pain, early morning stiffness and pain that persists for hours after ceasing walking. Venous claudication is rare and usually the patients will have a history of previous venous problems or signs of chronic venous insufficiency.

There is a small group of patients who have a non-atherosclerotic cause of their vascular intermittent claudication. They are often younger, have no other manifestations of cardiovascular disease and their symptoms may only occur after walking some distance. These patients should however be investigated further to exclude other rare causes of exercise induced ischaemia, which may need specific treatment. These include cystic advential disease, popliteal entrapment syndrome, congenital abnormalities such as persistent sciatic arteries and fibromuscular dysplasia.

Investigations

In some patients the diagnosis of intermittent claudication may remain uncertain. They may have other co-morbidities that make it difficult to determine the dominant cause of the symptoms or they may have non-compressible vessels. In these patients treadmill exercise testing by an experienced technician may be of value. Observation of the patient walking and determination of the distance walked on a treadmill may be helpful in determining the origin of the pain. However, relatively few patients will need this level of investigation. Treadmill walking (the distance to the onset of pain, the claudication distance, and the maximum distance they can walk, absolute walking distance) is most commonly used when new therapies are being evaluated.

If there still remains doubt as to the presence of PAD, such as in a patient with diabetes or if intervention is being considered, then colour flow Duplex (CFD) ultrasound scanning should be undertaken. CFD utilises the B mode ultrasound component to identify the vessel and then interrogates them with Doppler ultrasound to determine the velocity of blood flow through them. Direction of flow is colour coded on the display, which makes it easier and quicker to identify areas of disease due to turbulence or cessation of flow. This will display the extent of the PAD and also, using the Doppler component, give an objective evaluation of the haemodynamic severity of the disease based on the velocity shift across the diseased segment. Duplex is ideal for the infra-inguinal vessels but can be more difficult in the aorto-iliac segments. Usually an experienced ultrasonographer can get enough information to determine the extent and severity of the disease. Bubble contrast enhancing agents have been used but currently have not been found to be of great value in the investigation of PAD. Duplex ultrasound will confirm the diagnosis of PAD but will also usually give a strong indication of what interventions are likely to be applicable to an individual, e.g. angioplasty or bypass surgery. In many patients with clear Duplex scans no further imaging is required although some clinicians prefer more detailed imaging prior to intervention.

Depending on the pattern of disease and nature of the planned intervention more detailed information may be required. Digital subtraction angiography (DSA) is now rarely used for diagnostic imaging. It is invasive and requires a significant volume of contrast medium,

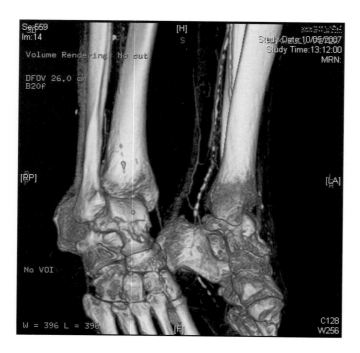

Figure 3.1 Computed tomography angiogram showing calf vessels of patient with diabetes. Calcification is clearly seen.

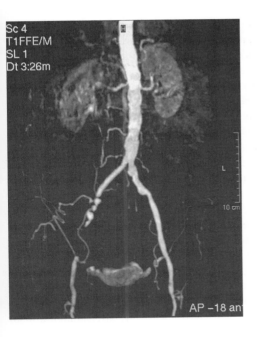

Sc 4
T1FFE/M
SL 1
Dt 3:26m

L

10 cm

AP –18 an

Figure 3.2 Magnetic resonance angiogram of patient with right iliac artery occlusion.

which is nephrotoxic. Multi-slice computed tomography angiography (CTA) is the preferred mode of imaging in many units (see Figure 3.1).

It is relatively non-invasive with very rapid acquisition times under 30 s. However an intravenous contrast medium is required and contrast induced nephropathy can occur, particularly in patients with impaired renal function. The radiation dose is also significant being 80–200 chest X-ray equivalents and, although for single studies this is not an issue, in patients having repeated scans this must be borne in mind. Image interpretation can pose problems, particularly with calcification in the vessel wall. Magnetic resonance angiography (MRA) is also widely used (see Figure 3.2).

Calcification does not cause the same problems for CTA but acquisition times are longer. Recognition of nephrogenic systemic fibrosis, which may be induced by the contrast agent gadolinium in patients with impaired renal function, has limited its role in these patients. Both of these techniques are ideal to use as outpatient investigations.

Management

The two aims of treatment are to reduce the cardiovascular risk and improve the walking ability of the patient.

Reducing cardiovascular risk

Smoking is the most important risk factor for the development of PAD and even passive smoking increases cardiovascular risk. Not only is disease progression and amputation more likely in smokers, but smoking increases the risk of hypertension and raised cholesterol. Excess cardiovascular risk is halved within one year of cessation and is the same as non-smokers within 5 years in those patients that successfully give up smoking. There is no strong evidence for the benefits of smoking cessation to the limb but some observational studies have suggested an improvement in walking distance and a reduction in amputation rates. Smoking cessation advice, when combined with nicotine replacement therapy, improves quit rates to around 30%. Recent UK legislation prohibiting smoking in public areas may also have an impact on the numbers of smokers.

The prevalence of diabetes is increasing across the world. Patients with type 2 diabetes have 3–5 times more chance of developing PAD. Also the effects of other risk factors such as hypertension and hypercholesterolaemia are amplified in patients with diabetes. Studies looking at tight diabetic control in type 2 diabetes have shown a reduction in cardiovascular events but the benefits of this were outstripped by the complications of hypoglycaemia. At present in patients with diabetes and PAD every attempt should be made to identify and reduce any other risk factors and diabetic control should be optimised for the individual patient. Patients with diabetes should also have regular checks of their feet for signs of neuropathy or PAD.

There is overwhelming evidence for the benefits of lowering cholesterol in patients with PAD. In the Heart Protection Study, patients with PAD and a total cholesterol over 3.5 mmol l^{-1} who took simvastatin (a HMG-CoA reductase inhibitor) had a 17.6% reduction in cardiovascular events compared to those on placebo [2]. There was also a reduction in the subsequent need for both cardiac and non-cardiac revascularisation procedures. Based on these results nearly all patients with PAD should be prescribed statin therapy. There is also emerging evidence that statins have a direct effect on atherosclerotic plaque, stabilising it and possibly causing plaque regression in high doses.

Up to 24% of the adult population are hypertensive and hypertension is associated with a threefold increase risk of PAD as well as being strongly associated with stroke and myocardial infarction. Treatment of hypertension will reduce stroke rates by 38% and cardiovascular deaths by 14%. In the Heart Outcomes Study, the angiotensin converting enzyme inhibitor, ramapril, demonstrated an advantage in reducing cardiovascular events, even in those patients whose blood pressure was not elevated [3]. However there are potential problems with the widespread use of ramapril in patients with PAD as many will have renal artery disease. At present in those with PAD and hypertension ramapril should be considered as the first-line treatment but there is not enough evidence to suggest widespread use in non-hypertensive patients.

The Antithrombotic Trialists' Collaboration meta-analysis found that antiplatelet agents (predominantly aspirin, a cyclo-oxygenase inhibitor) reduced the risk of cardiovascular events by 23% in patients with PAD [3]. A dose of 75 mg was as effective as higher doses. Approximately 20% of patients are unable to take aspirin largely due to gastrointestinal disturbance and it is emerging that a similar proportion of patients have aspirin resistance. In these patients normal doses of aspirin do not have the normal effect on patients. In these patients clopidogrel should be used. Clopidogrel is a theopyridine derivative that blocks ADP induced platelet activity. In the CAPRIE study, clopidogrel was shown to further reduce cardiovascular events compared to aspirin (particularly in the PAD group), with a relative risk reduction of 8.7%. However, as clopidogrel is more expensive the National Institute for Health and Clinical Excellence (NICE) recommends that it should be used only by patients who cannot take aspirin or by high-risk patients. Combination therapy of aspirin and clopidogrel should be considered very carefully. In the Charisma study patients on both drugs had a significantly greater risk of bleeding complications, which overall exceeded any apparent benefit.

A number of other lifestyle changes should be advocated. Weight reduction and regular exercise have proven cardiovascular benefit. They also have a positive effect on other risk factors. Omega 3 fatty acids (fish oils) appear to have some beneficial effects but their clinical role in PAD has not been established. Likewise antioxidants and other dietary additives have not been demonstrated to be of benefit.

Despite the overwhelming evidence for the benefit of risk factor management recent epidemiological studies have found that only around 30% of patients get adequate treatment for these.

Improving walking distance

In many patients confirmation of the diagnosis of intermittent claudication, reassurance of the natural history of the condition as regards the leg and risk factor management will be all that is required. The decision to directly attempt to improve walking distance is something that should be decided by the patient balanced by the impact of their symptoms on their day-to-day life compared to the chance of success versus the risks of treatment. Patients who have claudication are a heterogeneous group. Many will only be mildly troubled by their symptoms or have other significant co-morbidity that reduces their mobility. Others, however, may be severely restricted by their claudication, which can significantly alter their lifestyle. It is the role of the clinician to help the patient decide on the best therapeutic option for them based on the impact of their symptoms on their quality of life.

A number of vasoactive drugs have been promoted to increase walking distance. In the UK two drugs are currently used, naftidrofuryl and cilostazol. The benefit of naftidrofuryl on walking distance in claudication is variable and generally small. In a meta-analysis of eight studies cilostazol has been demonstrated to improve walking by 50% with some improvement in quality of life. Whether this is of benefit to individual patients or cost effective has not been established. In the UK cilostazol is generally used in patients when other physical interventions are not possible and the patients would benefit from some improvement in the walking distance. However, if symptoms do not improve after 6–8 weeks the drug should be discontinued.

The benefits of exercise have been realised for over a decade. Until recently no large randomised studies of exercise have been conducted but a meta-analysis of 21 studies suggested an improvement in walking distance of 124%. Supervised exercise with programmes requiring three sessions of 30 min per week seemed to be the optimum, but even upper limb exercises have been shown to improve walking. The main problem with this approach is making it appealing to patients and generally less than 30% of them will either want to try exercise or continue on a programme.

Two small randomised trials of angioplasty versus exercise showed the benefit of exercise in terms of walking distance. The recently published Mimic Trial compared best medical treatment (BMT) and exercise to BMT, exercise and angioplasty [5]. In this study of 144 patients with stable claudication they found a significant advantage for angioplasty above exercise and BMT alone, especially for patients with aorto-iliac disease. These results strongly suggest a broad approach to the treatment of patients with claudication and combining exercise with angioplasty, if indicated, to gain the maximum benefit.

Generally percutaneous angioplasty should be appealing for patients with intermittent claudication. It is relatively non-invasive, often can be done as a day case and significant complications occur in less than 3% and limb loss in around 0.3%. However re-stenosis rates, particularly in more distal disease, are significant and can be as high as 40% for distal superficial femoral artery disease. If patients with short stenoses or occlusion in the proximal vessels only are treated then about 50–60% of patients will be suitable. Stent placement after angioplasty may improve the initial technical success rates but has not been demonstrated to improve clinical outcome. Until recently the only evidence of comparison of angioplasty compared to exercise favoured exercise. This tended to restrict the use of angioplasty in the UK. It is likely that the findings of the Mimic Trial will change this.

Surgical reconstruction (bypass or common femoral endarterectomy) has been demonstrated to improve quality of life in patients with claudication. However, the risks of morbidity and mortality are significant. There are still a few patients with simple lesions who may be offered surgery. Usually for some reason they will not be suitable for endovascular treatment or will have had multiple re-stenoses after angioplasty. However, the expectation of a good result should be high and the patient should be fully aware of the potential risks.

Critical limb ischaemia (CLI)

A large number of patients who present with limb threatening ischaemia have not had a previous history of claudication. They are often less mobile so may not have precipitated any symptoms but often other factors, such as infection, cause a sudden deterioration. For this reason it has proved difficult to accurately define CLI. The Inter-Society Consensus for the Management of Peripheral Arterial Disease (TASC II) suggests that a patient with persistent pain, ulcers or gangrene, considered to be due to proven arterial disease, should be considered to have CLI [1]. This definition is based on previous attempts to define the condition in the Trans-Atlantic Inter-Society Consensus (TASC) of 2000. The diagnosis is usually confirmed by a low ankle blood pressure (under 50 mmHg) but this is not always the case in some patient groups, e.g. for diabetes. The need to intervene in patients with CLI is obviously much greater as a significant proportion will deteriorate and face limb loss without revascularisation.

Patients with CLI face an enormous cardiovascular risk and 50% will be dead within 1 year of diagnosis. It is important to recognise, and when possible correct, any associated risk factors. These patients also tend to be older and have significant co-morbidities that need to be optimised.

Options for revascularisation include angioplasty or surgery. Conventional transluminal angioplasty has limited results for more distal disease but the development of low profile catheters and stents for coronary artery work has improved outcomes. Sub-intimal angioplasty seems to have greater initial success but the medium-term patency rates tend to be variable. However, in many patients even if the original angioplasty site re-occludes, ulcers have often healed and it seems the angioplasty worked long enough to achieve wound healing.

Surgical bypass

Surgical bypass can either be inflow procedures to the femoral artery; anatomical bypasses, such as aorto-bifemoral bypass; or extra-anatomical bypasses, such as cross femoral bypass or axillo-femoral bypass. Distal bypass is technically demanding but if carried out in experienced units will achieve excellent results. A meta-analysis of infra-geniculate bypass in high-risk patients found limb salvage rates of over 78% at 5 years. The optimum bypass graft is autologous vein and if long saphenous vein is not available excellent results can be obtained using arm vein, short saphenous vein or the deep veins. Although moderate results can be obtained, there is little role now for the use of prosthetic grafts below the knee due to the high risk of infection.

In patients selected for surgery great care needs to be taken to identify the optimum run-off vessel and it is also important to carry out Duplex ultrasound scanning of he veins to ascertain if they will be suitable and to minimise the dissection required to harvest them. There is no clear advantage of *in situ* versus reversed vein techniques and it is really dependent on the experience of the surgeon.

Up to 30% of vein bypass grafts will develop stenoses and if left many will go onto occlude. It is not possible to detect these stenoses clinically and many patients are asymptomatic. Many units therefore carry out regular Duplex ultrasound surveillance of the grafts and correct any significant stenosis (greater than 50% or three times velocity shift across the narrowed segment). However, a randomised controlled study has brought this practice into question. Although the study found it was possible to detect stenoses, it found no difference in outcome between patients in surveillance and those simply followed up. As Duplex surveillance is time consuming and costly it was found not to be cost effective. Many units, however, continue to monitor these patients, arguing that there are other benefits, such as checking on risk factor management and long-term outcomes.

There are then a number of options available to re-vascularise a critically ischaemic limb. The TASC II document has classified lesion in the aorto-iliac and femoro-popliteal segment and reviewed the evidence for treatment options [1]. However, a randomised controlled study, the Bypass Versus Angioplasty in Severe Ischaemia of the Leg (BASIL) study, compared surgery versus angioplasty for the treatment of CLI and severe limb ischaemia [6]. This study found no difference in amputation free survival, which was 55% during the study period, between either treatment. There was also no difference in mortality, 3% and 5%, respectively, for angioplasty and surgery. However although there was an initial 20% failure rate from angioplasty, length of stay in hospital was much shorter, making angioplasty more economical.

There are a number of important points that arise from this study. First only 30% admitted to the units involved in the study were randomised, suggesting a large proportion were not re-vascularised. Also 37% died during the study period, largely from cardiovascular disease, emphasising the high cardiovascular event rate in these patients. Few patients were made worse by angioplasty, suggesting that in most of these patients who are elderly and frail it is worth trying angioplasty initially.

One group of patients in whom surgery is usually the optimum treatment are those with disease in the common femoral artery. Angioplasty here may put the profunda artery origin at risk and often these patients are treated by common femoral endarterectomy. There still remains some doubt over which is the optimum technique to re-vascularise the distal tissues in patients with diabetes and further studies are needed to determine this. The role of surgical profundaplasty (usually an endarterectomy of the common femoral artery into the profunda artery with patch closure) remains contentious. If no other options are available, or a distal procedure is not appealing due to poor quality distal vessels, it is worth attempting.

Amputation

Amputation is the only option possible in some patients. Extensive infection may require urgent intervention. If the patient is very sick then guillotine amputation of the infected tissue with subsequent conversion to formal amputation may be the best option. It will achieve

Table 3.1 Eight clinical features to look for in the diabetic foot

- Neuropathy
- Ischaemia
- Deformity
- Callus
- Swelling
- Skin breakdown/ulceration
- Infection
- Necrosis

control of sepsis and avoid infection of a definitive amputation stump. The patient can be returned to theatre when they are stable for conversion of the guillotine stump to the optimal formal amputation.

Primary amputation may also be required in patients in whom there is extensive tissue loss and no obvious method of re-vascularisation of the limb. Secondary amputation is required when a revascularisation attempt has failed to achieve tissue healing or relief of pain. Below-knee amputation has the advantages of greater mobility with a prosthesis due to preservation of the knee joint. However the primary healing rate of below-knee amputations is approximately 80% compared to 90% with above-knee amputation.

Selection of amputation level can be difficult. The presence of a good femoral pulse together with a well developed profunda femoris artery is encouraging for a below-knee amputation. The quality of the tissues in the leg, previous wounds and the presence of sepsis and the general condition of the patient also make a major contribution to the decision at what level to amputate. The use of measurements such as $TcPO_2$ at the level of amputation has been found to be helpful by some units but the general application of these techniques has not been widespread. Often the decision has to be made based on the clinical factors outlined above and the appearances of the tissues at the time of surgery.

Diabetic vascular disease

It is estimated that by 2010 there will be 221 million people diagnosed with diabetes worldwide [7] and in England the current prevalence is 3.75% [8]. In recent epidemiological studies it has been found that over 40% of patients presenting with PAD have diabetes and 20% of all hospital admissions for complications of diabetes are due to foot problems. An estimated 5% of patients with diabetes develop a foot ulcer every year and the lifetime risk of an ulcer is 15% [9]. The ultimate consequence of foot disease without adequate management is amputation; and the relative risk of amputation, associated with all types of diabetes, is 13 times compared to that of a non-diabetic [10]. It has been estimated that 85% of amputations could have been avoided with adequate care.

There are two main reasons why patients with diabetes are so prone to foot complications, neuropathy and ischaemia. Screening patients with diabetes is essential to detect early signs of neuropathy and PAD (Table 3.1). This can be simply done by the use of a 10 g monofilament test, peripheral pulse palpation and ankle blood pressure measurement. Patients who have any evidence of neuropathy or PAD should be given help and advice to detect problems early and seek help. There is encouraging evidence from some countries, such as Finland, that a multi-disciplinary approach to diabetic foot complications can reduce major amputation rates.

Neuropathy

1. Sensory neuropathy reduces the patient's ability to appreciate damage to the foot such as rubbing of ill-fitting footwear. Thus small lesions, such as from ill-fitting shoes, are not appreciated at an early stage by the patient. Also lack of proprioception means that when the patient is standing subtle movements in posture that would normally offload pressure do not happen.
2. Motor neuropathy results in reduced power of the short flexor muscles of the foot. The resulting in-balance between these and the long extensors results in an 'intrinsic minus' foot with clawing of the toes and prominence of the metatarsal heads. Abnormal weight bearing on the metatarsal heads (combined with reduced sensory proprioception) causes tissue damage and ulceration (Figure 3.3 and Table 3.1).
3. Finally autonomic neuropathy causes reduction in sweating and dry skin, which is more prone to cracking and damage. The failure of the autonomic system also has effects on the vasomotor tone in the skin circulation with abnormal arteriovenous shunting. All of these factors make the foot prone to damage and ulceration.

Ischaemia

Patients with diabetes have a fourfold increased risk of developing PAD and the resulting ischaemia is another factor predisposing the foot to injury and poor healing. Patients with diabetes and PAD have the greatest risk of suffering and amputation. There are also

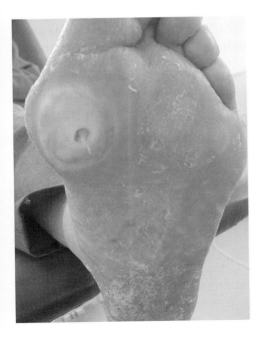

Figure 3.3 Typical neuropathic foot ulcer. The ulcer is surrounded by a ring of keratinised skin.

abnormalities of the microcirculation such as thickening of the basement membrane, increased capillary permeability and increased platelet adherence, which reduce tissue perfusion.

It has been estimated that of patients with foot complications approximately 10% will be due to ischaemia, 45–60% will be due to neuropathy and 25–45% will be a combination of the two (=neuro-ischaemia). However the final common presenting factor is often infection. The immunosuppressive effect of hyperglycaemia predisposes the patient with damaged ischaemic tissue to infection, which can be extensive.

Management of the diabetic foot

The first-line treatment of a patient with a diabetic foot complication is to ensure that their diabetes is controlled and this may require a sliding scale or correction of a keto acidosis. Treatment of infection involves cultures and local wound swabs followed by intravenous antibiotics. Units should have agreed regimens with their microbiology team, which will cover the common causative agents such as staphylococcus aureus, streptococcus, pseudomonas and anaerobic bacteria. Superficial wound swabs may fail to identify the causative organism and aspiration of tissue fluid using a 10 ml syringe and a green needle is advocated by some groups to obtain more accurate deep tissue cultures.

The extent of the infection is determined by careful inspection of the foot and palpation of the tissues. Tenderness or crepitus suggests extensive infection. Often infection of a digit will spread to the associated web space and infect the tissue between the metatarsals. This may only be apparent by a slight redness and tenderness over the dorsum of the foot. Plain X-rays should be undertaken. They may reveal osteomyelitis or gas in the tissues. Surgical drainage of any collection and removal of dead infected tissue should be undertaken within 24 hours of admission and further tissue sent for microbiological culture.

Once the situation has been stabilised by the above, full assessment of the neurological and vascular status of the limb can be undertaken. The absence of pedal pulses together with a low ankle blood pressure indicate a high-risk foot. Further investigation, starting with a Duplex scan and probably including a CTA, should be obtained. Unless the foot shows signs of healing revascularisation either by angioplasty or surgery should be performed.

Wounds on the foot should not be sutured but generally left to heal by secondary intention. Attempting to suture the skin may reduce skin edge blood flow and trap infected material, leading to abscess formation. Care should be taken to avoid oedema of the limb and the patients should rest with their leg elevated for the first few days. The use of negative pressure wound therapy has transformed management of these patients. Although the precise way in which it works is not clearly understood, negative pressure therapy will remove excess tissue fluid, increase microcirculatory blood flow beneath the wound and reduce the wound size. Patients can be mobilised early using total contact casts. A cast is placed on the lower limb with a window to allow inspection of any wound. These need to be expertly fitted as if there are abnormal areas of pressure the cast itself will cause damage.

Conclusion

PAD is a common problem and is strongly associated with cardiovascular risk. Despite overwhelming evidence for the benefit of the treatment of cardiovascular risk factors many patients remain undiagnosed and under-treated. Recent evidence has suggested that combining best medical treatment, exercise and intervention has the best results for symptomatic disease. Endovascular treatments seem to have the same result as surgical treatments in term of limb salvage. The commonest cause of amputation is diabetes, the prevalence of which is increasing. Evidence shows that early detection of foot problems in diabetes and a multi-disciplinary approach to the problem can reduce amputation rates.

References

1. Norgren L, Hiatt WR, Dormendy JA, Nehler MR, Harris KA, Fowkes FGR on behalf of the TASC II working group. Inter-Society Consensus for the Management of Peripheral arterial disease (TASC II). Norgren L, *J Vasc Surg* 2007; **45**: Supplement.

2. Heart Protection Study Group Collaborators Group. MRC/BHF heart protection study of cholesterol lowering with simvastatin in 20,536 high-risk individuals: randomised placebo controlled trial. *Lancet* 2002; **360**: 7–22.

3. The Heart Outcomes Prevention Evaluation Study Investigators. Effects of angiotensin-converting enzyme inhibitor, ramapril, on cardiovascular events in high-risk patients. *N Engl J Med* 2000; **342**: 145–53.

4. Antithrombotic Trialists' Collaboration. Collaborative meta-analysis of randomised trials of antiplatelet therapy for the prevention of death, myocardial infarction, and stroke in high risk patients. *BMJ* 2002; **324**: 71–86.

5. Greenhalgh RM, Belch JJ, Brown LC. The adjuvant benefit of angioplasty in patients with mild to moderate intermittent claudication (MIMIC) managed by supervised exercise, smoking cessation advice and best medical therapy: results from two randomised trials for stenotic femoro-popliteal and aortoiliac arterial disease. *European J Vasc Endovasc* 2008; **36**: 680–8.

6. Adam DJ, Beard JD, Cleveland T and BASIL Trial Participants. Bypass Versus Angioplasty in Severe Ischaemia of the Leg (BASIL): multicentre, randomised controlled trial. *Lancet* 2005; **366**: 1925–34.

7. Amos AF, McCarty DJ, Zimmet P. The rising global burden of diabetes and its complications: estimates and projections to the year 2010. *Diabet Med* 1997; **14** Suppl 5: S1–S85.

8. Scanlon P, Stratton I. Incidence and prevalence of diabetes. NHS Evidence – Diabetes June 2008. http://www.library.nhs.uk/diabetes.

9. National Institute for Health and Clinical Excellence (NICE) Guideline, Type 2 diabetes: prevention and management of foot problems. January 2004. Clinical guideline 10. http://www.nice.org.uk/CG010NICEguideline.

10. International Diabetes Federation. Position Statement – The Diabetic Foot. http://www.idf.org/Position_statementsdiabetic_foot.

4

Endovascular and surgical options for peripheral revascularisation

Colin Nice

Key points

- Risk factor optimisation and best medical therapy are the standard of care for all patients
- Severe acute ischaemia is best managed with surgery, there is a role for thrombolysis in less severe cases
- Thrombolysis requires intensive monitoring to identify and manage complications
- Surgical or endovascular revascularization is appropriate for patients with limiting claudication or critical limb ischaemia
- Non-invasive imaging should be used for procedural planning
- Bypass grafts with autologous vein produce the best long-term patency rates
- Endovascular procedures have lower mortality and morbidity rates than the equivalent surgery
- Stents and stent grafts improve endovascular results and are important for managing complications
- Patient fitness, co-morbidity and preference are as important as lesion characteristics in informing revascularization decisions
- Multi-disciplinary teams are best placed to manage individual patients in this rapidly evolving field

Background

Many patients with peripheral arterial disease (PAD) do not require any revascularization procedure. Identification and management of modifiable risk factors are effective in reducing the excess risk of cardiovascular mortality and preventing acute limb ischaemia due to disease progression. Also supervised exercise programmes can benefit those with intermittent claudication, a Cochrane review of randomised trials in patients with stable intermittent claudication suggested an improvement in walking distance of 150% with a regime of three sessions per week of walking to near maximum pain [1].

However, surgical and endovascular revascularization procedures produce substantial additional benefits when proficiently performed upon carefully selected and prepared patients. Treatment strategies addressing the differing aetiologies of chronic peripheral arterial disease and acute limb ischaemia determine the urgency, nature and effectiveness of attempted revascularization.

Postgraduate Vascular Surgery: The Candidate's Guide to the FRCS, eds. Vish Bhattacharya and Gerard Stansby. Published by Cambridge University Press. © Cambridge University Press 2010.

BASIL trial

The BASIL trial (Bypass Versus Angioplasty in Severe Ischaemia of the Leg) compared the outcomes of 452 patients presenting to UK centres with severe limb ischaemia [2]. Patients were randomized to either a surgery first ($n = 228$) or an angioplasty first ($n = 224$) strategy. Only 60% of participants received antihypertensive treatment, 54% received antiplatelet drugs and 34% were taking cholesterol lowering agents.

The primary endpoint was survival free from amputation for the trial limb. Trial duration was 5.5 years, with follow up ending when the endpoints of death or above-ankle amputation of the trial leg were reached.

At follow-up completion;

- 248 patients (55%) were alive without amputation of the trial leg;
- 38 (8%) were alive following amputation;
- 130 patients (29%) were dead without amputation.

A surgery first strategy was associated with a higher rate of early morbidity (57% versus 41%). Six-month amputation free survival was not significantly different between the treatment groups and health related quality of life (HRQL) was similar. At 2 years surgery was associated with a reduced risk of future amputation or death. A strategy of surgery first increased the hospital costs by about one third.

These results indicate that there is scope to substantially improve the medical treatment of risk factors. For patients with a short life expectancy an angioplasty first strategy reduces early morbidity and treatment costs but for relatively fit patients, expected to live beyond 2 years, a surgery first strategy is more durable and carries a reduced re-intervention rate, possibly outweighing the initial costs and increased short term morbidity.

Acute limb ischaemia

Acute limb ischaemia may be due to arterial occlusion arising from *in situ* thrombosis of established atheromatous plaques or embolization from remote sites. The majority of emboli are cardiogenic, resulting from atrial fibrillation or mural thrombus, complicating myocardial infarction. Aortic and popliteal aneurysms are other important causes and these should be sought with clinical examination and imaging.

Treatment decisions are often based on clinical assessment due to clinical urgency or limited availability of other imaging modalities.

Anticoagulation

Immediately following the diagnosis of acute limb ischaemia, anticoagulation with intravenous heparin should be commenced to prevent thrombus propagation. Daily assessment of activated partial thromboplastin time (APTT) ratio is required with a target ratio of 2 (range 1.5–2.5) considered optimal. This should be monitored at least daily and dose adjustments made according to local protocols. Intravenous fluid rehydration may be needed prior to and following endovascular revascularization to minimise the risk of contrast induced nephropathy (CIN).

Analgesia

Acute limb ischaemia causes severe pain. Lying flat may exacerbate symptoms and many patients are only able to tolerate a dependent limb position. Effective analgesia is needed to relieve this and also to permit the patient to lie still enough to allow surgical or endovascular procedures performed under local anaesthetic. Regional blocks of the femoral and sciatic nerve are promising techniques that alleviate ischaemic pain without the need for epidural or general anaesthetic [3].

Embolectomy

Surgical exposure and control of the common femoral artery can often be performed under local anaesthetic. Removal of emboli with balloon catheters may effectively restore limb perfusion. Associated fasciotomy may be required.

The chances of technical success are greatest with larger calibre arteries and cardiogenic emboli where the likelihood of an associated stenosis or occlusion is lower. Embolectomy is effective for supra-inguinal occlusive emboli as absence of a femoral pulse hinders vascular access for catheter delivered thrombolysis. Selective catheterization and embolectomy of below-knee vessels may prove impossible without fluoroscopic imaging and guidewire compatible embolectomy catheters.

Completion angiographic appearances indicate technical success, identify associated underlying lesions and determine the need for adjunctive procedures such as thrombolysis or angioplasty.

Following successful embolectomy, anticoagulation decreases the risk of recurrent embolization, particularly in those with atrial fibrillation. A target international normalised ratio (INR) of 2.5 (range 2–3) is optimal. If femoral embolectomy is unsuccessful then either on-table thrombolysis or surgical exploration of the distal popliteal artery or of the anterior tibial artery and tibio-peroneal trunk may be required.

Thrombolysis

Pharmacological thrombus dissolution is used to treat embolic occlusions or resolve *in situ* thrombosis and reveal the underlying stenotic lesions. In acute limb ischaemia thrombolysis delivered by an intra-arterial catheter within the thrombus is more effective and carries a lower risk of complications than systemic thrombolysis. Three main agents have been employed; they exhibit no major differences in efficacy:

- Recombinant tissue plasminogen activator (rTPA) is most widely used in the UK. This acts by converting plasminogen into plasmin and promoting fibrin degradation.
- Streptokinase induces antibody production, preventing repeat administration. It is ineffective in patients with prior streptococcal infections and is no longer widely used.
- Urokinase has similar efficacy to rTPA and has been favoured in the USA.

Concurrent administration of low dose heparin through the arterial sheath is used to prevent pericatheter thrombus formation. Newer classes of thrombolytic agents acting independently of the plasminogen system (alfimeprase and plasmin) offer the potential for more rapid lysis coupled with a lower risk of serious bleeding and an improved safety profile. Platelet GP2b/3a receptor antagonists, such as abciximab, produce a synergistic effect with thrombolytics, resulting in more rapid lysis but this may be at the expense of increased haemorrhagic complications. The role of these agents in PAD is still to be defined.

The efficacy of all thrombolytic agents diminishes rapidly and most units restrict usage to within 4–6 weeks of the presumed thrombus formation (usually a major symptomatic deterioration). Beyond this therapeutic window the low chance of successful lysis is outweighed by the relatively high complication rate.

In the acutely threatened ischaemic limb, emergency embolectomy is preferred to thrombolysis which can take up to 24 hours to substantially improve limb perfusion. The risks and benefits of thrombolysis must be carefully considered for each patient. Situations where thrombolysis is contraindicated include:

- active/recent bleeding;
- previous cerebral haemorrhage;
- surgery, major trauma or cardiopulmonary resuscitation within the preceding 2 weeks;
- proliferative diabetic retinopathy;
- recent ocular surgery or trauma;
- bleeding diathesis;
- pregnancy.

Prerequisites for successful thrombolysis are an informed, co-operative patient in whom the risk of inadvertent arterial sheath or catheter removal is low (the resulting haemorrhage may be very difficult to control) and careful supervision and monitoring, usually within a high dependency environment. Effective analgesia during this period may require intravenous opiates or specialist pain team input.

Several different thrombolysis regimes are described:

- Low dose regimes administer a continuous infusion typically for 24 hours or longer.
- High dose regimes involve an initial bolus followed by a high dose infusion with the aim of achieving faster thrombolysis during core working hours.

Both strategies are effective and confer similar limb salvage and complication rates. Persistent thrombotic occlusion resistant to embolectomy is often managed with intraoperative rTPA thrombolysis. A typical dosage regime is 15 mg diluted to 100 ml and delivered by infusion or repeated small bolus injections over 30 min.

Thrombolysis carries substantial risks. Thirty day mortality in a large UK based audit was 12.4% [4], with the majority of deaths attributable to myocardial infarction or stroke. Stroke occurs in approximately 3% of patients and may be haemorrhagic or thrombotic. Major arterial haemorrhage, requiring cessation of thrombolysis affects about 10% of patients. This is mostly from groin puncture sites but there is a significant risk of concealed retroperitoneal and intra-abdominal haemorrhage. Haemodynamic monitoring, frequent assessment of the puncture site, limb perfusion and neurological status are required to promptly detect serious bleeding and to minimise the duration of thrombolysis. Titration of thrombolytic dose to the results of coagulation studies is necessary to avoid excessive depletion of fibrinogen.

There should be a high index of suspicion for concealed arterial bleeding and a low threshold for performing CT examination to assess for cerebral or abdominal haemorrhage. Minor bleeding from the puncture site is common (20–40%) and can be managed by local compression and need not require thrombolytic cessation.

Distal embolization may produce a temporary deterioration in limb perfusion or be evident on check angiography. This usually resolves with continued thrombolysis or thrombus aspiration.

Surgery versus thrombolysis

Randomized controlled trials demonstrate no clear superiority for surgery or thrombolysis on 30-day limb salvage rates or mortality [5]. However, randomised trials include only those suitable for either treatment. Registry data shows that surgery is performed three to five times more frequently than thrombolysis.

Mechanical thrombectomy

A variety of adjunctive endovascular techniques involving mechanical thrombus aspiration or thrombectomy aims to promote faster thrombus resolution. They are often combined with thrombolysis. These add to the cost and complexity of treatment and are not currently widely used.

Unsalvagable limbs

Even with current techniques a significant proportion of ischaemic limbs cannot be saved. In these patients efforts must be directed towards pain management and resuscitation with prompt amputation and rehabilitation. Futile attempts at revascularization pose a major risk from rhabdomyolysis and hyperkalaemia.

Chronic limb ischaemia

In chronic arterial disease non-invasive imaging techniques including Duplex ultrasound, magnetic resonance angiography (MRA) and computed tomography angiography (CTA) have largely replaced catheter angiography for the majority of patients and allow accurate assessment of disease distribution. The haemodynamic significance of stenoses demonstrated by these techniques can be further evaluated with targeted Duplex ultrasound or translesional pressure gradients obtained with catheter angiography. Typical thresholds for treatment are a peak systolic velocity ratio (PSVR) of 2.5 for ultrasound and a 5–10 mmHg pressure gradient without vasodilatation or 10–15 mmHg with vasodilator administration measured at angiography.

Lesion prioritisation

When confronted with multiple lesions in a patient with chronic limb ischaemia, treatment of significant proximal lesions is undertaken first. Symptomatic improvement following angioplasty or stenting of aorto-iliac lesions frequently exceeds that of femoro-popliteal lesions and if a good response is achieved subsequent infra-inguinal revascularization may be unnecessary. Even when further surgical or endovascular procedures are required the optimization of arterial inflow increases the likelihood of technical success. It may be unnecessary or undesirable, due to severe potential complications, to treat all identified lesions and a staged approach with clinical review will optimise the risk/benefit balance for individual patients.

Surgical revascularization

Endarterectomy

Areas of bulky heavily calcified plaque respond poorly to angioplasty, which may fail to fracture the plaque. Stenting is similarly ineffective as stents lack sufficient radial force to overcome these lesions. For lesions in readily accessible surgical sites, such as the common femoral artery, endarterectomy is an effective treatment.

Surgical bypass

Infra-inguinal bypasses may be constructed from autologous vein or prosthetic graft such as woven Dacron or polytetrafluoroethylene (PTFE) There is a major advantage to using vein grafts with 5-year patency rates of 74–76% versus 39–52% for PTFE [6, 7]. In addition graft infection is reduced if autologous grafts are used. Most commonly the long saphenous vein (LSV) is used either as a reversed vein graft or an *in situ* vein graft, following valvotomy. There is no strong evidence that *in situ* grafts have better patency rates than reversed grafts. Narrow calibre and varicose veins are unsuitable and many patients may have already undergone LSV harvesting for prior lower limb or coronary revascularization. In these circumstances short saphenous vein, cephalic vein or superficial femoral vein are alternatives, with two more separate pieces being joined together if necessary (spliced vein graft). Preoperative Duplex ultrasound assessment reliably demonstrates suitable veins and avoids the unnecessary morbidity resulting from exploration of poor quality veins.

Anastomotic techniques

Venous cuffs or patches performed at anastomoses between prosthetic grafts and small (distal) arteries improve the patency of femoro-popliteal PTFE grafts performed below the knee or more distally but do not produce any benefit in above-knee grafts [8].

Aorto-iliac bypass

Surgical bypass with a prosthetic graft from the distal aorta to either the iliac or common femoral arteries is usually the preferred option for occlusive or diffuse stenotic disease. A variety of trans-peritoneal or extra-peritoneal approaches may be employed. The patency of aorto-bifemoral grafts is high (greater than 80% at 5 years).

Femoral-femoral crossover graft

Femoral-femoral crossover operations utilising prosthetic grafts are an alternative to aorto-iliac or aorto-femoral bypass for unilateral iliac occlusive disease. They are also employed following aorto-uni-iliac stent graft treatment of abdominal aortic aneurysms. As an intra-abdominal incision is avoided this is a less invasive option better suited to higher risk patients, although the majority will require either regional or general anaesthesia.

Axillo-bifemoral grafts

Axillo-bifemoral prosthetic grafts (Figure 4.1) are used as a less invasive alternative to aorto-iliac bypass procedures for occlusive disease or to treat aorto-iliac graft infection. Long-term graft patency rates for extra-anatomic bypasses are lower than those for aorto-bifemoral grafts and they are usually reserved for patients with critical limb ischaemia.

Femoro-popliteal bypass

Non-invasive imaging will confirm the adequacy of arterial inflow and determine whether there is sufficient outflow to promote graft patency. The proximal anastomosis is usually sited anteriorly on the common femoral artery. The distal anastomosis is in the popliteal artery and may be above or below the knee. Autologous vein grafts are preferred as they have the best long-term patency rates but prosthetic grafts may be necessary for patients with insufficient suitable vein. Five-year patency rates for above-knee and below-knee femoro-popliteal vein grafts are similar (62% and 68%, respectively). Prosthetic grafts perform much worse below the knee with 5-year patency falling from 43% above knee to 27% below. Many units restrict below-knee prosthetic grafts to patients with critical limb ischaemia.

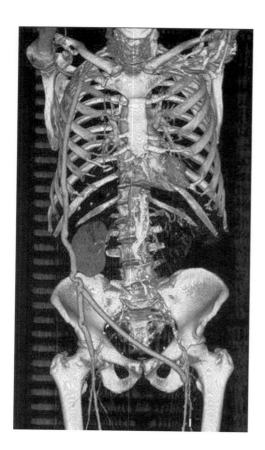

Figure 4.1 Computed tomography (CT) scan of right axillofemoral bypass.

Femoro-distal bypass

The quality of the outflow artery correlates with long-term graft patency rates. The choice of distal arterial anastomotic site (tibial or peroneal artery) does not appear to affect outcome and therefore the best quality artery with uninterrupted run off to the foot should be selected. Five-year assisted patency rates for vein grafts are approximately 60% and less than 35% for prosthetic grafts.

Endovascular techniques

Angioplasty

Angioplasty techniques use pressure controlled balloon inflation to fracture arterial plaque and remodel the artery. As the plaque is not removed this is most effective for short focal stenoses without heavy calcification. Excessively calcified lesions are resistant to angioplasty.

A recent randomised controlled trial demonstrated additional benefit of angioplasty over a supervised exercise programme and best medical therapy [9]. At 24-months post angioplasty absolute walking distance was improved by 78% for aorto-iliac lesions and 38% for femoro-popliteal lesions.

Procedural outline

- Patient symptoms, examination and pre-procedural imaging are reviewed.
- Arterial access site is planned (ultrasound guidance is a useful adjunct).
- Local anaesthetic infiltration.
- Arterial puncture and guidewire passage (Seldinger technique).
- Arterial sheath placed.
- Angiographic evaluation of lesion.
- Heparin anticoagulation.
- Guidewire passage across lesion (frequently requires a hydrophilic guidewire).
- Exchange for supportive guidewire.
- Angioplasty balloon placement and inflation.[1]
- Angiography to assess response.
- Repeat inflation or stenting if needed.
- Arterial puncture site compression/closure device.

Subintimal angioplasty differs from the usual intraluminal angioplasty because it is performed in the wall of the artery to create a new non-diseased channel whereas traditional angioplasty opens the narrowed lumen. This technique can be effective in recanalizing iliac, superficial femoral artery (SFA) and long below-knee occlusions. It involves intentional guidewire passage into the subintimal plane to create a channel that extends the length of the occlusion. The guidewire is then redirected back into the vessel lumen and the entire section angioplastied to create a new flow channel between the intima and media. Care must be taken to avoid major collateral vessels as occlusion of these can precipitate acute limb ischaemia. Heavily calcified vessels may prevent guidewire and catheter passage and it may be impossible to re-enter the vessel lumen.

Although procedures performed on crural arteries in patients with critical limb ischaemia achieve lower technical success rates, compared with those performed above the knee, this remains a valuable technique as many of this patient group are unfit for surgical revascularization. Long-term patency rates are a less important measure for this group as patient life expectancy is short and even a temporary increase in limb perfusion may be sufficient to achieve relief of rest pain, ulcer healing and limb salvage.

Complications of angioplasty

Arterial puncture site haemorrhage

This is potentially life threatening. Risk factors include:

- vessel wall calcification (loss of elastic recoil);
- hypertension;
- number of arterial puncture attempts;
- size of arterial sheath;
- anticoagulation.

Most risk factors can be controlled with manual compression, although this may need to be prolonged. Concealed retroperitoneal haemorrhage is a life-threatening emergency

---

[1] Medicines and Healthcare Products Regulatory Agency (MHRA) alert notice from May 2002 mandates use of a calibrated inflation device to minimise the risk of balloon rupture and embolization.

occurring within a few hours of the procedure. Pain, pallor, tachycardia, hypotension, flank tenderness or visible haemorrhage are all useful indicators of serious bleeding. Early detection prior to the onset of haemorrhagic shock is the aim and vigilant post-procedural monitoring in an appropriate environment is mandatory. Any clinical suspicion of serious bleeding should prompt emergency computed tomography (CT) examination and surgical exploration and repair if active bleeding is confirmed.

Arterial rupture

Iliac artery rupture is a rare but potentially fatal procedural complication. Female patients requiring angioplasty of heavily diseased, narrow calibre, external iliac arteries are most at risk. Severe pain unrelieved by angioplasty balloon deflation indicates likely rupture. Immediate angiography is required to confirm the site of rupture and then balloon inflation to tamponade the site is performed.

Urgent cross matching of blood is undertaken and experienced vascular, surgical and anaesthetic assistance urgently obtained. Once this team is assembled the tamponade balloon may be deflated. Minor ruptures may resolve with balloon tamponade alone but continued extravasation requires immediate placement of a covered stent placed across the rupture site. This usually resolves the problem but if not emergency surgery will be required. Rupture of infra-inguinal arteries seldom causes any major clinical problems.

Dissection

Arterial dissection is a frequent event during angioplasty. Usually this is minor and non-flow-limiting and no treatment is indicated. Flow restricting dissections may resolve with prolonged (5–15 min) balloon inflation or placement of an uncovered stent.

Distal embolization

Embolization may be caused by plaque fracture and detachment or by thrombus. Completion angiography of the distal vascular territory will detect this complication. If limb perfusion is maintained then further intervention is unnecessary. In cases where the limb is compromised then thrombus aspiration or thrombolysis are often effective but some patients will still need surgery. Symptomatic plaque embolization is more likely to require surgery.

Contrast induced nephropathy (CIN)

Following iodinated contrast administration there is frequently a transient deterioration in renal function which is maximal at 48 hours and has generally resolved by 5 days. Patients with normal pre-procedural renal function are unlikely to suffer clinical problems but for those with pre-existing renal impairment there may be an irreversible worsening of renal function. Adequate hydration in the peri-procedural period is essential to minimise this risk. Pre-treatment with n-acetylcysteine (NAC) may be beneficial. A meta-analysis showed a moderate reduction in CIN in patients pre-treated with NAC. The use of iso-osmolar contrast media lessens the degree of renal impairment in high risk patients with diabetes. The minimum possible contrast volumes consistent with high quality imaging should be used.

Carbon dioxide (CO_2) may be used as an alternative contrast agent to guide angioplasty in high risk patients. Infra-inguinal angioplasty performed solely with ultrasound guidance is a viable alternative for centres lacking the necessary equipment or experience in CO_2 angiography.

Stents

Stents are supportive frameworks that apply radial force to diseased arteries and promote vessel remodelling. Most are made of stainless steel or nitinol, a nickel-titanium alloy with the ability to regain its manufactured shape once deployed. Drug eluting stents, dissolvable and biodegradable stents all offer attractive theoretical benefits but are not part of current routine practice for peripheral arterial disease.

Stent deployment is by two basic mechanisms:

(1) Balloon expandable stents are securely mounted on a balloon angioplasty catheter by the manufacturer and deployed by pressure regulated balloon inflation. Advantages include their greater radial force and reliable accurate placement. Care must be taken when introducing balloon mounted stents through arterial sheaths and tight stenoses to prevent stent dislodgement.

(2) Self expanding stents are constrained by a low profile sheath and deploy when the covering sheath is withdrawn. They apply less radial force than balloon expandable stents and may require post-dilation. Some earlier versions shortened significantly upon deployment which hindered precise placement. Current devices are much less prone to this.

Continuous technological improvements mean that most stents can be delivered through a sufficiently small sheath to permit percutaneous procedures.

Aortic angioplasty

Infrarenal aortic atheroma and minor stenoses are common and often clinically insignificant. The small minority of lesions that produce significant haemodynamic effects may be treated with either aortic angioplasty or uncovered stent placement. Both methods result in excellent long-term patency rates.

Iliac stenting

Iliac artery angioplasty has high technical success rates and produces 5-year patency rates of approximately 70%.

Stent placement (Figures 4.2 and 4.3) either as a primary procedure or performed selectively following suboptimal response to angioplasty significantly reduces the failure rate of endovascular treatment. Although endovascular treatment for aorto-iliac occlusive disease carries lower risks than surgical revascularization a recent large UK registry recorded a 2% in-hospital mortality rate, with deaths mainly occurring in patients with critical limb ischaemia. Mortality for those with claudication was 0.2%.

SFA stenting

Previous attempts to stent SFA stenoses and occlusions failed. There was a very high incidence of early stent fractures and the majority of these subsequently occluded.

Fundamental stent re-design has produced a generation of devices better suited to the complex series of forces affecting the SFA. Recent trials suggest a much reduced early stent fracture rate with substantially improved vessel patency.

Two-year follow-up data comparing primary SFA stenting with a strategy of SFA angioplasty and selective stent placement for residual stenosis or dissection showed clinical

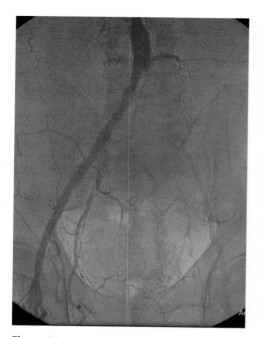

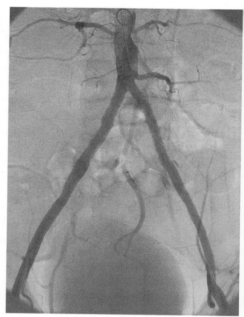

Figure 4.2 Angiogram showing a left common iliac artery occlusion.

Figure 4.3 Left common iliac artery occlusion treated with balloon expandable stent placement. A right-sided stent was also placed to preserve the right common iliac origin (same patient as Figure 4.2).

improvement and lower re-intervention rates with primary stenting. The current role of SFA stenting is as a 'bail out' procedure for significant residual stenosis or flow limiting dissection at the time of angioplasty. Longer-term data are needed before the substantial additional costs generated by a primary stenting policy can be justified.

Below-knee stenting

Treatment of short focal lesions of the tibial arteries with either coronary artery stents or dedicated below-knee stents is described. The majority of critically ischaemic limbs contain diffuse stenoses and long occlusions involving more than one run off vessel and are therefore anatomically unsuitable. There is currently very little evidence to support below-knee stent placement.

Stent grafts

Stent grafts, also referred to as covered stents, consist of a fabric covering (Dacron or PTFE) applied to a stent. The addition of the fabric covering increases the profile of the device and stent grafts require larger calibre arterial access than uncovered stents of the same diameter. Stent grafts allow endovascular treatment of arterial haemorrhage and exclusion of aneurysms whilst maintaining perfusion of the distal vascular bed.

Several case series describing stent graft treatment of long SFA lesions (mainly occlusions) suggest similar patency rates to prosthetic femoro-popliteal bypass procedures.

Great care must be taken to avoid covering the origin of profunda with the stent graft proximally. The distal extent of any stenting procedure must also be very carefully considered so that future surgical options are not compromised (i.e. conversion of an above-knee femoro-popliteal bypass into a below-knee femoro-popliteal or femoro-tibial bypass). Long-term antiplatelet therapy is recommended to maintain stent graft patency.

Hybrid procedures

Hybrid procedures typically consist of a surgical bypass combined with either angioplasty or stenting to optimise graft inflow or outflow. The order of these procedures requires careful consideration and the endovascular component is usually performed first to avoid compromising the inflow or outflow to a newly constructed graft by balloon inflation or haemostatic manoeuvres. A dedicated endovascular theatre is the optimal environment but satisfactory results can be obtained with a fluoroscopy compatible theatre table and portable image intensifier with vascular processing software including digital subtraction.

Radiation protection

Radiation protection legislation requires that all medical diagnostic and therapeutic procedures are justified and that exposures are As Low As Reasonably Achievable (the ALARA principle). Endovascular operators must be adequately trained in both the principles and practicalities of radiation protection. There is an individual legal responsibility to comply with local radiation protection policies and dosimetry monitoring arrangements.

Restenosis

Angioplasty or stent induced plaque fracture and vessel wall trauma induce a complex series of responses frequently leading to intimal hyperplasia and vessel restenosis. The incidence of restenosis varies between anatomical sites and small calibre vessels, long stenotic segments or occlusions are particularly prone.

The use of stent grafts may prevent tissue ingrowth and reduce restenosis rates. A variety of response modifying techniques aim to reduce or prevent restenosis. External beam radiotherapy significantly reduces restenosis and re-intervention rates in patients with a suboptimal response to SFA angioplasty requiring stent placement. Endovascular brachytherapy and the use of radioactive stents are also under evaluation.

Graft/stent surveillance

Occlusion of surgical bypass grafts and arterial stents is frequently preceded by progressive stenosis within or immediately adjacent to the graft or stent.

Retreatment at this stage is difficult and many units undertake graft and stent surveillance programmes in which significant stenoses identified with Duplex ultrasound are treated with the aim of avoiding graft or stent occlusion.

These programmes are resource intensive. Compliance rates with long-term follow up are low and patients still present requiring treatment for lesions occurring outside the surveillance zone (i.e. opposite limb).

The majority of re-interventions are required within the first year and it may be more cost effective to limit surveillance to one year or to stratify follow up according to early surveillance findings.

Upper limb revascularisation

Although less frequently affected than the lower limbs, revascularisation may be needed for either acute or chronic ischaemia involving the arms.

Surgical embolectomy or catheter delivered thrombolysis are the main options for embolic occlusions, with severity of ischaemia and local availability and expertise again the determining factors.

Chronic ischaemia associated with limiting symptoms may be treated by surgical bypass (carotid-subclavian or carotid-axillary) or by endovascular methods. Reduced upper limb pulses or asymmetric blood pressure measurements in the absence of limiting symptoms do not constitute an indication for revascularization.

Trauma from cervical or rudimentary first ribs in thoracic outlet syndrome (TOS) may cause subclavian arterial stenoses or aneurysm formation and distal embolisation. Revascularisation with autologous or prosthetic graft is combined with rib resection. Adjunctive embolectomy or thrombolysis may be needed for embolic presentations.

Additional considerations for upper limb endovascular procedures include

- The need for alternative arterial access sites (usually brachial artery), with associated risk of serious neurovascular complications (including median nerve compression) and higher incidence of arterial spasm.
- Manipulations around the aortic arch carry a risk of stroke. This must be explained to patients. Meticulous technique, avoidance of air bubbles in contrast media and measures to avoid peri-catheter thrombus formation are mandatory.
- Awareness of the vertebral artery anatomy and careful planning to avoid inadvertent embolisation or occlusion.

Evidence-based approach

The recently updated Transatlantic Inter-Society Consensus (TASC) Guidelines on the management of peripheral vascular disease are a collaboration involving international medical, vascular surgical, interventional radiology and cardiology societies [10]. Their recommendations are graded based upon the level of supporting evidence.

Lesions are stratified according to the results of surgical and endovascular revascularisation.

- Type A lesions give very good results with endovascular treatment and this is preferred.
- Type B lesions give good results with endovascular treatment and this is recommended unless there are adjacent lesions requiring surgical treatment.
- Type C lesions – surgical revascularization produces superior long-term results and endovascular methods should only be used in patients at high risk for surgery.
- Type D lesions respond poorly to current endovascular methods and surgical revascularization is preferred for fit patients.

These guidelines emphasise that 'patient's comorbidities, fully informed patient preference and the local operators long-term success rates must be considered when making treatment recommendations for type B and type C lesions.'

Decision making

The evidence base for these interventions continues to evolve and individual management decisions are best considered by a multi-disciplinary team experienced in best medical management, anaesthesia and able to offer the full range of surgical and endovascular techniques.

References

1. Watson L, Ellis B, Leng GC. Exercise for intermittent claudication. *Cochrane Database of Systematic Reviews* 2008, Issue 4. Art. No. CD000990. DOI: 10.1002/14651858.CD000990.

2. Adam DJ, Beard JD, Cleveland T and BASIL Trial Participants. Bypass Versus Angioplasty in Severe Ischaemia of the Leg (BASIL): multicentre, randomised, controlled trial. *Lancet* 2005; **366**: 1925–34.

3. Marcus AJ, Lotzof, K, Kamath et al. A new approach: regional nerve blockade for angioplasty of the lower limb. *Cardiovasc Intervent Radiol* 2006; **29**: 235–40.

4. Earnshaw JJ, Whitma B, Foy C on behalf of the Thombolysis Study Group. National Audit of Thrombolysis for Acute Limb Ischaemia (NATALI) clinical factors associated with early outcome. *J Vasc Surg* 2004; **39**: 1018–25.

5. Berridge DC, Kessel DO, Robertson I. Surgery versus thrombolysis for initial management of acute limb ischaemia. *Cochrane Database of Systematic Reviews* 2002, Issue 1. Art. No. CD002784. DOI: 10.1002/14651858.CD002784.

6. AbuRahma AF et al. Prospective controlled study of polytetrafluoroethylene versus saphenous vein in claudicant patients with bilateral above knee femoropopliteal bypasses. *Surgery* 1999; **126**: 594–602.

7. Green RM et al. Prosthetic above-knee femoropopliteal bypass grafting: five year results of a randomized trial. *J Vasc Surg* 2000; **31**: 417–25.

8. Stonebridge PA, Prescott RJ, Ruckley CV. Randomized trial comparing infrainguinal polytetrafluoroethylene bypass grafting with and without vein interposition cuff at the distal anastamosis. The Joint Vascular Research Group. *J Vasc Surg* 1997; **26**: 543–50.

9. Greenhalgh RM, Belch JJ, Brown LC et al. and Mimic Trial Participants. The adjuvant benefit of angioplasty in patients with mild to moderate intermittent claudication (MIMIC) managed by supervised exercise, smoking cessation advice and best medical therapy: results from two randomised trials for stenotic femoropopliteal and aortoiliac arterial disease. *Eur J Vasc Endovasc Surg* 2008; **36**: 680–8.

10. Norgren T, Hiatt, L, Dormandy, WR. Transatlantic Inter-Society Consensus for the Management of Peripheral Arterial Disease (TASC II). *J Vasc Surg* 2007; **45**: S5.

Section 2
Chapter

5

Final FRCS vascular topics

Abdominal aortic aneurysms

Vish Bhattacharya and Rob Williams

Key points

- An aneurysm is an abnormal focal dilatation of a vessel with a greater than 50% increase in its diameter
- Elastin degradation due to matrix metalloproteinases (mainly 2.9 and 12) in the aortic media is the most significant pathology
- Smoking, male gender, hypertension and genetics are the main risk factors
- The annual risk of rupture between 5 and 5.9 cm is 5%
- Contrast enhanced computed tomography (CT) is the gold standard for measuring size and morphology
- The UK Small Aneurysm Trial (UKSAT) helped reach a consensus about the minimal size of treatment, which is 5.5 cm
- The UK Endovascular Aneurysm Repair (EVAR) 1 (in fit patients) trial showed that the 30-day mortality for EVAR was 1.7% versus 4.7% for open repair, although by 4 years all-cause mortality was the same
- The EVAR 2 trial (in unfit patients) showed no difference in mortality between conservative management and stenting
- Fenestrated grafts allow stenting of juxtarenal aneurysms
- Stenting for ruptured aortic aneurysms has shown promising results and a UK trial is currently underway

Introduction

Abdominal aortic aneurysm (AAA) was first described around AD 100 by Roman physicians. In 1923, Rudolf Matas successfully ligated the aorta of a patient with an AAA. The intervening years have seen many advances and improvements in diagnosis and treatment, however ruptured AAAs still cause around 6000 deaths in England and Wales per annum [1].

Definition

An aneurysm is defined as an abnormal, focal dilatation of a vessel, with greater than a 50% increase in the diameter. The normal diameter for the abdominal aorta is up to 2 cm, therefore 3 cm is considered to be the minimum diameter of an AAA. All three vessel layers, the intima, media and adventitia, are intact. Aneurysms can be fusiform i.e. a cylindrical

Postgraduate Vascular Surgery: The Candidate's Guide to the FRCS, eds. Vish Bhattacharya and Gerard Stansby. Published by Cambridge University Press. © Cambridge University Press 2010.

dilatation of the whole vessel, or saccular, a focal bulge arising from the side of the vessel. Abdominal aortic aneurysms involve the abdominal aorta and can extend into the iliac arteries. Ninety per cent are infrarenal, the remaining 10% are para- or suprarenal.

Aetiology

Aneurysmal degeneration occurs most commonly in the elderly and is usually associated with atherosclerosis. In simplistic terms aging results in weakening of the aortic wall and aneurysmal dilation results. According to the Laplace law, luminal dilation results in increased wall tension and a cycle of progressive dilation and greater wall stress. The most marked pathological changes occur in the media and intima. The media is responsible for the majority of the tensile strength of the aortic wall. It is made of multiple layers of structural proteins, the bulk of which are collagen and elastin. Over time elastin fibre fragmentation occurs and the media degenerates. Collagen makes up about 25% of the wall of an atherosclerotic aorta and only 6–18% in aneurysms. Matrix metalloproteinase 2, 9 and 12 are found in increased amounts in the wall of aneurysms and cause degradation of the collagen and elastin matrix, causing a decreased amount of both in the wall of the aortic aneurysm. The smooth muscle cells in the media undergo a phenotypical change and are unable to maintain and protect the matrix. Changes in the adventitial layer are less marked, but inflammatory infiltrates are often present [2]. Inflammatory aneurysms will be mentioned later in this chapter.

Historically, aortic aneurysms were often referred to as 'atherosclerotic'. However, although atherosclerosis and aortic aneurysms share common risk factors and frequently occur concomitantly, aortic aneurysms primarily are the result of degeneration, which leads to a loss of aortic wall integrity. Subsequent enlargement and aneurysm formation predisposes the aorta to atherosclerosis and further degeneration of the aortic wall. It is likely that a combination of genetic predisposition, aging and damage to the aortic wall from risk factors, such as hypertension and smoking, are all involved.

Aneurysms can also be caused by infection (also known as mycotic aneurysms); there is normally a separate source of infection such as vertebral discitis rather than primary infection of the aorta. The classical syphilitic aneurysm is now rare. Other causes include trauma, arteritis, connective tissue disorders such as Marfan's, Ehlers–Danlos and Loeys–Dietz syndromes. These are probably degenerative aneurysms with more rapid progression due to underlying abnormalities. False aneurysms develop after dissection and lack of an intact intimal layer.

Various risk factors have been identified which can predispose an otherwise healthy individual to develop an AAA. The most important of these is tobacco smoking, which causes an eightfold increase in the risk of developing an aneurysm. There is an important genetic predisposition, although the exact association(s) has not been described. The familial association is strongest amongst men. Male siblings have an absolute risk of 20–30%. The other major risk factor is hypertension.

Most research is directed at degenerative aneurysms as these represent the largest and most important group; however the treatment techniques described will normally apply to aneurysms with other causes.

Inflammatory AAAs are defined by the presence of a thickened aneurysm wall, marked peri-aneurysmal and retroperitoneal fibrosis and dense adhesions to adjacent organs. They represent 3–10% of all AAAs and the triad of abdominal or back pain, weight loss and an elevated erythrocyte sedimentation rate (ESR) in a patient with an AAA is highly suggestive. The term periaortitis is used to describe the appearance of inflammatory tissue around the aorta, which enhances with intravenous iodinated contrast media and can therefore be picked up on CT scanning. The condition overlaps with, and is a variant of, retroperitoneal fibrosis and the precise aetiology remains elusive.

Operative repair of a large inflammatory AAA can be problematical. The duodenum can be stuck onto the neck of the AAA in a dense white sheet of inflammatory tissue, which will need to be separated by sharp dissection into the sac. If there is associated ureteric involvement and hydronephrosis prior ureteric stenting may be required and concomitant ureterolysis can be performed. Traditionally open repair has been preferred to stenting, particularly with renal involvement, as it has been thought that the inflammation in the retroperitoneum is more likely to resolve. However, there have been no randomised studies.

Epidemiology

Andominal aortic aneurysms are four times more common in men than women. The mean age for presentation is between 65 and 70 years, with an incidence of 2–6% in men over the age of 60. The prevalence of aneurysms increases with age. Caucasian men are more likely to be affected than other groups, with AAAs rare in Asian and African populations.

Natural history

Most AAAs behave in a relatively predictable manner until they rupture. Most gradually, but exponentially, increase in size until either the aneurysm ruptures or the patient dies of other causes. The annual rate of growth in diameter is generally around 10% of the sac diameter. Higher rates of growth are frequently related to either infected or inflammatory aneurysms and this is an indication for earlier and more urgent treatment.

The annual risk of rupture is directly related to, and increases with, the aneurysm size. Below 5 cm the risk is <2%, between 5 and 5.9 cm the annual risk of rupture is 5%; this increases to 6.6% for aneurysms from 6 to 7 cm and 19% for aneurysms over 7 cm [3]. Only 15% of patients with an AAA will rupture, the remainder will die of other causes.

Presentation

About 70 to 75% of aortic aneurysms are asymptomatic and are found either during routine physical examination or during imaging investigations for another problem. Aneurysms are commonly seen on abdominal ultrasound (US), computed tomography (CT) and magnetic resonance imaging (MRI) studies.

Aneurysms tend to become palpable on abdominal examination when they reach 5 cm or more in size. This figure varies greatly between patients depending on the size of the patient and the overlying soft tissue. Slim patients can often palpate their own normal aorta while obese patients can hide aneurysms much larger than 5 cm. Tumours adjacent to the aorta, unusual tortuosity and lumbar lordosis can cause the aorta to be pulsatile although only a true aneurysm will be expansile.

About 20% of patients present with a rupture. The classic triad of a rupture consists of mid abdominal or diffuse abdominal pain radiating to the back, shock and a pulsatile mass. The pain can be more severe in the back or flank and radiate into the groin, mimicking renal colic. Although a catastrophic event, the rupture can be contained in the retro-peritoneum with the contained haematoma tamponading the leaking aorta allowing time for assessment and treatment. Free intra-peritoneal ruptures are normally rapidly fatal. It is believed that only about 25% of patients survive a rupture due to high intraoperative and postoperative mortality. However this may be an overestimate of survival rate as many elderly patients who die in the community of undiagnosed ruptured AAAs do not have a post mortem and the deaths are falsely attributed to cardiac causes.

Imaging

Plain radiographs

Plain radiographs are of limited use for diagnosing or investigating AAAs. Vascular calcification can be seen in some instances allowing the aneurysm to be detected. Occasionally vertebral body erosion is caused by the pressure effect of a gradually expanding aneurysm. Plain radiographs are useful in the follow up of patients after endovascular repair of aneurysms as they allow detection of graft migration or graft deterioration as long as a standard projection is used.

Ultrasound

Many AAAs are found as incidental findings on abdominal US for other problems. With a few exceptions detection is easy, although obesity and gas within the bowel lumen can obscure the aorta. Abdominal ultrasound suffers from significant inter-observer errors so technique needs to be meticulous and consistent within a unit. Due to inherent errors in tranverse measurements on US most AAAs are measured in the antero-posterior (AP) plane. This rarely causes problems with fusiform aneurysms, but can lead to measurement errors with saccular aneurysms. Abdominal ultrasound is the mainstay of aneurysm surveillance for small aneurysms as it is quick, relatively cheap and risk free for the patients. Surveillance should generally be at 6–12-month intervals. Abdominal ultrasound can be used for follow-up surveillance of patients after endovascular repair, although there is debate over the reliability. Generally the aneurysm sac diameter is monitored and if concerns are raised then more advanced US techniques using colour Doppler and contrast enhanced US can be used to look for endoleaks. Ultrasound is unreliable for investigating ruptured aneurysms as the majority of patients who survive long enough to receive emergency medical care have a retroperitoneal rupture. The haematoma is often obscured by the bowel and other abdominal viscera.

Computerised tomography

Contrast enhanced CT has become the gold standard for diagnosing aortic aneurysms and assessing the size and morphology. Dedicated arterial phase images acquired on a multi-slice spiral scanner, with the slices reconstructed at thicknesses of 3 mm or less provide detailed information that allows treatment to be tailored to the patient. This is particularly important for planning endovascular treatment. Measurements are reproducible as long as the imaging protocol remains the same and detailed assessment of the aneurysm volume is possible, although unnecessary in the majority of cases. The incidence of non-aneurysm significant clinical abnormalities is reported to be up to 20%. CT is also the gold standard investigation for a ruptured aneurysm. Intravenous contrast is not required to visualise the haematoma but is necessary if the patient is being considered for emergency endovascular repair. Some clinicians are concerned that imaging introduces an unnecessary delay in treatment, which may increase the risk of death. Certainly if the patient is unconscious, profoundly hypotensive with strong clinical suspicion of rupture, then imaging in any form is not required.

CT is not without potential problems, the radiation dose is equivalent to around 5 years of normal background radiation and this carries a small but appreciable risk of causing malignancy. Repeated imaging increases this risk. The iodinated contrast media may cause anaphylactoid reactions and can precipitate acute renal failure particularly in diabetics with underlying renal disease. If contrast must be given then adequate pre-hydration is the most important step to reduce the effects.

Magnetic resonance imaging

MRI can, like CT, provide detailed information about the aneurysm. Magnetic resonance angiography protocols require intravenous (gadolinium based) contrast media to provide high quality information and care needs to be taken with interpretation as some sequences only display the vessel/aneurysm lumen and may underestimate the true size of the vessel. The resolution is generally less than that of CT and MRI is not commonly used for treatment planning unless there is a contraindication to contrast enhanced CT. MRI is susceptible to artefacts from metals (particularly ferro-magnetic) and pacemakers; some metallic implants are absolute contraindications to scanning. Gadolinium based contrast media should be used with care in patients with impaired renal function due to the risk of nephrogenic systemic fibrosis.

Intra-arterial angiography

Calibrated invasive angiography was the gold standard investigation used to plan endovascular repair. It has been superseded by CT scanning due to both the quality of information obtained and the inherent risks of the procedure. Intra-arterial angiography demonstrates the lumen of the aneurysm rather than the true diameter.

Screening for AAA

A Cochrane review has identified four controlled trials involving 127 891 men and 9342 women who were randomly assigned to aortic aneurysm screening using ultrasound or no screening [4]. Only one trial included women. Two of the trials were conducted in the UK, one in Denmark and one in Australia. The results provide evidence of a benefit from screening in men with a strongly significant reduction in deaths from AAA. The odds ratio (OR) for death was 0.60 (range 0.47 to 0.78, three trials) in men aged 65 to 83 years but was not reduced for women. From one trial there was also a decreased incidence of ruptured aneurysm in men but not women. Screening with ultrasound combined with elective treatment reduces mortality by 42% in the age group 65–74.

The UK screening programme has started and is being extended nationally. Men will be offered a single ultrasound scan at 65. Men over 65 will not be screened but will be offered a scan if they request one. Patients with an AAA will be offered either surveillance or treatment if the AAA is 5.5 cm or greater. It is envisaged that there will be about 70 screening centres covering the UK population of 60.2 million with each centre covering 800 000 to 1.2 million.

Treatment

The aim of treatment for AAA is to prevent death from rupture of the aneurysm. Surgery in a variety of forms has been the mainstay of treatment for many years. Early treatment involved ligating the aneurysm. Subsequently aneurysms were wrapped in various materials to stimulate fibrosis with only limited success. Albert Einstein had his AAA treated using this method in 1949 but subsequently died 5 years later when his aneurysm ruptured.

Surgery should be reserved for patients where the risk of rupture exceeds the risk of surgery, for all others conservative management with aneurysm surveillance and best medical therapy is indicated.

Aneurysm repair has a significant surgical mortality and small aneurysms have a low risk of rupture: the risk of treatment can outweigh the benefits. Two landmark trials (The UK Small Aneurysm Trial [UKSAT] [5] and the Aneurysm Detection and Mortality [ADAM] [6]) have helped reach consensus about the minimum size of aneurysm at which benefit of treatment outweighs the risks of surgical repair. The UKSAT randomized 1090 patients in 93 centres. About half received early surgery and the other half were under ultrasound surveillance between September 1991 and November 1995.

Overall the 30-day operative mortality was 5.5% in the early surgery group and 7.2% in the surveillance group where surgery took place when it expanded to 5.5 or at 1 cm per year or ruptured.

After 12 years mortality was 64% in the early surgery group versus 67% in the surveillance group. Sixty percent of all deaths were due to cardiovascular disease. A comparison with age- and sex-matched population showed a higher risk of death even after successful open repair in small aneurysms. There is evidence that patients with peripheral vascular disease including aortic aneurysms are under-treated with respect to cardiovascular risk reduction, even though the presence of an AAA carries a similar risk as an established diagnosis of coronary heart disease.

Similarly the US ADAM Study showed a lower mortality of 2.7% in the elective surgery group but also did not demonstrate a better survival in the early surgery group [6].

Elective aneurysm repair carries a significant risk of morbidity and mortality. The 30-day mortality from elective AAA repair in the UK currently stands at 7%. This is significantly higher than results reported by many other countries in Europe; however few countries have similarly robust methods of data collection.

Patient selection is critical so preoperative assessment and work-up is important. All patients should undergo standard assessment and risk scoring, including assessment of cardiac, respiratory, renal, diabetes and peripheral vascular disease. Preoperative assessment by a consultant vascular anaesthetist is recommended, normally with cardio-pulmonary exercise testing. All patients should be discussed in a multi-disciplinary environment. CT scanning should be used to assess suitability for endovascular repair if considered to be appropriate for the patient.

Open aneurysm repair

In 1951, Dubost performed the first successful open surgical repair of an AAA with a homograft. Open repair has evolved over the last six decades but the basic principles remain the same.

Blood should be cross-matched preoperatively, prophylactic antibiotics administered, nasogastric (NG) tube and bladder catheters inserted, large calibre venous access established. Both central venous pressure monitoring and invasive arterial monitoring are normally used. Normal body temperature is important for coagulation and metabolic function so all intravenous fluids should be warmed and the patient covered with a forced-air warming blanket.

For most infrarenal aneurysms the aneurysm is approached via an anterior midline abdominal approach. A retroperitoneal approach can be used, most commonly from the left for juxtarenal or suprarenal repairs as it allows better access to the suprarenal aorta. Shortly before proximal aortic control is obtained by clamping 5000 IU of heparin should be administered. Where possible the clamp should be placed on the infrarenal aorta to maintain kidney perfusion; this requires the identification of the left renal vein. Five per cent of individuals have a retro-aortic left renal vein, which can be vulnerable to iatrogenic trauma if not appreciated. Clamping of the suprarenal aorta increases the risk of both renal ischaemia and renal artery embolus. Suprarenal control will normally require division of the left renal vein. Supracoeliac control requires separation of the diaphragmatic crura and retraction of the left lobe of the liver. There is an increased risk of bowel ischaemia. The inferior mesenteric artery is sacrificed, although it is often already occluded due to thrombus in the aneurysm sac. Collateral supply to the distal large bowel from the internal iliac arteries may be important, so these vessels should be preserved where possible.

When proximal and distal control of the aorta has been obtained the aneurysm sac is opened and the aorta reconstructed using a graft. The grafts are normally made of Dacron or polytetrafluoroethane (PTFE). They may be soaked or impregnated with antibiotics or silver to reduce the risk of infection. The choice of graft configuration depends on the extent of the aneurysm. The most common grafts are either straight tubes or aorto-iliac bifurcated grafts.

Initial postoperative care normally requires intensive care facilities. Careful monitoring of fluid balance is needed and the fluid requirements in the first 24 hours can be high. The major risks in the early stages of recovery are of myocardial, visceral and limb ischaemia and infarction and renal failure related to embolic complications and hypotension and pneumonia. Longer-term complications include aortic pseudoaneurysms, wound and graft material infection, incisional hernias and erectile dysfunction in men. Most patients are discharged from hospital after a week.

Open repair has proved to be durable with a low rate of secondary interventions, although when infection or pseudo-aneurysms occur the mortality rate of secondary interventions is high.

Endovascular aneurysm repair (EVAR)

Endovascular repair has developed in response to the significant mortality and morbidity related to elective open repair. The rationale behind endovascular repair is the same as open repair, i.e. to prevent death from aneurysm rupture by excluding the aneurysm sac from the direct systemic circulation. Like open repair the endovascular technique involves using tubular fabric grafts to exclude the aneurysm sac. The major difference is the route by which the graft is inserted and secured.

In the late 1970s, Juan Parodi first proposed the concept of using an endovascular route to insert fabric grafts reinforced with metal stents. After more than a decade of engineering developments and animal experiments the first human implant was performed in 1990 on a patient unfit for open repair. The patient was a close friend of the president of Argentina; Parodi, who is Argentinean, was directly approached by the president and persuaded to perform the operation. The operation was a success and the patient lived for 9 years before dying from pancreatic carcinoma.

The early grafts were simple fabric tubes, reinforced with stents, which relied on radial force to maintain their position within the aorta. These proved vulnerable to migration and sometimes loss of the seal with the aortic wall. Over the next 29 years the grafts have evolved significantly. Most grafts are now modular bifurcated tubes with some form of active fixation at the proximal end to reduce the incidence of migration. The active fixation normally consists of a bare metal stent that extends into the suprarenal aorta or barbs/hooks that embed into the aortic wall. Some grafts use a combination of the two methods. The only other mechanism to prevent distal migration involves resting the flow-divider of the stent graft directly onto the aortic bifurcation. This requires a dedicated stent graft.

Preoperative work-up is generally identical to that required for open repair as rarely an endovascular repair may need to be converted to an open repair during the procedure. All patients considered for endovascular repair should have a planning CT scan to accurately assess the aortic morphology. The scan needs to be performed with contrast and timed for the arterial phase. The images need to be reconstructed at a maximum of 3 mm axial slices or 1.5 mm for fenestrated/branched grafts. The scan should extend from the level of the diaphragms to the groins. Around 25% of all pre-EVAR CT scans will have a significant unsuspected abnormality so they should all be formally reported by a radiologist. Planning for EVAR requires an understanding of how the images are acquired and how to make accurate measurements from the study. Ideally three-dimensional reconstructions should be performed to allow true axial measurements (related to the vessel, not the patient) and midline lumen measurements to be made. Accurate measurements of the vessel diameters are absolutely critical to the success of the procedure. Most manufacturers' stent grafts require measurements from the adventitial layer to the adventitial layer however some require intima–intima measurements. Accuracy is governed by both the operator and the patient. There is a variation of diameter of around 1 to 2 mm, depending on the phase of cardiac cycle when the scan was acquired. Length measurements do not need to be as accurate due to significant and unpredictable variability in the conformation of the grafts between patients. Fortunately the position of the stent graft can be adapted during the procedure.

Aortic morphology is perhaps the biggest limiting factor for EVAR. Each of the commercially available standard infrarenal stent grafts has different instructions for use (IFUs). Most grafts require a portion of infrarenal aorta measuring at least 10–15 mm long with a diameter of less than 30 mm to provide a proximal sealing zone. This is referred to as the proximal neck. This portion of vessel should be angulated relative to the aneurysm by less than 60°. The proximal neck should be relatively free of atheroma/thrombus. Both common iliac arteries should have relatively normal portions for the distal sealing zone, although the grafts can be extended into the external iliac arteries if required. The external iliac and common femoral arteries need to be large enough to allow the delivery system to pass through into the aorta. Most grafts require diameters of 7–8 mm. Iliac tortuosity alone tends not to cause major problems however extensive calcification (particularly in association with tortuosity) can cause major difficulties. These problems can normally be overcome and in extreme cases direct exposure of the iliac arteries can be useful. Strictly following the IFUs of the currently available, commercially produced stent grafts allows approximately 40–50% of all infrarenal AAAs to be treated with EVAR. Judicious use of more advanced techniques and a variety of stent grafts has meant that some enthusiastic high volume UK centres successfully treat 80–90% of AAAs using standard grafts and most of the remainder can be offered fenestrated or branched stent grafts if appropriate, although the evidence to support this approach is currently limited.

EVAR should generally take place in a theatre environment to reduce the infection risk to the minimum possible. Fortunately infection of the graft is very rare but it is a catastrophic complication. The quality of the fluoroscopic units used is critical to the success of the procedure. Ideally fixed high-specification angiographic fluoroscopy units should be used; however these are rarely found in a theatre environment and most centres use a mobile C-arm with angiographic capabilities and a high heat capacity to allow for prolonged screening. General purpose mobile fluoroscopic units are not suitable.

The procedure can take place under general, regional or local anaesthesia. The latter is uncommon as the patient may experience significant discomfort due to lower limb ischaemia while the delivery system occludes the femoral arteries. Most procedures start with surgical exposure of both common femoral arteries. Guidewires are passed into the thoracic aorta. An angiogram is performed to locate the renal arteries. The main body is deployed with the first covered stent placed as close to the lowest renal artery as possible. If a bifurcated device is used the contralateral limb is cannulated from the opposite groin and both stent graft limbs are extended down to the level of the iliac bifurcations. The proximal and distal seals and the junctions of the modular components can be balloon moulded to improve the seal. A completion angiogram is performed to confirm the patency of the renal and iliac vessels and to identify endoleaks.

Endoleaks

The term endoleak was coined to describe blood flow in the aneurysm sac despite the presence of a stent graft. An endoleak does not mean that the aneurysm itself has leaked. Endoleaks are classified by their source.

Type I

A type I endoleak is a failure of the seal between the stent graft and the artery wall. They are divided into proximal – where there is a leak between the main body of the stent graft and the infrarenal aortic neck and distal – where there is a leak between the stent graft limb and the iliac artery. The blood leaking into the sac is at systolic arterial pressure and results in a significant increase in the intra-sac pressure. The patient remains at significant risk of aneurysm rupture (some clinicians argue that the risk is higher than if the aneurysm had remained untreated) and the leaks must be treated at the earliest possible opportunity.

Treatment is normally endovascular. The simplest treatment involves using a moulding balloon to improve the contact between the stent graft and the arterial wall; this is commonly employed during the initial implantation procedure if a type I endoleak is seen on angiography. If the stent graft is not appropriately positioned in relation to the renal or iliac arteries it can be extended using additional pieces. If the stent graft is appropriately positioned but the leak persists then additional bare metal stents can be used to increase the radial force and improve the apposition to the arterial wall. A few papers have reported using coils or endovascular glue (either cyano-acrylate or ethylenevinylalcohol copolymer) to seal the leak, although there is scepticism among many clinicians as to the efficacy of this approach. Should these treatments fail the options involve surgery; either placing a band around the outside of the aneurysm neck to provide support for the stent graft. This can be done laparoscopically and does not involve opening the aneurysm sac. Otherwise the stent graft can be explanted and the aneurysm repaired in a conventional open fashion. This carries a significantly higher mortality than standard open repair and should not be undertaken unless all other options have been considered.

Type II

The infrarenal aorta supplies the lumbar arteries and the inferior mesenteric artery. In many AAAs these are occluded by atheroma; however they often remain patent. A type II endoleak is filling of the aneurysm sac from these side branches with blood flowing in a retrograde direction. They are often complex with blood flowing in through one branch and out through another. They are independent of the graft used and around 20% of patients will have a type II leak. They can be subtle and better quality imaging will discover more leaks. The majority are benign as they do not pressurise the sac to the same degree as a type I leak and around 60% will spontaneously thrombose by one year. A small proportion of all type II leaks will cause persistent sac expansion and these require treatment. Aneurysm rupture due to persistent type II endoleak is rare.

Treatment is normally endovascular. These endoleaks are analogous to arteriovenous malformations (AVMs) with inflow vessels, a central nidus and outflow vessels. Treatment should be aimed at occluding the cavity within the sac. This can be accessed via an endovascular route using microcatheters (often via the superior mesenteric artery [SMA]-marginal artery-inferior mesenteric artery [IMA]-aneurysm) or via a direct trans-lumbar route with CT guidance. The cavity can be occluded with a variety of embolic materials, taking care to avoid non-target embolisation of the outflow vessels. Simply occluding inflow or outflow vessels will lead to a recurrence rate of over 50%.

Type III

These leaks are due to either fabric defects in the graft material or dislocation/separation of the stent graft components. The former are normally due to manufacturing defects and are fortunately very rare, they present at the time of implant. The latter tend to occur much later as the aneurysm remodels and distorts the stent graft. The earlier generations of grafts were much more vulnerable to this phenomenon than the current grafts. Whatever the cause the implications are similar to type I endoleaks and they must be treated at the earliest safe opportunity.

Treatment is either endovascular, by relining the original graft with new component(s), or by surgical explantation.

Type IV

Immediately after implantation some graft material is porous, particularly while the patient is anticoagulated with heparin. These leaks are visible as a contrast 'blush' in the aneurysm sac on the angiogram. They are of no clinical consequence and generally resolve spontaneously.

Type V

Otherwise known as endotension, this is believed to be transmission of arterial pulse pressure into the aneurysm sac without a true leak of blood or fluid. This concept is controversial and many clinicians believe that endotension is in reality an endoleak of another type that is subtle and difficult to identify.

Follow up post EVAR

Current management of endovascular repair demands long-term follow up of the patients. This is due to the need for relatively frequent re-intervention (10–20%) to confirm and maintain graft integrity. Initial practice was to use interval CT scans to monitor the aneurysm sac size and to look for new endoleaks and plain X-rays to monitor the graft position and integrity. Many centres are now using ultrasound to monitor the sac size and are only using CT scanning if an increase in the aneurysm sac is recorded. Re-intervention is generally only indicated if the aneurysm sac size is increasing, the graft is migrating or if a type I or a type III endoleak is identified. Fortunately the newer generations of stent grafts appear to be much more robust than the previous models and the rates of graft migration and disintegration are significantly lower. The requirement for long-term follow up is one of the major reasons for the increased costs associated with EVAR compared to open repair. As ultrasound increasingly replaces CT and the grafts become more durable this cost difference decreases.

EVAR versus open repair

Initially it was hoped that endovascular techniques would allow patients who were medically unfit for open repair to be treated with less risk. Various trials have taken place to compare the outcomes of EVAR with open repair and with conservative management for unruptured aneurysms. The most important trials in the UK were the EVAR I and II trials.

EVAR I compared open repair with endovascular repair. It demonstrated that the 30-day mortality for EVAR was less than half that of open repair (1.7% versus 4.7%) [7]. Patients also recovered more quickly and were discharged from hospital much earlier. However by 4 years all cause mortality was virtually identical (~28%) suggesting that endovascular repair offers no long-term survival benefit. The EVAR group also had a significantly higher re-intervention rate (20% versus 6%), however the majority of these re-interventions were relatively benign.

EVAR II compared EVAR with conservative management for patients unfit for open repair. It demonstrated no significant differences in all-cause mortality between the treatment groups. By 4 years 64% of the patients had died [8]. The trial has been criticised for several reasons. The definition of unfit for open repair was loose and varied between recruiting centres. The crossover rate from conservative management to EVAR was high and these patients generally did well but were still analysed under intention to treat rules, thereby improving the outcome for the conservative management group. However, the conclusion seems to be that these patients are generally at high risk of death from many causes, whether or not the aneurysm is treated and intervention of any sort should only be offered after very careful consideration and after the patient's fitness has been optimised.

Open repair should still be considered the gold standard treatment for younger, fit patients because of the increased rate of secondary intervention with EVAR and the requirement for long-term follow up.

Fenestrated and branched grafts

Conventional endovascular repair is often limited by the aneurysm morphology. The most difficult problem to overcome is the length of the proximal neck.

Fenestrated grafts were developed to allow endovascular repair of AAAs with little or no normal aorta below the level of the renal arteries [9]. At their simplest the grafts have holes (fenestrations) that correspond with the positions of the renal arteries and/or the SMA to allow the covered portion of the stent graft to be placed more proximally. These are reinforced with either small bare metal stents or covered stents, which extend into the renal arteries. This helps to prevent migration and maintain alignment between the fenestrations and the renal arteries. The grafts are custom made for each patient and require very accurate planning.

Branched grafts come in two different forms. Iliac branch grafts are relatively simple bifurcated grafts that extend the limb on a standard stent graft. One branch sits in the internal iliac artery (IIA)and the other in the EIA. This allows treatment of aneurysms involving the distal common iliac artery (CIA) while maintaining patency of the IIA. The other type of branched graft is used to treat type intravenous aneurysms that involve the visceral segment of the aorta. These grafts have multiple branches for the visceral vessels. These grafts are in the early stages of development and are reserved for high volume, specialist canters.

Hybrid repairs

Type IV aneurysms can be treated by open repair, branched stent grafts or hybrid repairs. Hybrid repair involves extra-anatomical bypass to the visceral vessels; generally from the iliac arteries but occasionally from the ascending aorta. The origins of the visceral vessels are ligated and the aneurysm then repaired with a stent graft that covers the visceral segment of the aorta. The procedure can be performed in a single episode or staged. The complication rate can be high, particularly as the consequences of occlusion of the bypass grafts can be catastrophic.

Pharmacological management

No drug therapy has yet demonstrated a reduction in aneurysm size or mortality *in vivo* however various trails are ongoing. Doxycycline has been shown to down regulate the expression of metalloproteinase 9 in the aneurysm wall in humans [10]. Statins reduce aneurysm formation by their anti-inflammatory effect and this has been proven in human experiments. Curcumin has been shown to suppress the development of experimental aneurysms and reduce the expression of inflammatory cytokines, chemokines and proteinases that mediate aneurysmal degeneration [11].

Treatment of ruptured AAAs

Despite the development of EVAR, open repair remains the normal treatment for ruptured AAAs in most centres. The 30-day mortality for patients who get to the operating theatre alive is between 40–50%. Deaths are usually due to the physiological insult of hypotension/ischaemia to the heart, kidneys and other organs. Most patients require a prolonged period of intensive care. Endovascular aneurysm repair for ruptured AAAs is complicated by the need for planning and sizing of the stent graft. This inevitably takes time and delays surgery. Some patients will not be suitable for EVAR and will have had an unnecessary wait. However many clinicians feel that patients who are not stable enough to have a CT scan are highly unlikely to survive surgery of any sort and therefore the delay is acceptable. To provide an endovascular service requires provision of 24-hour CT scanning, 24-hour access to fluoroscopy, a large stock of stent graft sizes and, most critically, trained staff (either interventional radiologists or vascular surgeons) capable of performing the surgery. The most obvious benefit of endovascular repair is the ability to repair the aneurysm without opening the abdomen and de-tamponading the rupture. Control of the bleeding can normally be gained very rapidly by inflating a balloon in the descending thoracic aorta at the expense of renal ischaemia. The aneurysm can then be repaired in a relatively controlled manner. However, the patient may still require a laparotomy to treat abdominal compartment syndrome. There is little good evidence that EVAR for ruptured AAAs reduces the 30-day mortality. Some registries and single centre series report a benefit but no randomised clinical trial has been conducted to date [12]. However a UK trial is in the final stages of planning.

Conclusion

Abdominal aortic aneurysms still cause a significant number of deaths due to either rupture or complications of treatment. However recent advances raise the possibility that these deaths may soon be avoidable. Screening followed by endovascular repair when aneurysms are relatively small and easy to treat will hopefully virtually eliminate ruptures and perioperative deaths. In the longer term, promising advances in pharmacological therapy may prevent aneurysm growth and even allow healing and regression.

References

1. Office of Population Census and Surveys. *2000 Mortality Statistics.* London: Stationary Office; 2001.
2. Abdul-Hussien H, Soekhoe RG et al. Collagen degradation in the abdominal aneurysm: a conspiracy of matrix metalloproteinase and cysteine collagenases. *Am J Pathol* 2007; **170**: 809–17.
3. Szilagyi DE, Elliot JP, Smith RF. Clinical fate of the patient with asymptomatic abdominal aortic aneurysm and unfit for surgical treatment. *Arch Surg* 1972; **104**: 600–6.
4. Cosford PA, Leng GC. Screening for abdominal aortic aneurysm. *Cochrane Database of Systematic Reviews* 2007, Issue 2. Art. no. CD002945. DOI: 10.1002/14651858.CD002945.
5. UK Small Aneurysm Trial Participants. Long term outcome of immediate repair compared with surveillance for small abdominal aortic aneurysm. *N Engl J of Medicine* 2002; **346**: 1437–44.
6. The EVAR Trial Participants. Endovascular aneurysm repair versus open repair in patients with abdominal aortic aneurysm (EVAR trial 1): randomized control trial. *Lancet* 2005; **365**: 2179–86.
7. The EVAR Trial Participants. Endovascular aneurysm repair and outcome in patients unfit for open repair of abdominal aortic aneurysm (EVAR 2): randomized control trial. *Lancet* 2005; **365**: 2187–92.
8. Verhoeven EL, Muhs BE et al. Fenestrated and branched stent-grafting after previous surgery provides a good alternative to open redo surgery. *Eur J Vasc Endovasc Surg* 2007; **33**: 84–90.
9. Mosorin M, Juvonen J, Biancari F et al. Use of Doxycycline to decrease the growth of abdominal aortic aneurysms: a randomized double blind placebo controlled pilot study. *J Vasc Surg* 2001; **34**: 606–10.
10. Parodi FE, Mao D, Ennis TL, Pagano MB, Thompson RW. Oral administration of diferulolylmethane (curcumin) suppresses proinflammatory cytokines and destructive connective tissue remodelling in experimental abdominal aortic aneurysms. *Ann Vasc Surg* 2006; **20**: 360–8.
11. Hinchliffe RJ, Bruijstens L et al. A randomized trial of endovascular and open surgery for ruptured abdominal aortic aneurysm – results of a pilot study and lessons learned for future studies. *Eur J Vasc Endovasc Surg* 2006; **32**: 506–13; discussion 514–15.

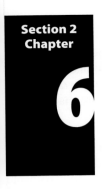

Final FRCS vascular topics

Thoracic, thoracoabdominal and suprarenal aortic aneurysms

Jenny Richards and Rod Chalmers

Key points

- Aneurysm disease affects the thoracic aorta much less commonly than the infrarenal aorta
- Most patients are asymptomatic but may have chest, back or abdominal pain
- Diagnosis is on computed tomography (CT) angiogram and the Crawford classification is used to describe the extent of the aneurysm
- Intervention is recommended if the aneurysm is >6 cm (or 5 cm in the presence of a connective tissue disorder or a family history of rupture)
- Open surgery remains the standard treatment for complex suprarenal, thoracic and thoracoabdominal aneurysms
- Specific complications incude risks of paraplegia and renal and visceral ischaemia
- Endovascular repair is suitable for descending thoracic aneurysms

Epidemiology

The incidence of aneurysmal disease affecting the suprarenal aorta and the thoracic aorta is difficult to estimate since it is a condition that is usually asymptomatic and rupture, which is often rapidly fatal, is commonly misattributed to other causes such as myocardial infarction or pulmonary embolism. The incidence is approximately 6 per 100 000 people per year. Males are affected about twice as commonly as females but interestingly the gender difference is less than for infrarenal aortic aneurysms, where the ratio is up to 7:1.

Natural history data are scarce, typically involving retrospective observation of patients not fit for open repair. In a series of 1600 cases the rupture risk for a 6 cm aneurysm of the thoracic aorta was 3.6% per year and for the composite endpoint of rupture/dissection/death the annual risk was 14.1%.

Aetiology and pathophysiology

The causes of descending thoracic aortic aneurysm (DTAA) and thoracoabdominal aortic aneurysm (TAAA) overlap significantly with those of infrarenal aortic aneurysm (described in Chapter 5). While atherosclerotic disease is still the most common cause of thoracic aneurysms other causes, including chronic dissection and connective tissue disease (e.g. Marfan's

Postgraduate Vascular Surgery: The Candidate's Guide to the FRCS, eds. Vish Bhattacharya and Gerard Stansby. Published by Cambridge University Press. © Cambridge University Press 2010.

syndrome) as well as infection, trauma and arteritis, account for a higher percentage of cases of thoracic than abdominal aneurysms. Aneurysmal tissue is characterised by deficiency of the tunica media of the vessel wall. Neovascularisation, inflammation and proteolytic digestion of the extracellular matrix are important processes, and biomechanical factors are also involved.

Presentation

The majority of DTAA and TAAA are asymptomatic. Those presenting to the vascular surgeon have either ruptured or have been detected as an incidental finding during an investigation for another indication. Patients may complain of chest, back or abdominal pain and if the aneurysm extends into the abdominal aorta may be detectable as an expansile mass on examination. Distal emoblisation can occur and usually manifests as 'trashing' of the lower limbs giving rise to the so called 'blue toe syndrome'. Other symptoms such as hoarseness, stridor, haemoptysis, haematemesis, nerve root pain and dysphagia aortica can result from compression or erosion of surrounding structures. The small proportion of aneurysms that are inflammatory can cause ureteric, bowel or venous obstruction, and occasionally a low-grade temperature and weight loss. Patients with a ruptured aneurysm will have sudden onset of severe chest, back or abdominal pain with syncope or profound cardiovascular collapse, and mottling of the lower limbs in particular. A retroperitoneal haematoma may be evident in a TAAA and superficial bruising is sometimes seen if the diagnosis is delayed.

Imaging and classification

A CT angiogram of the entire thoracic and abdominal aorta is required to define the extent of the aneurysm and its relationship to the key aortic branches. CT is also the investigation of choice for suspected rupture.

DTAAs commence beyond the left subclavian artery and terminate above the level of the diaphragm. TAAAs affect a variable length of the thoracic and abdominal aorta and are described according to the Crawford classification (Figure 6.1).

This practical classification system is useful for planning the surgical approach and for predicting complications. For example a laparotomy is often appropriate for type IV TAAA while an extensive thoracolaparotomy is required for aneurysms extending into the chest. Regarding complications, aneurysms affecting the visceral aorta carry a higher risk of renal and visceral ischaemia, and the risk of paraplegia is highest for the most extensive aneurysms and lower for those starting below the level of T6.

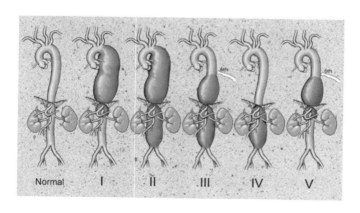

Figure 6.1 Modified Crawford classification of thoracoabdominal aneurysms. Safi HJ et al. Evolution of risk for neurologic deficit after descending and thoracoabdominal aortic repair. *Ann Thorac Surg* 2005; **80**: 2173–9; discussion 2179. Reproduced with permission.

Management

Based on what is known of the natural history of TAAA and DTAA, intervention is generally considered in medically fit patients when the descending thoracic component reaches 6 cm or the ascending aorta reaches 5 cm. A lower threshold of 5 cm may also be considered appropriate in patients with Marfan's syndrome or a familial tendency to rupture. Open surgical management of DTAA and TAAA is a major undertaking which, even with recent advances in perioperative care and surgical technique, is associated with a significant morbidity and mortality. There is an emerging and increasing role for the use of endovascular techniques in certain patients, which can reduce the surgical insult. Comprehensive preoperative assessment is essential.

Management of DTAA and TAAA disease is complex, but the frequency of cases is relatively low. Centralisation of services is essential and there is evidence that outcome is significantly better when patients are managed by high volume surgeons in high volume centres with dedicated vascular anaesthetists.

Non-operative management

Patients with an aneurysm below the diameter-threshold for intervention should remain in a surveillance programme with CT scans at appropriate intervals. These patients should receive standard cardiovascular best medical treatment including an antiplatelet agent and a statin (regardless of cholesterol) unless contraindicated, with careful control of blood pressure and blood sugar levels in diabetic patients. Patients who are not fit for surgical intervention can generally be discharged from the surveillance programme and be treated with best medical therapy in the community.

Preoperative assessment

The extent of the aneurysm and the relationship to key aortic branches is determined using CT scanning, which may also reveal surgically important anomalies such as a retro-aortic left renal vein, multiple renal arteries or a horseshoe kidney. From this information the nature of the operation and the risk of important complications can be gauged. The other side of the equation, how fit the patient is to withstand surgical intervention, is evaluated on the basis of a number of investigations.

It is important to obtain a full medical history and perform a thorough physical examination. In the assessment of cardiac function, the information available from a standard electrocardiogram (ECG) and echocardiogram is supplemented by some form of stress testing, either an exercise tolerance test or a stress echocardiogram. While an exercise bicycle or treadmill may be used for exercise testing, a treadmill is generally preferred since most patients are unused to cycling and quadriceps fatigue may limit exercise capacity. With continuous ECG monitoring the Bruce protocol involves up to 12 min of walking on a treadmill during which the speed and elevation are increased every 3 min, aiming to achieve 85% of the patient's maximum predicted heart rate. A positive test involves the development of angina-related symptoms, a fall in blood pressure or ECG changes including ventricular dysrhythmias or ST changes. Stress echocardiography may be preferred in patients with mobility difficulties and where motion affects data interpretation. During this examination echocardiography is performed during infusion of a pharmacological agent such as dobutamine, which has positive inotropic and chronotropic effects.

The focus of this test is the detection of wall motion abnormalities and assessment of their relationship to cardiac exertion, and is a sensitive way to detect stress-induced myocardial ischaemia. Cardiac catheterisation and angiography is performed selectively following non-invasive investigations. An assessment of pulmonary function is made using spirometry (FEV1, FVC and FEV1/FVC ratio). In addition a functional assessment, such as asking a patient to walk up a flight of stairs, is often informative. Cardiopulmonary exercise (CPX) testing is now available in a number of centres and gives detailed global information on the patient's cardiopulmonary performance during exercise. While exercising on a static bicycle ergometer, a closed breathing circuit is used to measure inspired and expired volumes and $pO2$ and $pCO2$ breath-by-breath. As the intensity of exercise increases the ECG is observed for ischaemic changes and the anaerobic threshold and oxygen consumption are calculated.

Renal function and hepatic function are assessed using standard blood laboratory measures. The patient's current level of mobility and independence and their mental resilience, although hard to assess objectively, are also important in their ability to rehabilitate following major surgery.

The results of all these investigations should be considered by a surgeon and anaesthetist with additional input from a radiologist in order that an appropriate management plan can be recommended to the patient. The patient's medications should be reviewed and consideration given to whether they can be optimised in advance of any surgical or endovascular intervention. In particular, consideration is given to antiplatelet, β-blocker and statin therapy.

Open surgical management

Type I, II, III and V thoracoabdominal aortic aneurysms

With the patient in the right lateral position an extensive thoracolaparotomy is made through the left 6th intercostal space with partial division of the anterior muscular part of the diaphragm, partial division of the left crus of the diaphragm and posterior division of the 6th rib to facilitate access. The left lung is partially deflated using a double lumen endotracheal tube and the aorta is exposed behind the left lung by division of the parietal pleura allowing control of the proximal aorta to be secured. The dissection is continued into the abdomen with medial visceral rotation of the left colon, left kidney and spleen being performed through the left paracolic gutter to expose the entire length of the aorta in the abdomen. The iliac arteries are dissected out and the left femoral artery is exposed through a separate incision to accommodate the bypass circuit. Following full heparinisation left heart bypass is established with the afferent limb in the left pulmonary vein or left atrium and the efferent limb in the femoral artery. For a type II TAAA the aorta is crossclamped distal to the left subclavian and in the mid-descending aorta (above T6). The aorta is opened longitudinally between the clamps and transected proximal to the aneurysm. The proximal end of a Dacron graft of appropriate diameter is anastomosed using a continuous prolene suture, and Teflon pledgelets and cyanoacrylate glue can be used to reinforce this suture line. The graft is clamped just beyond the anastomosis and the aortic clamp is replaced in a supracoeliac position. The thoracic aorta is opened along its length and large intercostals arteries, usually between T8 and L1, are selected for anastomosis to the graft on a patch. Occasionally a jump graft is required if vessels are widely spaced. Remaining small intercostal arteries are oversewn. The graft clamp is replaced beyond the intercostal patch restoring in-line flow to the spinal artery for the remainder of the procedure. The infrarenal aorta is then clamped and the renal, supracoeliac and superior mesenteric arteries are anastomosed to the graft on a patch using a jump graft to incorporate the left renal artery if necessary. Flow to the visceral vessels is restored while the distal anastomosis is performed.

By using a serial clamping technique the ischaemic insult to the spinal cord and viscera is minimised compared to clamping the entire aorta for the duration of the procedure. Prior to closing, the patient is actively warmed since normothermia is important for achieving haemostasis. The surgical techniques and adjuncts that can be used to reduce the complication rate are discussed below.

Descending thoracic aneurysms

An aneurysm of the descending thoracic aorta is repaired through a left-sided thoracotomy without the need to open the abdomen. Otherwise the technique for open repair is similar to that described for the thoracic component of an extensive TAAA. As discussed below DTAA are readily amenable to endovascular repair, which has now largely superseded open repair in this setting.

Aneurysms involving the aortic arch

Complete replacement of the ascending aorta and arch mandates hypothermic cardioplegic circulatory arrest and cardiopulmonary bypass, and lies within the remit of the cardiothoracic surgeon. However, the vascular surgeon is frequently faced with an aneurysm of the descending aorta, which also involves part of the aortic arch or which allows insufficient space to clamp the aorta distal to the left subclavian artery. Endovascular stenting of the arch would interrupt the blood supply to the brain if the proximal landing zone were to occlude the left carotid artery and the left vertebral artery, which is a branch of the left subclavian artery. In this situation a staged procedure should be performed involving a carotid-carotid bypass and a carotid-subclavian bypass before the aneurysm is repaired endovascularly.

Type IV thoracoabdominal and suprarenal aneurysms

The surgical approach for type IV and suprarenal aneurysms is similar and generally involves a midline laparotomy or 'roof-top' incision, although some surgeons prefer a thoracolaparotomy through the 8th, 9th or 10th interspace. The retroperitoneal space is accessed though the left paracolic gutter and the viscera (descending colon, spleen and left kidney) are mobilised and rotated medially to reach the aorta. The left crus of the diaphragm is partially divided but the diaphragm itself is left intact. A Dacron graft is used to replace the abdominal aorta. A bevel at the proximal end allows incorporation of the renal and visceral vessels on a patch. The size of the patch should be minimised to reduce the chance of further aneurysm formation so if the vessels are widely spaced any outlying vessels are anastomosed using a jump graft. Cerebrospinal fluid (CSF) drainage and other adjuncts are not necessary for the repair of type IV and suprarenal aneurysms.

Type IV and suprarenal aneurysms are less amenable to endovascular repair than infrarenal and descending thoracic aneurysms due to the difficulty in preserving the visceral vessels (see below). A hybrid approach can be used but does not offer improved outcomes in most patients compared to standard open surgery. In a hybrid approach the coeliac, superior mesenteric and renal arteries are revascularised in a retrograde fashion using a graft from one of the iliac arteries prior to placement of an endovascular stent-graft to exclude the aneurysm.

Endovascular management

Endovascular strategies offer a minimally invasive alternative to open surgical management with the particular advantage of reducing cardiorespiratory complications. Descending thoracic aneurysms are particularly amenable to a wholly endovascular approach since there is no involvement of the arch or visceral vessels. Branched and fenestrated grafts open up the possibility of treating aneurysms involving the arch and visceral vessels but these techniques are still being evaluated and currently are only available in a small number of centres with a particular interest in endovascular aneurysm treatment. Encouraging results have been achieved in small case series but, while early technical success rates are high, target vessels remain at risk from stent migration, fracture and kinking [1]. Such grafts are individually made for elective patients but cannot be obtained in time for patients requiring urgent intervention. Wholly endovascular techniques undoubtedly reduce the cardiopulmonary complications associated with open repair but the risk of paraplegia remains, re-intervention may be necessary, long-term durability results are awaited and annual post-procedure CT surveillance is required [1]. The stent graft industry is continuously developing improved devices that make increasingly complex lesions accessible to endovascular approaches. Hybrid procedures, combining endovascular exclusion of the aneurysm with open surgical revascularisation of aortic branches covered by the stent, have also been advocated but again accrual of outcome data is ongoing. Hybrid procedures have been used with particular success to treat arch aneurysms when accompanied by an open debranching procedure of the arch.

Complications and adjuncts

The morbidity and mortality associated with repair of extensive aneurysms has been reduced to acceptable levels over recent years with a better understanding of the pathophysiology of complications leading to modifications to the perioperative strategy [2]. Despite this, however, it is unsurprising that the complication rate, as a product of the magnitude of the operation and the level of comorbidity present in the DTAA/TAAA patient population, remains significant. Table 6.1 shows the incidence of the major complications associated with thoracic and thoracoabdominal aneurysm repair reported in two large contemporary case series.

Reducing the overall risk

Preoperative assessment is necessary to stratify the risk of complications on an individual patient basis and to select patients suitable for intervention. Centralisation of services for managing DTAA and TAAA is vital in order that experienced surgical, anaesthetic, critical care and theatre teams can be assembled along with the wide range of facilities and equipment that they require.

Intraoperatively systemic heparinisation is preventative against myocardial infarction, minimises the risk of embolisation, preserves the microcirculation and reduces the risk of thrombosis of key branches, particularly intercostal arteries, during clamping. Moderate

Table 6.1 Contemporary results of open repair of thoracoabdominal aneurysms

	Conrad et al. (2007) [4]	Coselli et al. (2007) [3]
Number of patients (dates)	445 (1987–2005)	2286 (since 1986)
Crawford extent I/II (%)	41.8	64.2
Ruptured (%)	11.4	6.1
Death (<30 day) (%)	8.3	6.6
Major paraplegia (%)	9.5	3.8
Renal failure (requiring dialysis) (%)	4.6	5.6
Cardiac complications (%)	14.7	7.9
Pulmonary complications (%)	49	32.1

permissive hypothermia (32–34 °C) reduces the metabolic demands of the viscera and the spinal cord, thereby increasing their tolerance to ischaemia. Unlike repair of the ascending aorta and aortic arch, full hypothermic circulatory arrest is rarely required for DTAA and TAAA repair. Left heart bypass is used for extensive repairs (Crawford extent I and II) enabling retrograde aortic perfusion, facilitating cooling/re-warming and reducing spinal cord and visceral ischaemia. Left heart bypass also allows patients with cardiac disease to tolerate proximal aortic clamping more readily by offloading the left side of the heart. Serial aortic clamping (as described above) involves moving the clamps distally along the aorta as the operation progresses and reduces the ischaemic insult and subsequent reperfusion injuries. Additional strategies are directed at reducing the incidence of specific complications.

Reducing cardiac and respiratory complications

The aetiology of cardiac and respiratory complications following DTAA and TAAA repair is multifactorial involving, in particular, existing comorbidities, a large surgical incision involving the thoracic cavity and fluid replacement to compensate for significant blood loss. Unfortunately there is limited potential to modify these factors, which is the reason that cardiopulmonary complications remain problematic in extensive aortic surgery and is why the possibility of endovascular repair is so attractive. Nonetheless identification of risk and optimisation of function preoperatively are important. Limitation of the incision to a laparotomy for type IV repair avoids the need to enter the thorax. Chest drains are placed routinely when the chest has been entered. Prompt extubation reduces ventilator-associated pneumonia and respiratory muscle wasting, and early tracheostomy placement in selected patients facilitates weaning.

Reducing the risk of paraplegia

The risk of paraplegia was much higher (in the region of 16%) before the introduction of modern adjuncts, but remains higher for type II aneurysms (6.3–14.5%) than for less extensive type IV aneurysms (2.9–3.8%) [3]. This is directly related to the length of aorta that is replaced and the risk of paraplegia is also increased following previous aortic surgery or dissection. The blood supply to the spinal cord is from multiple sources including the vertebral arteries, anterior segmental medullary arteries (intercostal and lumbar) and the internal iliac arteries, all of which contribute to the anterior spinal artery. The artery of Adamkiewicz is the largest contributor to the anterior spinal artery and is generally a left-sided intercostal artery but may sometimes arise from the right or from a lumbar artery.

Reimplanation of the major segmental arteries, ideally including the artery of Adamkiewicz, is thought to be important in reducing the risk of paraplegia. While some surgeons advocate preoperative mapping of the spinal cord blood supply using MRI, most would select one to three large pairs of intercostal vessels (usually between T6 and T12) intraoperatively for reattachment. Serial clamping and left heart bypass reduce spinal cord ischaemia during extensive repair but despite this some degree of spinal cord ischaemia is inevitable. Placement of a CSF drain allows monitoring of CSF pressure during the operation and postoperatively. CSF is actively drained during aortic cross clamping and passively drained for 48 hours postoperatively allowing decompression of the vertebral foramen in the event of spinal cord swelling. Since CSF drainage carries the risks of infection and haematoma formation it is reserved for extensive aneurysm repairs. Spinal cord perfusion is further optimised by maintaining the mean arterial pressure >80 mmHg and avoiding hypotensive, vasodilating drugs where possible. Motor evoked potentials can be used to detect spinal cord ischaemia during cross-clamping and following reimplanation of vessels. Postoperatively, rather than being fully sedated, even intubated patients are nursed in a rousable state to facilitate assessment of the neurological function of the lower limbs and detection of signs of delayed-onset spinal cord ischaemia.

Reducing the risk of renal and gastrointestinal tract ischaemia

Left heart bypass, moderate systemic hypothermia, heparinisation and serial clamping all contribute to a reduced risk of visceral ischaemia. Additionally a trial of renal cooling comparing renal perfusion with normothermic blood and 4C crystalloid fluid found the latter to be advantageous in reducing renal complications. Retrograde aortic perfusion on left heart bypass maintains the blood supply to the abdominal viscera during surgery on the proximal aorta. When the clamps are replaced on the infrarenal aorta, selective visceral perfusion can be maintained using individual balloon perfusion catheters in the ostia of the visceral vessels. Some surgeons use renal cooling and selective visceral perfusion routinely whilst others use these measures selectively in patients perceived to have a higher than average risk of complications.

Reducing complications of blood loss and coagulopathy

Significant blood loss occurs during the repair of extensive aneurysms and massive heterologous transfusion is associated with a number of complications including coagulopathy, hypothermia and transfusion reactions. The use of a cell saver and autologous transfusion reduces heterologous transfusion requirements. Near-patient testing of coagulation, such as thromboelastography, can be used to detect impending coagulopathy before it becomes evident clinically. It also enables identification of the specific part of the coagulation cascade that is deficient so that treatment can be targeted and timely, before bleeding complications become problematic.

References

1. Greenberg RK, Lytle B. Endovascular repair of thoracoabdominal aneurysms. *Circulation* 2008; **117**: 2288–96.

2. Coselli JS, LeMaire SA. Tips for successful outcomes for descending thoracic and thoracoabdominal aortic aneurysm procedures. *Semin Vasc Surg* 2008; **21**: 13–20.

3. Coselli JS, Bozinovski J, LeMaire SA. Open surgical repair of 2286 thoracoabdominal aortic aneurysms. *Ann Thorac Surg* 2007; **83**: S862–S4; discussion S890–S2.

4. Conrad MF, Crawford RS, Davison JK, Cambria RP. Thoracoabdominal aneurysm repair: a 20-year perspective. *Ann Thorac Surg* 2007; **83**: S856–S61; discussion S890–S2.

Aortic dissection

Jenny Richards and Rod Chalmers

Key points

- Aortic dissection may be defined as acute (<2 weeks since symptoms) or chronic (>2 weeks since symptoms)
- Acute aortic dissection is associated with hypertension and pre-existing disease of the aortic wall
- Patients usually present with severe, tearing chest and back pain
- Diagnosis is with transoesophageal echocardiogram and computed tomography (CT) angiogram
- The Stanford or DeBakey classifications are used to describe the pattern of dissection
- Type A dissections require early surgical treatment. The in-hospital mortality is high but the prognosis is very good in patients surviving to discharge from hospital
- Type B dissections are treated medically in the first instance. The in-hospital mortality is much lower but complications may occur following discharge
- Chronic type B dissection may result in aortic dilatation and rupture so surveillance is required
- Endovascular strategies have a role in some situations for acute type A dissection and acute type B dissection, but the role in chronic type B dissection is unclear

Epidemiology

Aortic dissection occurs with an incidence of approximately 3 per 100 000 per year. Accurate estimates are difficult due to the high out-of-hospital mortality for this condition and the low post-mortem rate in most countries. It affects males twice as commonly as females and the risk increases with age. Interestingly, as with a number of other cardiovascular conditions, it demonstrates circadian variation with a peak incidence early in the morning and during the winter. This pattern correlates with times of peak blood pressure.

Aetiology

Factors predisposing to aortic dissection involve pre-existing degenerative, genetic or inflammatory conditions that weaken the aorta and primary or secondary causes of hypertension. Table 7.1 shows the factors that have an association with aortic dissection.

Postgraduate Vascular Surgery: The Candidate's Guide to the FRCS, eds. Vish Bhattacharya and Gerard Stansby. Published by Cambridge University Press. © Cambridge University Press 2010.

Table 7.1 Factors associated with aortic dissection

- Increasing age
- Male sex
- Diabetes mellitus
- Pre-existing aortic disease e.g. aneurysmal disease, atherosclerosis, arteritis
- Connective tissue disorders e.g. Marfan's syndrome, Ehlers–Danlos syndrome
- Congenital anomalies e.g. bicuspid valve, aortic hypoplasia
- Hypertension primary or secondary e.g. pregnancy, cocaine use, weightlifting
- Iatrogenic e.g. cardiac catheterisation and intervention, coronary artery bypass grafting, valve replacement
- Trauma e.g. deceleration injury
- Previous aortic surgery
- Family history

Pathophysiology

A breach in the aortic intima allows blood to track within the media of the vessel wall, creating a true lumen and a false lumen. This entry tear usually lies in the ascending aorta, aortic arch or just distal to the left subclavian artery. Dissection results from a combination of the stress applied to the aortic wall due to high, fluctuating blood pressure and disease processes, which damage and weaken the vessel wall. It is now recognised that the breach in the intima may be caused by a penetrating atherosclerotic ulcer or alternatively an intramural haematoma resulting from disruption of the vasa vasorum, which may subsequently penetrate into the lumen. Although initially benign, intramural haematoma regresses in only 10% of patients while 28–45% progress to aortic dissection, 20–45% rupture and more proximal lesions are particularly prone to complication [1]. In a smaller number of patients the intimal injury is traumatic or iatrogenic. Intimal disruption initiates the dissection and proximal and/or distal propagation follows and is facilitated if the media has been weakened by enzymatic (e.g. matrix metalloproteinases) degradation of the extracellular matrix. Blood may travel within the false lumen along a variable length of the aorta and its branches. The exit tear may re-enter the true lumen connecting it with the false lumen or it may rupture outwards, with the latter resulting in rapid death. End-organ ischaemia occurs as branches become thrombosed or perfusion may be dynamically influenced as the true lumen is variably compromised by changes in flow in the false lumen during the cardiac cycle and as arterial pressure fluctuates.

Presentation

The classical presentation of acute aortic dissection is with sudden onset of extremely severe chest pain, often described as 'tearing' in nature, located anteriorly radiating to the neck or back and migrating as the dissection propagates. While pain is prominent in the majority of patients, a proportion will complain of less severe pain or no discomfort at all and, in fact, lack of pain is a predictor of poor outcome, perhaps because diagnosis is delayed. Where chest pain is present the diagnosis is often confused with acute myocardial infarction although, if a detailed history is taken, the sudden onset and nature of the symptoms may be used to distinguish the true cause. The two may also occur together if the coronary arteries are affected by the dissection. The integrity of the aortic valve may be disrupted causing acute aortic regurgitation and, if the dissection communicates with the pericardium, tamponade may result. Patients with a type A dissection are often hypotensive while hypertension is typical in type B dissection.

As the false lumen extends it may compromise some of the key branches of the aorta, impairing end-organ perfusion and precipitating organ dysfunction or failure. Symptoms include myocardial ischaemia (coronary arteries), cerebrovascular accident (carotid and vertebral arteries), spinal cord ischaemia (intercostals and lumbar arteries), renal dysfunction (renal arteries), mesenteric ischaemia (coeliac and mesenteric arteries) and limb ischaemia (subclavian and iliac arteries), which often become evident in serial fashion as the dissection extends. On examination pulses may be weak, asymmetrical or absent, and again may disappear serially with progression of the dissection.

Diagnosis and classification

Sudden death may occur but in those surviving to present to the emergency department, rapid diagnosis is important to plan treatment. Plain radiography and electrocardiogram (ECG) are commonly performed in patients presenting with acute chest pain but, while they may show some non-specific changes consistent with aortic dissection, neither is diagnostic. A plain radiograph of the chest may be normal in a third to a half of patients [2] or reveal mediastinal widening, an abnormal contour of the aortic arch or a haemothorax. Electrocardiogram is often normal but may show signs of myocardial ischaemia or left ventricular strain/hypertrophy.

An echocardiogram and cross-sectional imaging (either magnetic resonance imaging [MRI] or CT) are needed to confirm the diagnosis and the extent of the dissection proximally and distally. Whilst transthoracic echocardiography (TTE) has the advantage of being rapid and non-invasive in unstable patients, transoesophageal echo (TOE) has a higher sensitivity and specificity. CT or magnetic resonance angiography with contrast yield additional information about organ perfusion and the relative flow in the true and false lumens and, unlike echocardiography, both have the advantage of imaging the entire thoracic cavity if an alternative diagnosis is possible. The performance of CT and MRI are comparable in diagnosing and excluding aortic dissection. The advantage of CT is that it is more widely available and the scanning time is short. The use of MRI for long-term surveillance to avoid an accumulating ionising radiation dose is beneficial.

Acute dissection is defined as being within 2 weeks of the onset of symptoms and after this time becomes chronic. The Stanford and Debakey classifications are useful for stratifying risk, predicting complications and planning treatment. The Stanford classification distinguishes dissections affecting the ascending aorta (type A) from those which affect only the descending aorta (type B). The Debakey classification further subdivides dissections affecting the ascending aorta into those affecting the descending aorta as well (type I) and those only affecting the ascending aorta (type II). Debakey type III is equivalent to Stanford type A (Figure 7.1).

If the ascending aorta is affected the patient may experience cardiac, cerebral and upper limb complications since the coronary, carotid and subclavian arteries are at risk. Dissections of the descending and abdominal aorta cause complications related to spinal cord, visceral and limb ischaemia. Considering treatment, type A dissections generally require surgical intervention while type B dissections can be managed medically in the majority of patients.

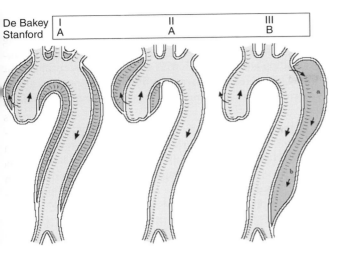

Figure 7.1 Stanford and Debakey classification of aortic dissections.
Erbel R et al. Diagnosis and management of aortic dissection. *Eur Heart J* 2001; **22**: 1642–81. Reproduced with permission.

Management

The management of aortic dissection depends upon the extent and location of the dissection and the stability and comorbidities of the patient [6]. Due to the nature of this condition there is a paucity of high-level evidence to support practice but the International Registry of Aortic Dissection (IRAD) has gathered valuable information about the trends and outcome of recent practice [1, 4]. In addition the European Society of Cardiology taskforce produced guidelines for the management of aortic dissection [2].

Type A

Type A dissections account for around two thirds of all cases of dissection [3]. Urgent surgery is almost always required for type A dissections unless the patient is moribund or has significant pre-existing co-morbidities. Untreated type A dissections have a mortality in the region of 1–2% per hour for the first 24 hours, amounting to 50–75% by 2 weeks. With medical management alone the mortality of type A dissections in the IRAD database was 56% [1]. Surgical management involves sealing off the entry point to decompress the false lumen and reduce the risk of propagation of the dissection. Since the entry tear usually lies in a diffusely diseased part of the aorta, this generally involves resection of the aorta at the site of the entry tear and reconstruction using a short graft (e.g. Dacron) through a median sternotomy approach with hypothermic cardioplegic circulatory arrest and cardiopulmonary bypass. When the entry tear lies in the arch, reconstruction or reimplantation of the innominate, carotid and subclavian vessels will be necessary. If there is incompetence of the aortic valve this may have to be reconstructed or, more commonly, replaced with a prosthesis. The ostia of the coronary arteries may also require reconstruction or coronary artery bypass grafting. The operative mortality for dissections of the ascending aorta is in the region of 16%, higher (31.4%) if the patient is shocked before surgery [1].

The false lumen may extend for a variable distance into the descending aorta but due to the morbidity associated with replacing long segments of the aorta, including the visceral vessels, this is usually avoided in the first instance where possible. The operation on the ascending aorta effectively converts this situation into a type B dissection, which can then be managed medically as described below. While there is not yet an established role for endovascular management of type A dissections, there is interest in using a hybrid approach combining open surgery for the ascending aorta and arch with endovascular stenting of the descending aorta. This approach may be useful for patients with malperfusion syndromes, intractable pain, uncontrolled hypertension or continued propagation or expansion of the false lumen.

An elephant trunk procedure is used when it is anticipated that the descending aorta will need to be replaced subsequently. The ascending aorta and the arch are replaced with a tube graft. The arch vessels are re-implanted into the graft on a single patch. Rather than cutting the graft to length the distal end is left long and projects into the descending aorta enabling a staged procedure to be performed. At a later date an open surgical approach to the descending aorta can be used with the proximal anastomosis being made to the elephant trunk, or the elephant trunk can be used as the proximal landing zone for an endovascular stent graft. The advantage of this is that it avoids the need to graft directly onto diseased and fragile aortic wall.

Type B

Type B – uncomplicated

The outcome for type B dissection is much more favourable than for type A dissection with a 30-day survival rate of 89% [1]. Operative management is extremely hazardous and is avoided if possible [5]. Aggressive medical management involving analgesia and control of hypertension and heart rate is important. Patients should be admitted to a coronary care or intensive care unit for close monitoring of blood pressure, end organ function and any evidence of progression such as escalating or intractable pain or development of new symptoms. Intravenous β-blockers (e.g. esmolol, labetolol), unless contraindicated, are used in the first instance to reduce systolic blood pressure to 100–120 mmHg. Rate-limiting calcium channel blockers (e.g. diltiazem) are an alternative for patients intolerant of β-blockers, and a nitrate infusion may be used if either of these agents is insufficient in isolation. In the longer term, angiogenesis-converting enzyme (ACE) inhibitors may have the additional advantage of promoting remodelling of the aortic wall but the evidence for this has not yet been accumulated.

Type B – complicated

In the International Registry of Acute Aortic Dissection (IRAD) database, 17.2% of patients with type B dissection required surgical intervention during the acute phase [6]. Indications for surgery were rupture (23%), further propagation of the dissection (52%), uncontrolled hypertension (15.5%), intractable pain (14.1%), malperfusion of the viscera (23.9%) or limbs (15.5%) or a combination of these factors. The exact procedure is tailored to the anatomy of the dissection for a given patient. Graft replacement of the descending aorta is the most common open surgical procedure (69.3% of surgically managed acute type B dissections in the IRAD series [9, 6]), which may be performed in conjunction with replacement of the arch and fenestration, stenting or bypass for compromised vessels. The requirement for surgical intervention was associated with high mortality (29.3%), particularly if required during the first 2 days [6] and there has therefore been considerable interest in the possibility of employing endovascular techniques in the management of complicated acute type B dissection. From the EUROSTAR/United Kingdom registry 131 patients with aortic dissection were treated with 89% primary technical success, a paraplegia rate of <1% and a mortality rate of 8.4% at 30 days and 10% at one year [7]. In the IRAD database endovascular treatment was associated with better short-term outcomes than open surgical treatment for acute type B dissection [1]. Long-term follow-up data are awaited. In this context a stent graft may be used to occlude the entry tear and bare metal stents hold the true lumen open and compress the false lumen, which may improve dynamic malperfusion phenomena. Compromised vessels may also be targeted directly with bare metal stents to restore flow. In the longer term it is possible that endovascular occlusion of the false lumen will promote thrombosis, thus encouraging remodelling of the dissected wall and reducing the risk of late expansion and rupture. There is currently no definite evidence to support prophylactic placement of bare metal stents for this purpose.

Type B – chronic

Accurate data on the outcome of patients with chronic dissection are sparse and 5-year mortality is estimated at 50%, suggesting that medical management alone is suboptimal. The European Society of Cardiology recommends regular surveillance at 1, 3, 6, 12 months and annually thereafter to monitor for expansion of the affected aorta [2]. Thresholds for intervention are recommended at 5 cm for the ascending aorta and 6 cm for the descending aorta [2]. The IRAD database showed partial thrombosis of the false lumen to be an independent predictor of risk of death at 3 years [1]. Surgical management involves graft replacement of the entire aorta as described for open thoracoabdominal aneurysm repair. While early technical success can be achieved using endovascular repair, evidence to support or refute a role for endovascular treatment of chronic type B dissection is currently limited but early results do not appear to be as encouraging as for acute dissection.

Complications

The main complications of type A dissection repair are cardiac, stroke and death. The complications of intervention for type B aortic dissection are similar to those described for open repair of extensive TAAA but patients with a history of dissection are at higher risk of paraplegia, renal failure and death.

While acute type A dissection has a high in-hospital mortality (33%) among patients who survive to discharge, the 1- and 3-year survival rates are 96% and 91%, respectively [1]. In contrast 90% of patients with acute type B dissection survive to discharge but amongst those surviving to be discharged from hospital the 1- and 3-year survival rates are 78% and 76%, respectively [1].

References

1. Tsai TT, Trimarchi S, Nienaber CA. Acute aortic dissection: perspectives from the International Registry of Acute Aortic Dissection (IRAD). *Eur J Vasc Endovasc Surg* 2009; 37: 149–59.

2. Erbel R et al. Diagnosis and management of aortic dissection. *Eur Heart J* 2001; 22: 1642–81.

3. Golledge J, Eagle KA. Acute aortic dissection. *Lancet* 2008; 372: 55–66.

4. Trimarchi S et al. Contemporary results of surgery in acute type A aortic dissection: the International Registry of Acute Aortic Dissection experience. *J Thorac CardiovascSurg* 2005; 129: 112–22.

5. Akin I, Kische S, Ince H, Nienaber CA. Indication, timing and results of endovascular treatment of type B dissection. *Eur J Vasc Endovasc Surg* 2009; **37**: 289–96.

6. Trimarchi S et al. Role and results of surgery in acute type B aortic dissection: insights from the International Registry of Acute Aortic Dissection (IRAD). *Circulation* 2006; **114**: 357–64.

7. Leurs LJ et al. Endovascular treatment of thoracic aortic diseases: combined experience from the EUROSTAR and United Kingdom Thoracic Endograft registries. *J Vasc Surg* 2004; **40**: 670–9; discussion 679–80.

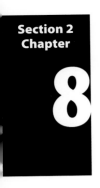

Section 2
Chapter

Final FRCS vascular topics

Popliteal artery aneurysms

Robert Davies, Asif Mahmood and Rajiv Vohra

Key points

- Popliteal artery aneurysm is the most common lower limb aneurysm
- Lower limb arterial aneurysms rarely occur in isolation
- The majority present either as an incidental finding or as lower limb ischaemia
- Aneurysm rupture is rare, but life and limb threatening when it occurs
- All symptomatic popliteal and femoral artery aneurysms should undergo repair
- Asymptomatic popliteal artery aneurysms >2 cm in maximum diameter should be considered for elective repair
- Asymptomatic femoral artery aneurysms >2.5 cm in maximum diameter should be considered for elective repair
- Adequate imaging of the proximal and distal vasculature is vital for successful repair

Introduction

Popliteal artery aneurysms are the second most common peripheral arterial aneurysm and together with femoral artery aneurysms represent the vast majority of true lower limb arterial aneurysms. They frequently occur in association with aortic aneurysms and are often identified as an incidental finding during routine examination or radiological imaging. However, they may present with lower limb thromboembolism or rupture and thus their identification and subsequent management is vitally important to the patient's quality of life and life expectancy.

Pathophysiology

The majority of popliteal artery aneurysms (PAAs) develop secondary to a systemic atherosclerotic disease affecting the medial layer of the artery and are often associated with aneurysms elsewhere. In early retrospective studies in which PAAs were detected clinically or with the use of angiography rather than Duplex scanning, the incidence of PAAs in patients with aortic aneurysms was between 3.2 and 3.9%. However, more recent prospective studies have shown the incidence to be two to three times greater than this. Conversely, if a PAA is detected, concomitant aortic and femoral aneurysms are present in up to 50% and 40% of cases, respectively. It is also important to examine and image the contralateral popliteal artery, as 50% are bilateral[1].

Postgraduate Vascular Surgery: The Candidate's Guide to the FRCS, eds. Vish Bhattacharya and Gerard Stansby. Published by Cambridge University Press. © Cambridge University Press 2010.

Table 8.1 Presentation of popliteal aneurysms

Presentation	%
Limb ischaemia	55
Asymptomatic	37
Rupture	1.4
Local compression	6.5

Causal explanations for the preponderance of the popliteal artery to become aneurysmal include fixation at the adductor hiatus and exposure to repetitive trauma with the use of adductor magnus or extrinsic compression from knee flexion and extension. Uncontrolled hypertension is associated with aneurysm expansion. Non-atherosclerotic causes of aneurysmal change are rare and include inflammatory and connective-tissue disorders such as Marfan's syndrome and Behçet's disease. Aneurysmal changes can also be seen after post-stenotic blunt and penetrating trauma. Mycotic aneurysms in the popliteal fossa have also been rarely reported.

Symptoms and signs

Most occur in men with a median age of 60 to 65 years at the time of diagnosis. Approximately 63% (Table 8.1) are symptomatic at presentation with asymptomatic aneurysms detected on palpation or surveillance Duplex ultrasound scan (DUS) of the popliteal fossae in patients with diagnosed aortic, iliac, femoral or contralateral PAAs.

A pulsatile mass on palpation of the popliteal fossa must be differentiated from other vascular lumps such as pseduoaneurysm from trauma or anastomotic dehiscence after bypass surgery. Venous aneurysm and non-vascular lumps with transmitted pulsation arising from the soft tissues such as Baker's cyst, bursae, tumours and lymph nodes are also included in the differential diagnoses.

The most common complication of popliteal aneurysms is thrombosis, embolism or a combination of both. This may result acutely with either intermittent claudication or as an acutely ischaemic leg, threatening the limb unless revascularisation is rapidly undertaken. Because of the need for aneurysm ligation during surgery and greater risk of embolism during intra-arterial thrombolysis it is important to differentiate acute ischaemia with popliteal aneurysm from ischaemia from other causes of thrombosis and embolism.

A more insidious presentation is that of gradual onset of claudication or chronic critical limb ischaemia with rest pain and tissue loss. Silent thrombosis and embolism is also possible; clinically detected by impalpable pedal pulses and reduced ankle brachial pressure index (ABPI), this is one of the indications for surgery. Large aneurysms may compress neighbouring structures such as the popliteal vein and/or tibial nerve. The former may be mistaken for other causes of lower limb oedema and venous hypertension while the latter may be misdiagnosed as a primary neurological disorder. Rupture is the most unlikely presentation of popliteal aneurysms but may threaten life as well as limb from the blood loss.

Investigation

Information is required regarding the extent of the aneurysm, the state of inflow and run-off vessels due to coexistent disease. In the case of aneurysms that are producing compression symptoms, information about the anatomy of the aneurysm, including diameter, extent and

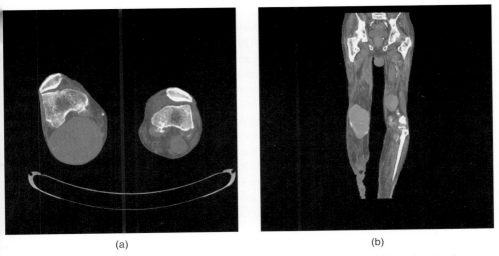

(a)   (b)

Figure 8.1 (a) Cross-sectional view of bilateral popliteal aneurysms. (b) Coronal view of bilateral popliteal aneurysms.

effect on neighbouring structures is required. Duplex ultrasound scan provides excellent information regarding inflow, outflow, diameter and presence of sac thrombus. Although angiography will show the state of the run-off, it adds little to anatomical evaluation. Fusiform aneurysms tend to involve the whole length of the popliteal artery and may have stenotic or occluded segments in addition to the aneurysmal disease and may also affect the superficial femoral artery. Sacular aneurysms, on the other hand, are more localised, affecting mainly the mid-popliteal artery. In cases where there are compression symptoms, assessment of the surrounding structures may be carried out with computed tomography (CT) angiography or magnetic resonance imaging (MRI) (Figures 8.1(a) and (b)).

Management
When to repair

All patients with symptomatic aneurysms require intervention for the relief of symptoms and prevention of limb loss. The indications for surgery in asymptomatic popliteal aneurysm remain controversial with no randomised controlled trials available to establish clear indications for intervention. Enthusiasts of surgery argue that since up to 100% of asymptomatic aneurysms will develop thromboembolic complications within 5 years without surgery, with an associated amputation rate of <67%, intervention is always recommended [1, 2]. In one prospective study, 18 of 58 aneurysms that had been treated conservatively developed complications [1]. Better graft patency and limb salvage have been noted for asymptomatic rather than symptomatic aneurysms. In fact, the results for reconstruction for popliteal aneurysm are better than for occlusive disease [3]. This may be related to better run-off, use of shorter length grafts or reduced thrombogenicity of blood in these patients compared with occlusive disease. Some surgeons favour an expectant policy with the use of thrombolysis if required. Schellack et al. showed that only 2 of 26 (8%) aneurysms developed thromboembolic complications at a mean follow up of 37[4]. Bowyer et al. reported good results with intra-arterial thrombolysis for asymptomatic aneurysm presenting with acute ischaemia [5].

Most of these studies have been retrospective with risk factors for complications being a diameter greater than 2 cm, presence of aneurysm sac thrombus and signs of silent embolism i.e. loss of pedal pulses or lowering of ABPI. Varga et al. attempted to identify indications for the management of asymptomatic aneurysm in a prospective multi-centre study but the numbers with small aneurysms (<2 cm) were insufficient to establish risk of complications with conservative treatment in this group [1]. In another prospective study, Galland et al. showed that those with a diameter of less than 3 cm were unlikely to thrombose [6]. Conversely, it has been shown that enlarging diameter of the sac does not increase the risk of thromboembolism. Also, some small aneurysms (<2 cm diameter) may have disproportionate amounts of thrombus in the sac with a greater risk of embolism. Thus we advocate elective surgical repair for all asymptomatic PAAs ≥2 cm in maximum diameter or those PAAs ≥1.8 cm with high thrombus content in suitable patients.

Surgical approaches

The most widely utilised surgical technique for repair of PAA is proximal and distal aneurysm ligation combined with long saphenous vein bypass through a medial approach. The advantages of this approach are the ability to expose the crural vessels and harvest the long saphenous vein from the same incision. However, the disadvantage is the potential for continued sac expansion post repair. In our series, 15% of PAA repairs treated by ligation and bypass demonstrated sac perfusion at a median of 75 months after primary PAA repair. Forty per cent of these patients presented with symptoms, including one rupture [7]. This complication of the ligation and bypass technique has been reported by others and is thought to be secondary to patent collaterals, similar in endovascular terms to a type II collateral endoleak. This imparts near systemic arterial pressure within the excluded sac, causing expansion with the possibility of subsequent rupture or neurovascular compression.

Some authors advocate a posterior approach with interposition grafting in the presence of compressive features or focal PAAs (Figure 8.2). This involves an 'S' shaped incision in the popliteal fossa with dissection of the aneurysm from other popliteal structures followed by inlay grafting

The advantage of this approach is the direct visualisation of the geniculate arteries allowing them to be oversewn thereby preventing aneurysm sac reperfusion. Furthermore, the sac may be excised, which is especially important in cases of neurovascular compression. This technique is not generally suitable for PAAs extending proximal to the adductor hiatus or where crural vessel exposure is required. Thus we advocate interposition grafting as the operation of choice for focal, large PAAs that do not extend above the adductor hiatus.

Conduits

Although the autologous vein is the conduit of choice, the conduit for grafting depends on the availability of a suitable vein, the presence of infection and the length of the graft required. Hence, for mycotic aneurysms, prosthetic conduits should be avoided.

Inlay grafting requires a small length of graft and as such prosthetic conduits such as polytetrafluoroethane (PTFE) have been shown to produce adequate results, although a venous conduit is recommended if the distal anastomosis is on the distal below-knee popliteal artery.

For bypass grafts below the knee, a thorough search for a vein using a combination of preoperative vein mapping and on-table exploration of the leg veins (saphenous trunks) usually allows several segments of composite spliced vein to be anastomosed together to

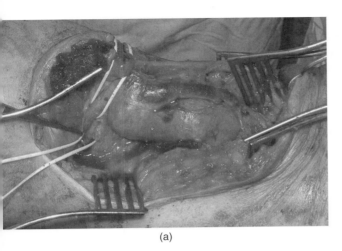

Figure 8.2 (a) Posterior approach to large popliteal aneurysm. (b) Vein inlay graft repair of large popliteal aneurysm.

(a)

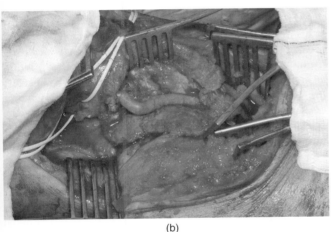

(b)

form a suitable conduit if a single length of vein is not available. Arm vein can be utilised if the saphenous vein is not available. In our series the long-term results using this approach are comparable to ligation and bypass with a trend for superior primary patency rates. The second best option is the use of a composite-sequential conduit with above-knee prosthetic conjoined by a three-panelled anastomosis to the above-knee popliteal artery and vein traversing the knee. [7]. A prosthetic graft with the addition of a venous cuff or fistula remains the least attractive option due to the relatively poor results in terms of graft patency, limb salvage and risk of infection.

Management of thromboembolism

The acutely ischaemic leg from popliteal aneurysm remains a challenge because of the poor limb salvage achieved. A multi-disciplinary approach involving a vascular surgeon and interventional radiologist is required. Treatment options include intra-arterial thrombolysis alone, thrombolysis to remove clot in the aneurysm sac and run-off followed by surgery or intraoperative lysis with thromboembolectomy followed by reconstruction. The treatment depends on the degree and duration of ischaemia and co-morbidities. In a chronically ischae-mic leg, it is unlikely that lysis or embolectomy will clear a well packed clot in the run-off and therefore a crural or pedal bypass remains the most realistic option. Interventional radio-logical techniques include preoperative intra-arterial thrombolysis and aspiration embolec-tomy. First described by Schwarz et al. in 1984, thrombolysis can be successfully used as the primary intervention [8]. In a unit favouring conservative treatment of all asymptomatic aneurysms, Bowyer et al. reported successful thrombolysis in six of nine patients with acute thromboembolic complications [5]. Limb salvage was achieved in all nine cases, including those with failed lysis requiring additional procedures such as lumbar sympathectomy and angioplasty. The combination of preoperative lysis, followed by surgery, was shown to be effective by Carpenter et al., who reported a limb salvage rate of 100% with combination treatment in comparison to 57% for surgery alone [9]. However, details of run-off clearing procedures were not given in this study. Preoperative intra-arterial thrombolysis should not be considered in every case, especially in the presence of neurological signs, as it is associ-ated with a poor outcome. Immediate surgery is required in this situation. Preoperative lysis is also associated with a risk of distal embolism of 13% in popliteal aneurysms, compared to 2% in patients with acute ischaemia due to occlusive disease. Not all cases are successful and lysis may not be effective in dislodging well-packed clot or cholesterol emboli ('trash') with clearance rates of only 58–66%. The theoretical risk of stroke as well as systemic bleed-ing has been reduced when a low dose lytic agent has been used in the on-table technique. Intraoperative thrombolysis may be delivered either trans-femorally, via the popliteal artery or from the ankle routes with the latter two routes being favoured in cases of a threatened limb with more rapid clearance of run-off being achieved with the catheter being closer to the run-off. Isolated limb perfusion may also give good results and limit side effects by reducing the dosage of lytic agent reaching the systemic circulation. Methods for improving the removal of distal thrombus include popliteal trifurcation embolectomy and ankle level micro-embolectomies. The embolectomy catheter may not pass easily from the popliteal artery all the way down the calf vessels for mechanical reasons such as angulations or due to the nature of occlusive disease. In these circumstances, embolectomy of the crural and pedal vessels via arteriotomy at the ankle may successfully retrieve clot in the crural or pedal vessels that is otherwise inaccessible. In this technique the anterior tibial, posterior tibial or both arteries are exposed by small separate ankle incisions and opened transversely using loupe magnification and a micro-knife. Proximal and distal embolectomy can be carried out using a size 2 balloon catheter, directed proximally to the popliteal trunk and distally into and around the pedal arch. Adjunctive thrombolysis may also be used in cases of incom-plete embolectomy. In our series, of the 17 patients with acute ischemia, limb salvage was achieved in 14 with an aggressive management with thromboembolectomy in 12 and bypass grafting in 6. This was combined with thrombolysis in a few. Acutely ischemic limbs had a cumulative 5-year secondary patency of 80% and a 30-day mortality of 11.8% [7].

The endovascular era

In recent years endovascular repair has been increasingly employed as a valid alternative to open surgical repair. Reported benefits include significant reduction in operation time, blood loss, perioperative morbidity and postoperative hospital stay compared with conven-tional surgical repair [8, 9]. However, to date, only one randomised controlled trial (RCT) and three case series with more than 10 PAAs are reported in the literature (Table 8.2).

Table 8.2 Summary of results of endovascular treatment of popliteal artery aneurysms (PAAs)

Author	No. of PAAs	Mean (months) follow up	Primary patency		Secondary patency		Occlusions
			1 year	2 years	1 year	2 years	
Tielliu et al. [10]	57	24	80%	77%	90%	87%	12 (21%)
Mohan et al. [11]	30	24	80%	75%	89%	83%	6 (20%)
Antonello et al. [12]	15	46	87%	80%	100%	100%	1 (6.7%)

The experience of the Padua group who presented data on 30 PAAs randomised to surgical (15 PAAs) or endovascular repair (15 PAAs) suggests comparable short-term patency rates between surgical and endovascular repair. However the study was significantly compromised by its power limitation and short follow up. The largest cohort by Tielliu et al. (57 endovascular repairs) reported inferior primary and secondary patency rates (80% and 90% at 1-year follow up, and 77% and 87% at 2-year follow up) compared to surgical repair [10]. Multivarate analysis demonstrated treatment with clopidogrel in the postoperative period was the only predictor of success. Endovascular PAA repair is associated with a risk of stent occlusion of 6.7–44% at 2-year follow up, with 67–100% occurring within the first 6 months postoperative. Despite this the limb salvage rate is 100% with the majority of stent occlusions being successfully treated by intra-arterial thrombolysis with residual claudication symptoms. Endovascular PAA repairs are also at risk of endoleak and stent migration. Tielliu et al. reported two type I endoleaks secondary to late stent migration in short sealing zones that were successfully repaired with graft extension. In the same series, early stent migration caused disconnection of two overlapping stents, resulting in a type III endoleak requiring a secondary intervention. Of particular interest is the lack of a type II endoleak in Tielliu et al.'s series, which in open surgical repair is believed to account for the high rate of sac reperfusion. This lack of type II endoleak may well represent diagnostic error as one aneurysm sac subsequently showed evidence of enlargement during follow up. Mohan et al. reported two type II endoleaks in their series [11].

Despite the inferior patency rates and risk of stent-related complications associated with endovascular repair, proponents argue that this is offset by the benefits gained from a minimally-invasive procedure in a population with significant co-morbidity and reduced life expectancy. In our series the 5- and 10-year patient survival rates were 81% and 64%, respectively. For the majority of patients in this series, endovascular repair would not represent a sufficiently durable procedure.

References

1. Varga ZA, Locke-Edmonds JC, Baird RN. A multicenter study of popliteal aneurysms. *Joint Vascular Research Group. J Vasc Surg* 1994; **20**: 171–7.
2. Dawson L, van Bockel JH, Brand R, Terpstra JL. Popliteal artery aneurysms. Long-term follow-up of aneurysmal disease and results of surgical treatment. *J Vasc Surg* 1991; **13**: 398–407.
3. Shortell CK, DeWeese JA, Ouriel K, Green RM. Popliteal artery aneurysms: a 25-year experience. *J Vasc Surg* 1991; **14**: 771–6.
4. Schellack J, Smith RB, Perdue GD Jr. Non-operative management of selective popliteal aneurysms. *Arch Surg* 1987; **122**: 372–5.

5. Bowyer RC, Cawthorn SJ, Walker WJ, Giddings AEB. Conservative management of asymptomatic popliteal aneurysm. *Br J Surg* 1990; **77**: 1132–5.

6. Galland RB, Magee TR. Management of popliteal aneurysm. *Br J Surg* 2002; **89**: 1382–5.

7. Davies RS, Wall M, Rai S et al. Long-term results of surgical repair of popliteal artery aneurysm *Eur J Vasc Endovasc Surg* 2007; **34**: 714–8.

8. Schwarz W, Berkowitz H, Taormina V, Gatti J. The preoperative use of intraarterialthrombolysis for a thrombosed popliteal artery aneurysm. *J Cardiovasc Surg (Torino)* 1984; **25**: 465–8.

9. Carpenter JP, Barker CF, Roberts B, Berkowitz HD, Lusk EJ, Perloff LJ. Popliteal artery aneurysms: current management and outcome. *J Vasc Surg* 1994; **19**: 65–73.

10. Tielliu IF, Verhoeven EL, Zeebregts CJ, Prins TR, Span MM, van den Dungen JJ. Endovascular treatment of popliteal artery aneurysms: results of a prospective cohort study. *J Vasc Surg* 2005; **41**: 561–7.

11. Mohan IV, Bray PJ, Harris JP et al. Endovascular popliteal aneurysm repair: are the results comparable to open surgery? *Eur J Vasc Endovasc Surg* 2006; **32**: 149–54.

12. Antonello M, Frigatti P, Battocchio P et al. Open repair versus endovascular treatment for asymptomatic popliteal artery aneurysm: results of a prospective randomised study. *J Vasc Surg* 2005; **42**: 185–93.

Final FRCS vascular topics

Femoral artery aneurysms

Robert Davies, Asif Mahmood and Rajiv Vohra

Key points

- Lower limb arterial aneurysms rarely occur in isolation
- The majority present either as an incidental finding or as lower limb ischaemia
- Aneurysm rupture is rare, but life- and limb-threatening when it occurs
- All symptomatic femoral artery aneurysms should undergo repair
- Asymptomatic femoral artery aneurysms >2.5 cm in maximum diameter should be considered for elective repair

True femoral aneurysms

Incidence

Femoral artery aneurysm (FAA) is the second most common peripheral artery aneurysm after popliteal artery aneurysms. They most often occur in male patients over 65 years with an age-adjusted incidence of combined femoral and popliteal artery aneurysms of 7.39 per 100 000 population in the USA; male-to-female ratio of 10:1 [1]. Patients with FAAs demonstrate a high incidence of cardiovascular disease and associated risk factors, including hypertension, smoking and hypercholesterolaemia. Diabetes mellitus appears to be protective for femoral artery aneurysm. Although FAAs predominantly occur in association with atherosclerotic disease, there are reports available in the English literature suggesting an association with vasculitides and connective tissue disorders.

FAAs rarely occur in isolation and are frequently associated with a contralateral aneurysm or/and aneurysmal disease affecting the aorta or other peripheral arteries. In a cohort of 100 patients with FAAs Graham et al. reported 72% were bilateral, 85% were associated with aorto-iliac aneurysms and 44% were associated with popliteal artery aneurysms [2]. Alternatively, the incidence of FAAs in patients with abdominal aortic aneurysms is ≈5%.

Pathophysiology

The pathophysiological conditions predisposing to the development of FAAs are poorly understood. It has been postulated that, in conjunction with weakening of the arterial wall by atherosclerosis, turbulent flow plays an important part. Constriction at the level of inguinal ligament may promote the development of poststenotic dilatation with resultant turbulent flow and pressure fluctuations affecting the common femoral artery. This localised change in

Postgraduate Vascular Surgery: The Candidate's Guide to the FRCS, eds. Vish Bhattacharya and Gerard Stansby. Published by Cambridge University Press. © Cambridge University Press 2010.

flow dynamics causes the arterial segment to vibrate, clinically evident as a bruit, weakening the arterial wall predisposing it to aneurysmal change [2, 3]. This would be consistent with the clinical finding that femoral artery aneurysms classically affect the common femoral artery (CFA) in isolation without extending proximal to the inguinal ligament.

Symptoms and signs

Of patients with FAAs 30–40% are asymptomatic at the time of diagnosis with an incidental finding of a smooth, fusiform and pulsatile mass. However, the majority of patients with FAAs present with localised symptomatology or lower limb claudication/rest pain. In 20% of patients localised pain in the groin or anterior thigh is the sole symptom.

Slowly enlarging FAAs may cause chronic compression of the adjacent neurovascular structures. Up to 10% of patients demonstrate changes attributable to lower limb chronic venous hypertension secondary to chronic femoral vein compression. However, chronic dysthesia or paraesthesia, resulting from femoral nerve compression, is uncommon unless associated with spontaneous FAA rupture.

Femoral artery aneurysms may be complicated by acute or chronic thromboembolism or rupture in as many as 50% of cases at the time of initial presentation. The incidence of FAA thrombosis varies in the literature although the incidence of chronic and acute thrombosis appears to be similar. Acute thrombosis complicates up to 16% of femoral artery aneurysms at the time of presentation. Patients present with an acutely ischaemic lower limb (Rutherford classification IIb or III), clinically mimicking a femoral artery embolus. Inflow into both the superficial femoral artery and profunda femoris artery is disrupted, thereby dramatically reducing any potential source of collateral flow. Chronic thrombosis may mimic peripheral occlusive disease in presentation, particularly as a high number of patients have concomitant atherosclerotic cardiovascular disease.

Symptomatic distal embolisation is less common with a reported incidence of 2–8% [1, 2]. This may not reflect the true incidence as a large proportion of distal emboli are clinically silent. The majority of reports cite femoral artery aneurysm rupture as occurring less frequently than thrombosis or distal embolisation with an incidence of <15%. This may partly reflect the 'protective' nature of the tough femoral sheath [2].

Classification

Femoral artery aneurysms can be classified into type I and II according to the involvement of the superficial femoral artery (SFA) and profunda femoris artery (PFA). Type I involves the CFA in isolation, type II involves the CFA and one or both of the SFA and PFA.

Investigation

Only 20% of femoral artery aneurysms are reliably identified on clinical examination alone. Those measuring < 2 cm are particularly unlikely to be identified by routine physical examination. A high index of suspicion is required depending on the circumstances in which the patient presents. All patients with abdominal aortic aneurysms or peripheral artery aneurysms should undergo formalised imaging assessment of their lower limb vasculature. Conversely, all patients with femoral artery aneurysms should undergo formalised assessment of their abdominal aorta and popliteal arteries.

Modern Duplex ultrasonography (DUS) is an adequate screening tool in both emergency and elective settings. High quality images can be obtained of the aneurysm sac size, thrombus content and morphology, while other vascular beds can be screened for aneurysmal or occlusive disease.

Upon confirmation of the diagnosis a suitable imaging modality is required to accurately quantify the extent of thromboembolic disease locally and distally as well as any concomitant aneurysmal disease identified by DUS. This should be dictated by the patients' clinical picture. In those patients suitable for elective investigation percutaneous angiography remains the gold standard. Computed tomography and magnetic resonance angiography are providing an increasingly accurate crural vessel assessment and thus are an alternative to percutaneous angiography, particularly in those in whom aorto-iliac disease is suspected. In the patient with an acutely ischaemic limb, lengthy preoperative investigation should not prevent a limb-saving operation from being performed expeditiously. In these situations the use of on table angiography is the key.

Management

It is generally accepted that all medically fit patients with symptomatic aneurysms or aneurysms complicated with thromboembolism or rupture should be offered primary surgical repair. Aneurysms that are enlarging on serial imaging should also be considered for elective surgical repair.

The treatment of asymptomatic aneurysms remains controversial. Conflicting evidence regarding the safety of conservative management exists in the literature. Proponents of a conservative management strategy cite the lack of evidence between aneurysm size and the development of ischaemic complications. Furthermore, the risk of developing limb-threatening complications in an asymptomatic aneurysm with conservative treatment at 2-year follow up is less than 5% [2]. Most vascular surgeons would consider a femoral aneurysm measuring >2.5 cm, or enlarging on serial imaging, for elective repair.

Surgical approach

The majority of type I femoral aneurysms are best repaired with a straight interposition graft anastomosed proximally at the external iliac-common femoral artery junction and distally to the common femoral artery bifurcation. This is performed from within the aneurysm with the redundant sac plicated over the graft. The conduit utilised is dependent on individual surgeon preference, but unless there is a suspicion of infection, autologous conduit offers no benefit over prosthetic. A variety of configurations have been utilised for type II femoral aneurysms, often based around the concept of an interposition graft extending distally into either the SFA or PFA with re-implantation of the remaining artery, with or without an interposition graft.

Often femoral aneurysms occur in conjunction with aorto-iliac and popliteal aneurysmal or occlusive disease. In these situations the type of repair needs to be tailored to the anatomy of the presenting pathology. In particular the most pressing disease needs to be dealt with first whilst simultaneously planning for any second- or third-stage procedures.

Outcome

Perioperative mortality rates following femoral artery aneurysm repair are low although rise to 5% when undertaken concomitantly with other aneurysm repairs [2]. Five-year patency rates in asymptomatic patients approaches 90%. Patients presenting with lower limb claudication or rest pain/gangrene have worse patency rates at 5 years [2].

Profunda femoris artery aneurysms

Isolated profunda femoris artery aneurysms (PFAas) are rare and account for < 3% of femoral aneurysms. Three-quarters of patients have aneurysmal disease affecting one other vascular bed, most often the popliteal artery [4]. Due to the difficulty in identifying isolated profunda femoris aneurysms at clinical examination, spontaneous rupture rates are higher than for other peripheral aneurysms, with up to 50% of patients presenting with rupture. Diagnosis is predominantly by DUS and formal assessment of the aorta-iliac and popliteal arteries is recommended to identify concomitant aneurysms.

There is no current evidence regarding the optimal size at which PFAas should be repaired, however many surgeons recommend considering repair for those >2 cm in an otherwise fit patient. Those medically unfit for repair should be evaluated regularly with DUS to assess for aneurysm expansion.

The primary aim of treatment is to prevent rupture. However one series reports ipsilateral SFA occlusion in 45% of cases, therefore maintaining PFA blood flow is important [4]. Vessel reconstruction with an interposition graft or aneurysm ligation and autologous bypass is recommended.

Femoral artery pseudoaneurysms

Pathophysiology

Femoral artery pseudoaneurysms (FApAs) develop as a result of high pressure blood flow through an arterial wall defect that becomes constrained by the perivascular soft tissue or surrounding haematoma. Unlike a true aneurysm, the wall consists of thin fibrous tissue and not all three tunica layers.

Iatrogenic, postcatheterisation pseudoaneurysm formation is the commonest cause (Table 9.1) with a reported incidence of 1–6% in prospective sonographic studies [5, 6]. Infection, particularly in the drug abuser population, and anastomotic leakage may lead to FApA formation. At a median follow up of 8 years, 2.5% of all femoral anastamoses and 8% of aortobifemoral bypasses are complicated by FApA formation [7, 8].

Symptoms and signs

FApAs may present as a pulsatile groin mass that may or may not be painful. Enlargement may cause compression of the adjacent femoral nerve or vein with resultant paraesthesia/dysthesia or symptoms/signs of venous hypertension, respectively. Mycotic aneurysms present as a painful, erythematous groin mass with or without purulent/sanguinous discharge.

Investigation

Duplex ultrasonography is the initial investigation of choice with a reported sensitivity and specificity of >90%. Computed tomography angiography may be utilised as an adjunct to ultrasound scan (USS), particularly in the assessment of patients with anastomotic pseudoanuerysms, in whom complex reconstructive surgery may be required.

Treatment

Most small postcatheterisation pseudoaneurysms have an indolent clinical course with the majority undergoing spontaneous thrombosis. Pseudoaneurysm size and anticoagulation

Table 9.1 Factors predisposing to postcatheterisation pseudoaneurysm formation

- Anticoagulation
- Hypertension
- Haemodialysis
- Obesity
- Sheath size >7 French
- Cannulation of superior femoral/profunda femoris artery
- Simultaneous puncture of artery and vein
- Heavily calcified arteries
- Short vessel compression time postcatheterisation

Toursarkissian B, Allen BT, Petrinec D, Thompson RW, Rubin BG, Reilly JM, Anderson CB, Flye MW, Sicard GA. Spontaneous closure of selected iatrogenic pseudoaneurysms and arteriovenous fistulae *J Vasc Surg* 1997; **25**: 803–8.

status of the patient are the two most important predictors of spontaneous thrombosis. Toursarkissan et al. reported 87% of FApAs <3 cm having undergone spontaneous thrombosis at a mean follow up of 23 days[9]. Thus it is acceptable to initially treat a small pseudoaneurysm (<3 cm) conservatively with serial DUS evaluation. However the economic burden of such an approach can be prohibitive and many institutions advocate active treatment of all FApAs, irrespective of size.

The advent of minimally invasive percutaneous treatment methods has limited the indications for open surgical repair to those FApAs that are either rapidly expanding, infected, causing neurovascular compression, causing skin necrosis or have undergone failed percutaneous treatment. The presence or absence of infection dictates surgical technique. For mycotic pseudoaneurysms surgery is aimed at excising infected tissue whilst endeavouring to preserve the distal circulation. This may require the use of autologous arterial bypasses routed outside the field of infection. In cases of gross suppurative infection primary ligation of the femoral vessels may become necessary with a 30% risk of subsequent amputation. Non-infected pseudoaneurysms are repaired primarily with interrupted non-absorbable sutures or with a vein patch-angioplasty, depending on the size of the arterial defect.

In recent years minimally invasive methods of treating FApAs, and particularly postcatheterisation FApAs, have been trialled. Ultrasound guided compression was the first to gain widespread acceptance with success rates between 63 and 100% [10]. Patients receiving anticoagulation with pseudoaneurysm sizes >3 cm are predictors of the failure of ultrasound-guided compression. Complications including rupture, femoral vein thrombosis and acute limb ischaemia have been reported in 2–4% of patients [10]. Ultrasound guided percutaneous thrombin injection into the pseudoanuerysm sac is now in widespread usage with reported success rates of >90%. This may be performed in combination with an intra-arterial balloon protection device to prevent spillage of thrombin into the native vessels, particularly in pseudoaneurysms with side necks. Complications including distal embolisation and anaphylaxis are reported in <4% of cases.

References

1. Lawrence PF, Lorenzo-Rivero S, Lyon JL. The incidence of iliac, femoral, and popliteal artery aneurysms in hospitalized patients. *J Vasc Surg* 1995; **22**: 409–15.

2. Graham LM, Zelenock GB, Whitehouse WM Jr et al. Clinical significance of arteriosclerotic femoral artery aneurysms. *Arch Surg* 1980; **115**: 502–7.

3. Gow BS, Legg MJ, Yu W, Kukongviriyapan U, Lee LL. Does vibration cause poststenotic dilatation in vivo and influence atherogenesis in cholesterol-fed rabbits? *J Biomech Eng* 1992; **114**: 20–5.

4. Harbuzariu C, Duncan AA, Bower TC, Kalra M, Gloviczki P. Profunda femoris artery aneurysms: association with aneurysmal disease and limb ischemia. *J Vasc Surg* 2008; **47**: 31–4.

5. Katzenschlager R, Ugurluoglu A, Ahmadi A. Incidence of pseudoaneurysm after diagnostic and therapeutic angiography. *Radiology* 1995; **195**: 463–6.

6. Lumsden AB, Miller JM, Kosinski AS. A prospective evaluation of surgically treated groin complications following percutaneous cardiac procedures. *Am Surg* 1994; **60**: 132–7.

7. Marković DM, Davidović LB, Kostić DM et al. False anastomotic aneurysms. *Vascular* 2007; **15**: 141–8.

8. Biancari F, Ylönen K, Anttila V et al. Durability of open repair of infrarenal abdominal aortic aneurysm: a 15-year follow-up study. *J Vasc Surg* 2002; **35**: 87–93.

9. Toursarkissian B, Allen BT, Petrinec D etal. Spontaneous closure of selected iatrogenic pseudoaneurysms and arteriovenous fistulae *J Vasc Surg* 1997; **25**: 803–8.

10. Morgan R, Belli AM. Current treatment methods for postcatheterization pseudoaneurysms. *J Vasc Interv Radiol* 2003; **14**: 697–710.

Carotid, subclavian and vertebral disease

A. Ross Naylor

Key points

- The extracranial arteries are prone to involvement with a number of important atherosclerotic and non-atherosclerotic conditions
- The provision of best medical therapy should not be delegated to the most junior member of the team. It is an essential component of care
- Patients with symptomatic carotid disease benefit from very rapid intervention. Investigative strategies and rapid access to the operating theatre should be geared to ensuring all patients are treated within 2 weeks of suffering their index symptom
- Relatively few patients with asymptomatic carotid disease benefit from intervention (especially females and patients aged >75 years). It is essential that trials identify high-risk subgroups
- The role of several technical aspects of carotid surgery has been guided by large randomised trials
- Patients with symptomatic vertebral stenoses may have a much worse prognosis than was previously thought

Radiation arteritis

Demographics

Despite the widespread use of radiotherapy in the treatment of head and neck cancers, there is still insufficient data regarding the incidence of symptomatic radiation arteritis.

Pathology

- Acute phase: fibrin deposition/endothelial swelling followed by intimal necrosis.
- Subacute phase: endothelial regeneration with destruction of the internal elastic lamina. Inflammatory cell infiltration of the media and adventitia.
- Chronic phase: intima becomes thickened with a tendency towards accelerated atherosclerosis. The media and adventitia become progressively fibrotic.

Clinical features

False aneurysm or vessel rupture (acute/subacute phase), stroke due to carotid/vertebral thrombosis, or upper limb ischaemia following subclavian thrombosis (sub-acute phase). In

Postgraduate Vascular Surgery: The Candidate's Guide to the FRCS, eds. Vish Bhattacharya and Gerard Stansby. Published by Cambridge University Press. © Cambridge University Press 2010.

the chronic phase (where radiation arteritis co-exists with atherosclerosis) thromboembolic stroke/transient ischaemic attack (TIA) or upper limb claudication (subclavian stenosis/occlusion) can occur.

Investigation

First line is Duplex ultrasound. Computed tomography angiography (CTA) or magnetic resonance imaging (MRI)/contrast enhanced magnetic resonance angiography (CEMRA) should also be performed in order to evaluate the full extent of the arteritic process (proximally and distally) and to evaluate the status of the circle of Willis and to exclude recurrent malignant disease.

Management

Management decisions must take account of (1) the overall health status of the patient and (2) whether there is ongoing malignant disease, acute/chronic nature of arteritic process, age of patient, mode of presentation, presence of tracheostomy, likelihood of cranial nerve injury, likelihood of compromising skin flaps, ongoing embolisation using transcranial Doppler (TCD).

In general, asymptomatic stenoses should probably be treated conservatively, unless there is a non-functioning circle of Willis. Symptomatic lesions should be considered for intervention (autologous reconstruction/carotid stenting). Stenting is currently the preferred option (especially in patients with a tracheostomy), although surgery may be safer in patients with crescendo symptoms and evidence of spontaneous embolisation on TCD.

Prognosis

Little quality data are available regarding the prognosis in untreated patients.

Fibromuscular dysplasia [1]

Demographics

Fibromuscular dysplasia (FMD) is found in 0.5% of patients undergoing angiography for symptomatic cerebral vascular disease, while 10% of patients suffering a carotid dissection will have FMD in the contralateral internal carotid artery (ICA). Fibromuscular dysplasia is bilateral in up to 60% of patients, 25% of patients with carotid involvement will have renal artery FMD. One quarter of FMD cases involve the vertebral arteries, while up to 50% of patients with carotid/vertebral FMD will also have an intracranial aneurysm.

Pathology

Fibromuscular dysplasia is a non-inflammatory, non-atheromatous segmental disorder. There are three main subtypes based upon involvement of media, intima or adventitia. Intimal fibroplasia (<10% of FMD cases) causes band-like narrowing or long smooth stenoses and carries a poorer prognosis. Medial dysplasia (90% of FMD cases) causes a beading appearance and is subdivided into medial fibroplasia (75–85%), perimedial fibroplasia (<10%) and medial hyperplasia (<5%). Adventitial fibroplasia is seen in <1% of cases and is characterised by dense collagen formation.

Clinical features

There are a wide spectrum of features, ranging from being asymptomatic (the majority) to subarachnoid haemorrhage, embolic TIA/stroke, neurovascular hypertension or features suggestive of carotid dissection (see later).

Investigation

Duplex remains the first-line investigation, but it cannot image the distal ICA/vertebral arteries. If there is any clinical or Duplex suspicion of FMD, CTA/CEMRA should be performed (preferably including the renal vasculature). The intracranial circulation should also be imaged to exclude an aneurysm.

Management

There is no Level I, Grade A evidence to guide practice. Asymptomatic patients should probably be treated conservatively and be subject to serial surveillance. Carotid/vertebral angioplasty is now the first-line treatment for patients with symptomatic FMD, with stenting being reserved for patients with either a poor technical result or secondary dissection.

Prognosis

Multi-focal intimal fibroplasia carries the worst prognosis; medial dysplasia carries a reasonably good prognosis. It is important, however, to remember that more than one vascular bed can be affected with FMD and do not ignore the possibility of there being an intracranial aneurysm.

Carotid artery dissection

Demographics

Carotid dissection (CD) causes relatively few strokes, but traumatic CD complicates about 1% of all head injuries and about 25% of trauma patients with an unexplained focal neurological deficit will have a dissection.

Pathology

Carotid dissection occurs spontaneously (Marfan's/FMD), it can follow iatrogenic injury (cannulation, angioplasty) or follow trauma (forced lateral rotation and hyper-extension, which causes the ICA to be crushed between the skull base and the transverse process of C2). The plane of dissection usually starts 2–3 cm beyond the origin of the ICA, but then extends over a variable distance towards the skull base. Type 1 lesions cause a minor intimal irregularity or stenosis <50%. Type 2 lesions are either associated with false aneurysm formation or a stenosis >50%. In type 3 lesions, the dissection can cause complete vessel occlusion through compression of the true lumen by a thrombosed false lumen.

Clinical features

Ipsilateral headache and/or neck pain occur in 80% of patients. Ocular signs and symptoms are present in about 60% (miosis, painful Horner's syndrome, hemianopia, ischaemic optic neuropathy) along with III, IV or VI nerve palsies. Stroke and TIA may also complicate a dissection (thrombosis or distal embolisation from the false lumen).

Investigation

Awareness of the potential diagnosis is integral to instituting effective treatment. Duplex is generally limited by its inability to image the upper reaches of the carotid and vertebral arteries. Here CTA or CEMRA is the investigation of choice and is also useful for serial surveillance of small false aneurysms.

Management

There is little Level I, Grade A evidence. Traditionally, the majority of patients with CD have been managed conservatively with bed rest and anticoagulation (heparin followed by warfarin). Evidence suggests that a significant proportion will recanalise and clinically improve. A few symptomatic patients have undergone attempts at surgical revascularisation, but this has now been replaced by endovascular technology (covered stents, etc.), which also lessens the likelihood of cranial nerve injury.

Prognosis

Stroke following undiagnosed CD carries a high risk of morbidity and mortality. The key to minimising stroke risk is early awareness and rapid institution of anticoagulation.

Giant cell arteritis (GCA) [2]

Demographics

This is the most common vasculitis in the Western world and seen predominantly in women aged >50 years (mean age of presentation is 75). Over one-third of GCA patients will have polymyalgia rheumatica at the time of diagnosis. Giant cell arteritis predominantly affects large (thoracic aorta) and medium-sized vessels (extracranial carotid branches, subclavian, axillary and vertebral).

Pathology

An infiltrate of lymphocytes and macrophages involving the entire vessel wall is typically seen. The characteristic feature is fragmentation of the internal elastic lamnia. Giant cells are often present.

Clinical features

Three syndromes may co-exist:

1. Systemic inflammatory syndrome: non-specific constitutional symptoms including arthralgias, myalgias, anorexia, weight loss and night sweats.
2. Cranial arteritis: localised vasculitis of the carotid and vertebral arteries causing headache/facial pain, scalp tenderness, jaw claudication, hoarseness and visual loss.
3. Large vessel vasculitis: symptoms secondary to stenotic/occlusive disease of the subclavian and axillary arteries (arm claudication, Raynaud's phenomenon).

Giant cell arteritis involvement of the thoracic aorta predisposes to aneurysm formation. Cerebrovascular events (stroke/TIA) occur in 3–4% of GCA patients and follow inflammatory occlusion of the vertebral/carotid arteries. Episodes of transient visual loss precede permanent visual loss in 50% of untreated patients within 7 days and are usually due to inflammatory occlusion of the short posterior ciliary arteries, causing ischaemia of the optic disc and choroids.

Investigations

Temporal artery biopsy should be performed as soon as possible (it will be negative in 50% of patients with large vessel vasculitis). Duplex ultrasound will identify stenoses/occlusions, but CEMRA or CTA is preferred in order to evaluate aortic arch and major branch vessels (looking for bilateral patterns of disease, thoracic aneurysm) as well as excluding intracranial vasculitis. Laboratory investigations should include erythrocyte sedimentation rate (ESR) (85% of GCA patients will have an ESR >50 mm h^{-1}), C-reactive protein (CRP) (98% sensitivity for active GCA), thrombocytosis (present in 48% of biopsy-positive patients) and normocytic normochromic anaemia.

Management

High-dose steroid therapy (intravenous or oral), which is then gradually reduced over 6–12 months with titration against CRP and other inflammatory markers.

Prognosis

Visual loss persisting for >24 hours tends to be permanent. High dose steroid therapy is then aimed at preventing visual loss in the other eye. Patients with thoracic aneurysm require serial monitoring.

Takayasu arteritis (TA) [3]

Demographics

Pan-arteritis of unknown aetiology occurs, affecting the aorta and its main branches and seen predominantly in young females, especially from the Orient. Overall incidence is about 2.6 cases per million per year.

Pathology

The inflammatory process starts with inflammatory infiltration (lymphocytes and occasional giant cells) around the vasa vasorum, extending transmurally. If disease progression is rapid, aneurysm formation becomes more likely. In the later stages of the condition, there is progressive fibrosis, leading to occlusion (hence the term 'pulseless' disease). The common carotid arteries are involved in 65–75% of cases, the subclavian arteries in 50–75%, while the vertebral arteries are involved in 6–10%.

Clinical features

The American College of Rheumatology has determined that a diagnosis of TA requires at least three of the following six criteria to be met: (1) age at onset <40 years; (2) claudication of extremities; (3) decreased brachial artery pulse; (4) blood pressure difference >10 mmHg between arms; (5) bruit over subclavian arteries or aorta; and (6) arteriogram abnormality.

Given the large number of arteries that can be subject to aneurysm formation, stenosis or occlusion, the mode of presentation will vary considerably. In the early stage most complain of constitutional symptoms (fatigue, malaise etc.). In the second stage, symptoms are related to the increasing inflammatory reaction: (1) systemic inflammatory response (fatigue, fevers, extremity pain, headache, rashes); (2) vascular insufficiency (claudication, arm numbness, TIA/stroke/amaurosis fugax); or a combination of (1) and (2). In the final 'burned out' stage of the disease, the inflammatory reaction is replaced with transmural fibrosis.

Investigations

Laboratory investigations (ESR, thrombocytosis, anaemia) show whether there is an underlying inflammatory reaction and also monitor the effect of treatment. Conventional angiography has been replaced with CTA and CEMRA for evaluating the anatomical extent of the inflammatory process. These imaging modalities also permit evaluation of aortic aneurysm formation and measurement of arterial wall thickness and extent of oedema, which can also be used for monitoring the effect of treatment.

Management

High-dose steroid therapy (intravenous then oral) is used, which is reduced over 6–12 months with titration against CRP and other inflammatory markers. If it proves difficult to reduce the steroid dose or adverse side effects occur, methotrexate, cyclophosphamide and azathioprine are alternative immunosuppressive agents. Patients with renovascular hypertension require aggressive treatment and patients should receive antiplatelet therapy unless contraindicated. There is relatively limited experience with angioplasty or stenting in TA. Surgical revascularisation of the carotid, subclavian and vertebral arteries is also rarely required. If revascularisation becomes necessary, try to avoid this in the acute phase of the condition. It is also important to perform an inflow from the aorta rather than the subclavian artery.

Prognosis

Provided medical treatment is initiated early, approximately 90% of patients will survive 5 years.

True and false aneurysms

Incidence

Aneurysms of the carotid, vertebral and subclavian arteries comprise <2% of all arterial aneurysms.

Pathology

The prevalence of true or false aneurysms will reflect differing patient populations. South African studies tend to describe aneurysms in predominantly young men with infection (HIV, tuberculosis). In metropolitan areas, many will be secondary to trauma (gunshot, knife), while in studies reporting outcomes from urban populations, the majority of true aneurysms are classed as 'atherosclerotic'. While the commonest cause of a false aneurysm is prosthetic patch infection after carotid endarterectomy.

Clinical features

The commonest clinical feature is a pulsatile neck mass, followed by detection of a cervical bruit. Aneurysm rupture is extremely rare. By contrast, TIA/stroke is a relatively common presentation (presumably secondary to thromboembolism), as are cranial nerve signs/symptoms due to direct compression. Patients with false aneurysms will present with related symptoms and signs (e.g. history of recent trauma, evidence of prosthetic patch infection).

Investigation

The majority presenting with pulsatile neck 'masses' will have coiling/ectasia of the common carotid or innominate arteries. Accordingly, the first-line investigation is Duplex ultrasound. Thereafter, investigations are directed towards determining the likely underlying cause (FMD, trauma, etc.) as management strategies will vary. Second-line investigations include CTA or CEMRA, which can rapidly image other arteries (e.g. renal arteries in suspected FMD). They will also provide information regarding the feasibility of endovascular treatment.

Management

Management will depend upon the underlying aetiology, urgency of symptoms and the level/distal extent of the aneurysm. Operative strategies include: (1) proximal/distal ligation; (2) open reconstruction (venous bypass, partial aneurysm excision, patch angioplasty, prosthetic bypass, resection and end-to end-bypass); and (3) endovascular repair (stent graft exclusions, carotid stenting augmented with coil exclusions, endovascular balloon occlusion). In the carotid and vertebral circulations, ligation should only be considered if reconstructive options have been excluded. Inflation of an endovascular balloon within the artery under local anaesthesia may assist in determining whether ligation will be tolerated.

Prognosis

Most patients with carotid (vertebral) aneurysms will become symptomatic with time. Surgery, however, carries the risk of procedural stroke and cranial nerve injury in 5–7% of patients. Management decisions must therefore balance the risks and benefits associated with intervention, which may mean adopting a more conservative strategy in selected asymptomatic patients with small distal ICA aneurysms.

Carotid body tumour [4]

Demographics

The carotid body is a collection of chemoreceptor cells responsible for detecting changes in blood oxygen/carbon dioxide levels and pH, and is located within the adventitia of the carotid bifurcation. Carotid body tumours (CBTs) may be sporadic or familial. Familial CBTs (10% of all CBTs) are more common in females and are more likely to be bilateral. Carotid body tumours represent <1% of all neck tumours.

Pathology

Carotid body tumours are highly vascular tumours derived from the neural crest ectoderm and are the commonest type of cervical paraganglionoma (glomus vagale, glomus jugulare, glomus tympanicum). Most present in the fourth/fifth decades and cause characteristic splaying of the bifurcation. By contrast, glomus vagale tumours (second commonest) cause splaying of the ICA and ECA above a normal bifurcation. Approximately 5% of CBTs are bilateral, 5% will be locally malignant and 5% systemically malignant.

Clinical features

Asymptomatic neck swelling is the most common feature. Larger lesions cause pain, cranial nerve palsies (XII, IX, X) and rarely a Horner's syndrome. Stroke and TIA are unusual, while some will present with a neuroendocrine-mediated syndrome with flushing, dizziness, arrhythmias and hypertension.

Investigations

Consider CBT in all patients with lateral neck swellings and definitely before any decision is made to undertake an open biopsy. Duplex ultrasound will show the characteristic blush of hypervascularity within a splayed carotid bifurcation. Cross-sectional imaging will provide information regarding the upper and lower limits of the lesion, which is useful in planning resection strategies (i.e. do you need to plan for a high approach to the carotid artery). Computed tomography and MRI are also useful in excluding bilateral lesions. Radionuclide imaging and conventional angiography are not routinely necessary.

Management

Resection is the main treatment strategy and is typically described as being performed in a subadventitial plane. A conservative approach is indicated in elderly patients with small lesions. Occasionally, it may be preferable to resect the tumour and carotid bifurcation (adherent tumour, carotid injury, suspicion of malignancy) and perform an interposition bypass. Perioperative bleeding may be reduced by preoperative embolisation of ECA feeding vessels or insertion of a covered stent within the first few centimetres of the ECA. This strategy is probably only necessary in large lesions.

Prognosis

Resection carries a 1% mortality rate and a 2–3% risk of stroke. Cranial nerve injuries are not uncommon, but tend to be transient. Provided a macroscopically complete excision has been performed, the risk of recurrence is <5%.

Carotid occlusive disease

Demographics

Stroke (responsible for 12% of UK deaths) is defined as a focal (occasionally global) loss of cerebral function, which lasts for >24 hours and has a vascular cause. A TIA carries a timescale of <24 hours. The incidence of first-ever stroke is 2.4/1000, but increases with age. The annual incidence of TIA is 0.5/1000.

Pathology

Approximately 80% of all strokes are ischaemic (20% are haemorrhagic), while approximately 80% of ischaemic strokes affect the carotid territory. The main causes of carotid territory ischaemic stroke include thromboembolism of the ICA and/or middle cerebral artery (50%), small vessel occlusion of the deep penetrating end-arteries (25%), cardiogenic embolism (15%), haematological disorders (myeloma, polycythaemia, thrombocytosis) in 5%, whilst 5% have a miscellany of causes (tumour, arteritis, oral contraceptive, etc.). Risk factors for stroke include hypertension, ischaemic heart disease, smoking, hyperlipidaemia, TIA, diabetes and hyperfibrinogenaemia. The commonest single cause of ischaemic, carotid territory stroke is thromboembolism from an atherosclerotic plaque at the origin of the ICA. The carotid bifurcation is prone to atherosclerosis, particularly on the outer aspect of the bulb. Some of these plaques then undergo an acute change (plaque rupture, intraplaque haemorrhage), which predisposes towards overlying thrombus formation and embolisation to the brain.

Clinical features

Asymptomatic disease

Of the population 10% will have an asymptomatic >50% ICA stenosis, but only 1% will have a stenosis >70%. Asymptomatic stenoses are usually detected by auscultation of a bruit, with the patient complaining of pulsatile tinnitus or by ultrasound. However, the term 'asymptomatic' may be misleading as many patients do not consider a transient episode of hand paraesthesia or weakness to be important and it could go unreported. Similarly, because 33% of our lives are spent sleeping, nocturnal TIAs will go unreported. Approximately 25% of asymptomatic patients will have ischaemic brain injury on CT/MRI.

Symptomatic disease

'Classical' carotid territory symptoms include: hemisensory/motor signs; higher cortical dysfunction (dysphasia, visuospatial neglect); and monocular blindness. There has previously been a tendency to ascribe a diagnosis of 'non-hemispheric' symptoms to patients with blackouts, isolated diplopia, isolated vertigo, isolated dizziness, presyncope and syncope. In practice, these should never be considered to be carotid (or vertebrobasilar in origin) unless they coexist with more typical symptoms.

Investigations

Baseline investigations include biochemistry, lipids, glucose, full blood count, plasma viscosity, chest X-ray and electrocardiogram (ECG). More specialised investigations (thrombophilia screening, autoantibodies, homocysteine levels, echocardiography and 24-hour tapes) should be reserved for selected cases.

Routine catheter angiography (previously the gold standard) is not now indicated (radiation, 1–2% stroke risk), having been replaced by non-invasive alternatives. Table 10.1 summarises the sensitivity and specificity for Duplex, CTA (excluding multislice CT), MRA and CEMRA from a recent systematic review [5]. Overall, CEMRA emerged as the best investigation, but it remains limited by accessibility and the potential for gadolinium-induced nephrogenic systemic fibrosis. In practice, each imaging modality has an important role because investigations in patients being worked up for carotid endarterectomy (CEA) are different to those should the patient be considered for carotid artery stenting (CAS).

Table 10.1 Results of a meta-analysis of the accuracy of non-invasive imaging for all stenosis groups and imaging modalities

Stenosis group (%)	Imaging	Sensitivity	Specificity (%)
70–99	US	89	84
	CTA	77	95
	MRA	88	84
	CEMRA	94	93
50–69	US	36	91
	CTA	67	79
	MRA	37	91
	CEMRA	77	97
0–49, 100	US	83	84
	CTA	81	91
	MRA	81	88
	CEMRA	96	96

US, ultrasound; CTA, computed tomography angiography; MRA, magnetic resonance angiography; CEMRA, contrast enhanced magnetic resonance angiography.
Wardlaw JM, Chappell FM, Stevenson M et al. Accurate, practical and cost-effective assessment of carotid stenosis in the UK. *Health Technol Assess* 2006; **10**: no. 30. Department of Health Crown copyright material is reproduced with the permission of the Controller of the HMSO and Queen's Printers for Scotland. Document available at: http://www.hta.ac.uk/fullmono/mon1030.pdf. Reproduced with permission.

Duplex remains the first-line investigation. In centres with internal validation, it is acceptable for surgery to be performed on the basis of ultrasound provided the first scan has been corroborated by a second (using a different technologist). In other hospitals, Duplex findings are corroborated with either CTA or MRA, especially if there is any question of inflow/outflow disease or excessive calcification. The most important advantage of CEMRA and CTA is that it can simultaneously image the arch, great vessel origins, distal ICA and intracranial circulation (a prerequisite for CAS). The main disadvantage of CEMRA and CTA is that neither are as accessible as Duplex. Unless hospitals are prepared to provide more 'single visit' facilities for CT and MRI, Duplex will remain the first-line investigation.

Management

Table 10.2 summarises what is currently considered to be 'optimal medical therapy' in patients presenting with symptomatic and asymptomatic carotid disease [6]. In addition to risk factor control and initiating medical therapy, selected patients will benefit from a more invasive intervention (CEA or CAS).

Symptomatic carotid disease

Table 10.3 summarises the 5-year findings from the Carotid Endarterectomy Trialists Collaboration (CETC) who combined data from the European Carotid Surgery Trial (ECST), North American Symptomatic Carotid Endarterectomy Trial (NASCET) and Veterans Adminstration (VA) trials (>6000 patients), having remeasured the pre-randomisation

Table 10.2 European Stroke Initiative recommendations for what constitutes 'best medical therapy' in patients with asymptomatic and symptomatic carotid disease [6]

	Level of evidence	
Treatment	Asymptomatic	Symptomatic
BP<140/90 mmHg or <130/80 mmHg in diabetics	I	I
Glycaemic control to prevent other diabetic complications	III	III
Statin therapy	I	I
Stop smoking	II	II
Avoid heavy consumption of alcohol	I	I
Regular physical activity	II	II
Low salt, low saturated fat, high fruit and vegetable diet rich in fibre	II	II
If BMI elevated, reduce weight	II	II
HRT should not be used for stroke prevention in women	I	I
Aspirin	To prevent MI level IV	I
Aspirin and dipyridamole	Not recommended Level IV	I
Clopidogrel	Not recommended Level IV	I

BMI, body mass index; HRT, hormone replacement therapy; MI, myocardial infarction.

Table 10.3 Effect of delay to surgery on overall benefit conferred by carotid endarterectomy

Stenosis group	Delay (weeks)	ARR (%)	NNT	Strokes prevented per 1000 CEAs at 5 years
50–69	<2	14.8	7	148
	2–4	3.3	30	33
	4–12	4.0	25	40
	>12	−2.9	Nil	Nil
70–99	<2	30.2	3	302
	2–4	17.6	6	176
	4–12	11.4	9	114
	>12	8.9	11	89

Data recalculated from the Carotid Enarterectomy Trialists Collaboration (CETC) [8] and excludes patients with 'near occlusion'. ARR, absolute risk reduction in 5-year risk of ipsilateral stroke conferred by carotid endarterectomy (CEA) over best medical therapy. NNT, number needed to treat to prevent 1 ipsilateral stroke at 5 years. Strokes prevented is the number of ipsilateral strokes prevented at 5 years by performing 1000 CEAs.

angiograms using the NASCET method [7]. Carotid endarterectomy conferred no benefit in symptomatic patients with 0–50% stenoses. A small, but significant benefit was seen in patients with 50–69% stenoses, while maximum benefit was present in those with more severe degrees of stenosis.

Secondary analyses from ECST, NASCET and the CETC have provided information regarding which patients gain most (and least) benefit from intervention. Markers of increased benefit include (1) males versus females, (2) increasing age, especially >75 years, (3) hemispheric versus ocular symptoms (4) cortical versus lacunar stroke, (5) increasing medical co-morbidity, (6) very recent symptoms, especially the first 2 weeks, (7) irregular versus smooth plaques, (8) increasing degrees of stenosis (not subocclusion) (9) contralateral occlusion, (10) tandem intracranial disease and (xi) a failure to recruit intracranial collaterals. Patients with subocclusion (string sign) derived no apparent benefit from intervention.

One of the most striking predictors of benefit is speed to treatment. It has previously been taught that the 7-day risk of stroke after TIA/minor stroke is 1–2% (2–4% at 30 days). These data, along with a perception that procedural risks increase the quicker one intervenes, have made surgeons reluctant to intervene quickly. However, recent evidence suggests that the 7-day risk of stroke may be as high as 8%. Table 10.4 summarises CETC data regarding outcomes stratified for delays to surgery and show (unequivocally) that any delay significantly reduces the long-term benefit accrued to the patient [8].

There has also been controversy about how long CEA should be delayed after suffering a stroke (traditionally 6–8 weeks). Evidence now suggests that expedited surgery can be undertaken safely in patients who meet the following criteria: rapid neurological recovery/neurological plateau, no carotid occlusion, Rankin 0–2 in terms of disability, area of infarction less than one third of the middle cerebral territory, no intracranial haemorrhage and patients should be lucid and able to give informed consent.

Carotid artery stenting has now emerged as an alternative to CEA in the management of symptomatic carotid disease. The 2007 Cochrane Review of 12 published randomised trials observed that while the prevention of cranial nerve injury significantly favoured CAS, stenting was associated with a significantly higher 30-day risk of death/stroke. The International Carotid Stenting Study (ICSS) was a multicentre randomised controlled trial in 1713 patients. The results showed that stenting was associated with twice as many stokes when compared to surgery (7.7% vs 4.1%, 65 vs 35, $p = 0.002$), most of these strokes in the stenting group were, however, non-disabling stoke, death of periprocendural myocardial infarction (MI) was higher in the stentin group (8.5% vs 5.2%, 72 vs 44, $p = 0.006$) [9]. The Carotid Revascularisation Endarterectomy Stenting Trial (CREST) results were recently published. In this trial symptomatic and asymptomatic carotid artery 2502 stenosis patients were randomised to stenting and surgery and were followed up for two and half years. There was no significant difference in the rate of stroke, MI or death. However, during the periprocedural period there was a higher risk of stroke with stenting and a higher risk of MI with endarterectomy. Younger patients had slightly fewer events with stenting and older patients fewer events with surgery [10].

Asymptomatic carotid disease

Table 10.3 summarises outcomes from Asymptomatic Carotid Artery Stenosis (ACAS) and Asymptomatic Carotid Surgery Trial (ACST) who compared CEA with best medical therapy in asymptomatic patients with 60–99% stenoses. The 'headline' conclusion was that

Table 10.4 Five-year prevention of 'any' stroke in the symptomatic and asymptomatic randomised trials comparing carotid endarterectomy (CEA) with medical therapy

| Trial | Stenosis | n | 30-day CEA risk | 5-year risk | | ARR | RRR | NNT | Strokes prevented per 1000 CEAs |
				Surgery	Medical				
Symptomatic trials*									
CETC	<30	1 746	No data	18.36	15.71	−2.6	n/b	n/b	None at 5 years
	30–49	1 429	6.7	22.80	25.45	+2.6	10	38	26 at 5 years
	50–69	1 549	8.4	20.00	27.77	+7.8	28	13	78 at 5 years
	70–99	1 095	6.2	17.13	32.71	+15.6	48	6	156 at 5 years
	string	262	5.4	22.4	22.30	−0.1	n/v	n/b	None at 5 years
Asymptotomatic trials**									
ACAS	60–99	1 659	2.3	17.5	12.4	+5.1	29	20	51 at 5 years
ACST	60–99	3 120	2.8	11.8	6.4	+5.4	46	19	54 at 5 years

* Data derived from the Carotid Endarterectomy Trialists Collaboration (CETC) [7], which combined data from ECST, NASCET and the VA trial. All pre-randomisation angiograms were remeasured using the NASCET method.

** ACAS data cited here are for the 5-year risk of 'any' stroke, in order to permit direct comparison with ACST.
n/b, no benefit conferred by CEA; ARR, absolute risk reduction; RRR, relative risk reduction; strokes prevented per 1000 CEAs, number of strokes prevented at 5 years. by performing 1000 CEAs; NNT, number of operations to prevent one stroke at 5 years.

CEA conferred a significant reduction in the 5-year risk of stroke. More importantly, ACST showed that CEA conferred a significant reduction in fatal/disabling stroke and that it was not beneficial in patients aged >75 years. Neither ACAS nor ACST showed any relationship between stenosis severity or bilateral severe disease and 5-year stroke risk. Note that the data published in Table 10.3 are slightly different to those normally published as they specifically refer to the 5-year risk of 'any stroke'. The 5-year risks of ipsilateral stroke in ACAS were 11.0% (medical) and 5.9% (surgical).

The management of patients with asymptomatic carotid disease continues to arouse controversy, largely because it is still not possible to identify who benefits most (and least) from intervention. For example, neither trial showed that women gained significant benefit from CEA (ACST only demonstrated benefit if the operative risk was excluded). Moreover, cost-effectiveness analyses suggest that up to 94% of patients ultimately undergo an unnecessary intervention, whilst incurring massive costs to health systems [11]. Finally, there is emerging evidence that the natural history risk of stroke is diminishing with time, presumably due to improvements in 'optimal medical therapy'. It is imperative, therefore, that we identify high risk cohorts in whom to target therapy. At present, it is not appropriate to offer CAS to otherwise normal risk asymptomatic patients without participation in randomised trials.

Performance of CEA

Carotid endarterectomy has been subject to more scientific scrutiny than any other surgical procedure, including a number of randomised trials aimed at evaluating different aspects of the procedure. The principal findings will be summarised below.

- The Aspirin and Carotid Endarterectomy (ACE) trial showed that low-dose aspirin (75–300 mg) conferred significant reductions in early and late death/stroke compared with higher doses (650–1300 mg). This trial was performed in response to a NASCET subgroup analysis suggesting the converse to be true. Low-dose aspirin is currently the preferred choice and should not be stopped perioperatively.

- The GALA trial showed that there was no evidence that performing CEA under general or locoregional anaesthesia influenced outcome, quality of life, hospital stay, intensive therapy unit (ITU) stay or costs. Surgeons and anaesthetists may use either anaesthetic technique according to their preference.

- A Cochrane meta-analysis of six randomised trials showed that routine patching conferred a threefold reduction in the 30-day risk of death/stroke and thrombosis and a similar reduction in late stroke/restenosis compared with routine primary closure. No trial has compared selective with routine patching. The evidence favours a policy of routine patching over routine primary closure and there is no evidence that patch type (vein/prosthetic) influences outcome.

- A meta-analysis of five randomised trials showed that provided the arteriotomy is patched, eversion endarterectomy does not confer any additional benefit over traditional endarterectomy.

- A meta-analysis of two randomised trials showed that routine shunting conferred a non-significant 25% reduction in the 30-day risk of death/stroke compared with no shunting. These studies were, however, methodologically flawed and this remains an unresolved issue. It is intuitively hard to defend a policy of 'never shunting'. Unless surgeons are prepared to perform CEA under locoregional anaesthesia, there is no safe or reliable way of predicting who needs a shunt.

Subclavian occlusive disease
Pathology
The commonest cause of occlusive/stenotic disease of the subclavian artery is atherosclerosis, usually at its origin. Other important conditions include arteritis (GCA and TA), thoracic outlet compression, occasionally FMD and rarely aneurysms of the subclavian artery.

Clinical features
Acute obstruction (embolus/thrombosis) of the subclavian artery may cause acute ischaemia of the upper limb, as well as a posterior circulation stroke due to compromised flow in the ipsilateral VA. The more common presentation is pain in the forearm with exercise (claudication) or dizziness while using the ipsilateral limb. The latter condition (subclavian steal syndrome) is due to a temporary reduction in flow in the posterior cranial circulation due to reversed flow in the ipsilateral vertebral artery (VA) during arm exercise. A related condition (coronary steal syndrome) is now being increasingly reported with the trend towards using the internal mammary artery as a conduit for coronary bypass. In the presence of a proximal subclavian stenosis/occlusion, there may be reversed flow in the internal mammary artery graft during arm exercise, which can be sufficient to precipitate angina or breathlessness.

Investigations
Duplex remains the first-line investigation (it is very accessible and cheap), supplemented by CTA or CEMRA. Patients suspected of having arteritis or FMD require additional investigations (see earlier).

Management
Risk factor modification and statin/antiplatelet therapy should be instituted. A significant proportion of patients with subclavian occlusive disease can be managed conservatively, especially if it is discovered as an incidental (asymptomatic finding). The decision to intervene must be based on the mode of presentation and extent of disability (pain, employment, etc.) in the context of the potential risks (surgery and angioplasty carry a small but significant risk of stroke). Compelling indications include severe arm pain with exercise that compromises employment, vertebrobasilar symptoms at presentation, subclavian steal syndrome and coronary steal syndrome. Less compelling indications include mild dizziness with head movement and minor forearm claudication (especially in the non-dominant limb). In the past, surgical revascularisation was the cornerstone of management (carotid-subclavian bypass, transposition), but many centres now increasingly use angioplasty +/- stenting as the first-line option. There is no Level I Grade A evidence to guide practice in this situation. In general, surgery carries a slightly higher initial risk but probably offers better long-term durability. Conversely, endovascular interventions are less invasive (and less risky), but long-term patency rates may be slightly poorer.

Vertebral occlusive disease
Demographics
Approximately 20% of all ischaemic strokes are vertebrobasilar.

Pathology

The commonest aetiology is atherosclerosis, but dissection, arteritis and FMD must be considered in patients with appropriate symptoms. In a recent population-based study of CEMRA imaging in 151 patients presenting with vertebrobasilar symptoms, approximately 26% were found to have significant disease (>50% stenosis) in the vertebral or basilar arteries [12]. Of those with demonstrable disease, 62% were located in the extracranial VA, 11% were located in the intracranial VA, while 8% of lesions were found in the basilar artery. Interestingly, in those patients presenting with vertebrobasilar symptoms and who had a significant with extracranial VA stenosis, 69% had their stenoses either at the origin or near to the origin of the VA, while 31% had lesions in the upper third of the VA.

Clinical features

'Classical' vertebrobasilar symptoms include; bilateral sensory/motor symptoms and signs, hemisensory/motor symptoms and signs (seen in 10% of vertebrobasilar events), bilateral visual loss (cortical blindness), dysarthria, nystagmus, and problems with gait and stance. Patients with isolated non-hemispheric symptoms (without other more definite vertebrobasilar symptoms) should not be considered to have suffered posterior circulation-based symptoms. Similarly, it has become conventional to make a diagnosis of 'positional' vertebrobasilar ischaemia in patients who develop symptoms (dizziness, vertigo) on lateral or flexed head movements. Recent evidence suggests that the vast majority of these patients do not have a vertebrobasilar cause for their symptoms. Such a diagnosis should only be made after comprehensive investigation as most will have inner ear pathology.

Investigations

Duplex ultrasound remains the first-line investigation but it is limited by its ability to fully evaluate the extracranial VA. Transcranial Duplex can image the intracranial VA and basilar arteries, but it is usually preferable to undertake either CEMRA or CTA. This will provide comprehensive information regarding the arch, subclavian/vertebral origins as well as the intracranial vessels and circle of Willis. The other advantage of CT and MRI is that it will provide valuable information regarding structural cranial abnormalities (tumour, infarction, A-V malformation). However, extracranial and transcranial Duplex is an excellent method for seeing whether head movements cause any change in flow in the extracranial VA or posterior cerebral artery.

Management

Most centres in the UK have relatively little experience of treating isolated vertebral and basilar artery stenoses. In the past, the mainstay of management was medical therapy or surgery (vertebral patch angioplasty, transposition to the carotid artery and proximal/distal bypass). Modern endovascular technological advances now offer an alternative means of treatment (angioplasty, stenting), which is emerging as the new first-line intervention in most centres. All patients will, of course, require optimisation of risk factors, and antiplatelet/statin therapy.

Prognosis

It was previously thought that patients with vertebrobasilar symptoms faced a lower risk of late stroke than those with carotid artery disease. However, emerging data from population-based studies suggest that this assumption may be erroneous. The Oxford group have recently shown that 46% of patients with a recently symptomatic VA stenosis suffered either a recurrent TIA or stroke in the first 90 days after presentation [12]. This compares with only 21% in similar patients with no VA stenosis.

References

1. Olin JW. Recognizing and managing fibromuscular dysplasia. *Cleveland Clin J Med* 2007; **74**: 273–82.

2. Kawasaki A, Purvin V. Giant cell arteritis: an updated review. *Acta Ophth* 2009; **87**: 13–32.

3. Johnston SL, Lock RJ, Gompels MM. Takayasu arteritis: a review. *J Clin Pathol* 2002; **55**: 481–86.

4. Sajid MS, Hamilton G, Baker DM on behalf of the Joint Vascular Research Group. *Eur J Vasc Endovasc Surg* 2007; **34**: 127–30.

5. Wardlaw JM, Chappell FM, Stevenson M et al. Accurate, practical and cost-effective assessment of carotid stenosis in the UK. *Health Technol Assess* 2006; **10**: no. 30. Available at: http://www.hta.ac.uk/fullmono/mon1030.pdf.

6. The European Stroke Initiative Executive Committee and the EUSI Writing Committee. European Stroke Initiative Recommendations for Stroke Management – Update 2003. *Cerebrovasc Dis* 2003; **16**: 311–37.

7. Rothwell PM, Eliasziw M, Gutnikov SA et al. for the Carotid Endarterectomy Trialists Collaboration. Analysis of pooled data from the randomised controlled trials of endarterectomy for symptomatic carotid stenosis. *Lancet* 2003; **361**: 107–16.

8. Rothwell PM, Eliasziw M, Gutnikov SA, Warlow CP, Barnett HJM for the Carotid Endarterectomy Trialists Collaboration. Endarterectomy for symptomatic carotid stenosis in relation to clinical subgroups and timing of surgery. *Lancet* 2004; **363**: 915–24.

9. International Carotid Stenting Study Investigators. Carotid artery stenting compared with endarterectomy in patients with symptomatic carotid stenosis. *Lancet* 2010; **375**(9719): 985–97.

10. Brott TG, Hobson RW, Howard G et al. Stenting versus endarterectomy for treatment of carotid artery stenosis. *N Engl J Med* 2010; **363**(1): 11–23.

11. Naylor AR, Gaines PA, Rothwell PM. Who benefits most from intervention for asymptomatic carotid stenosis: patients or professionals? *Eur J Vasc Endovasc Surg* 2009; **37**(6): 625–32.

12. Marquardt L, Kuker W, Chandratheva A, Geraghty O, Rothwell PM. Incidence and prognosis of >50% symptomatic vertebral or basilar artery stenosis: prospective population based study. *Brain* 2009; **132**: 982–8.

11

Diagnosis and management of thoracic outlet syndrome

Hassan Badri and Vish Bhattacharya

Key points

- Thoracic outlet syndrome (TOS) can be neurogenic, venous or arterial
- Neurogenic TOS is the commonest presentation, seen in 90% of cases
- Arterial presentation is very rare but may be more dramatic with digital gangrene
- TOS is due to extrinsic compression from fibrous bands, cervical rib or first rib
- Physical examination may be helpful with the Roos test being positive in the majority
- Plain X-rays, Duplex and magnetic resonance angiography (MRA) may be helpful but the diagnosis is mainly clinical
- Electrophysiology testing is non-specific although median antebrachial nerve response has recently shown to be useful
- Removal of fibrous bands, cervical ribs and the first rib may be needed along with anterior scalenectomy
- Arterial reconstruction of the subclavian artery may be required

Introduction

TOS is one of the most controversial clinical entities in medicine. This is partly because there is no definitive diagnostic test and debate continues as to whether the syndrome even really exists in some of its forms! Its incidence has been estimated at 5:100 000 per year in the UK although the true figure is still unknown [1].

The thoracic outlet is the region at the top of the rib cage between the base of the neck and the axilla through which the brachial plexus and the subclavian vessels travel. The first channel is the interscalene triangle, which is bordered by the scalenus anterior, scalenus medius and the medial border of the first rib (Figure 11.1). This is followed by the costoclavicular space, bordered anteriorly by the middle part of the clavicle and posteriorly by the first rib and the scapula. The last channel is the subcoracoid space below the coracoid process deep to the pectoralis minor tendon.

Thoracic outlet syndrome refers to a variety of complex disorders in the upper extremity caused by damage to the brachial plexus, or the subclavian artery or vein, as they pass through the thoracic outlet tunnels described above. Thoracic outlet syndrome is more

Postgraduate Vascular Surgery: The Candidate's Guide to the FRCS, eds. Vish Bhattacharya and Gerard Stansby. Published by Cambridge University Press. © Cambridge University Press 2010.

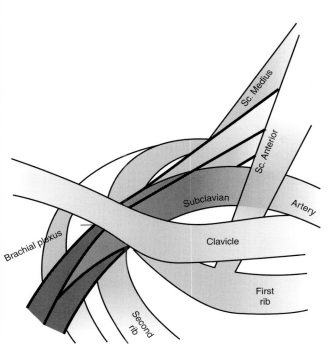

Figure 11.1 Anatomy of the thoracic outlet showing structures in the interscalene triangle.

common in women and in the age group between 30 and 50 years but can occur in all ages, including in children.

Pathophysiology/causes

Anatomical factors such as cervical ribs, fibrous bands, repetitive injuries or whiplash causing scarring of the scalenus anterior muscle can lead to TOS. However, in many cases no specific anatomical factor can be identified.

Cervical ribs are seen in 0.1% of adults and only 5–10% of these are symptomatic. Fifty per cent of cervical ribs are bilateral (Figure 11.2). Fibrous bands, which traverse the thoracic outlet, are the most common congenital anomaly causing TOS and will not be seen on plain X-ray and may not be seen with magnetic resonance imaging (MRI) either. Anomalous muscular insertions and muscle hypertrophy have also been known to cause TOS. Malunion and formation of prominent callus after clavicle fractures have also been reported to cause TOS. Pancoast tumours, enlarged regional lymph nodes and developmental changes in the cervical spine are rare causes of TOS [2].

Clinical presentation

Clinical features differ according to the compressed structure/s in the thoracic outlet tunnel. Hence, there are four main clinical syndromes described:

1. neurogenic TOS (NTOS);
2. arterial TOS (ATOS);
3. venous TOS (VTOS);
4. non-specific (combined) TOS, which is a mixture of any combination of the above three.

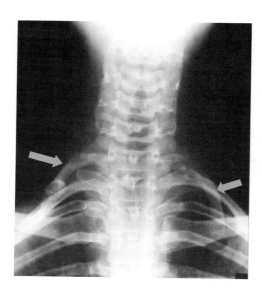

Figure 11.2 Bilateral cervical ribs.

Neurogenic TOS (NTOS)

This is the commonest form of TOS (90%) and patients usually present with symptoms in the ulnar nerve distribution (C8, T1 nerve roots). Pain, especially with activities with the arms raised, is an early and very common presentation. The pain may radiate to the axilla, shoulder, back of neck or down the arm. Paraesthesia is usually felt on the medial aspect of the arm, forearm and hand. There may be tenderness over the scalene muscle and reproduction of symptoms on provocation tests as below. Often there are associated vasospastic-type symptoms, such as coldness or Raynaud's, which may lead to an erroneous suspicion that there is arterial involvement.

Adson test

In this test the patient takes a deep breath and extends his neck and rotates the head towards the side being examined. The test is positive if the radial pulse is abolished or patient's symptoms are replicated. Another variant is described where the manoeuvre results in paraesthesiae in the hand. This test is reported to be 76% specific and 79% sensitive [3] although diagnostic decisions are rarely based on this test alone.

Roos test (Elevated Arm Stress Test, EAST)

This is a more reliable test for screening for TOC. In this test the patient abducts both arms at 90° from the body with the elbows bent and opens and closes the hands repeatedly for 3 min. It is positive if the patient's symptoms are reproduced. This test has been found to be 84% sensitive and 30% specific [3].

Motor weakness of the intrinsic muscles, innervated by the ulnar and median nerve, is a late finding. Fine hand movement and hand grip may become clumsy. Patients often complain of occipital headaches. Muscle wasting is usually a late presentation and may be noted in the thenar muscles and the abductor thumb muscles. Vasomotor disturbances include bluish red discolouration and blanching of the hand. Intermittent attacks of cyanosis or pallor of the hand usually accompanies emotional disturbances and exposure to cold.

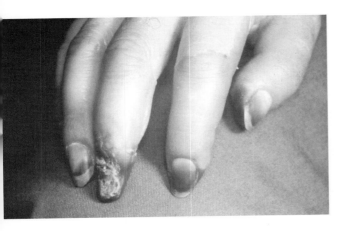

Figure 11.3 Distal embolization due to arterial thoracic outlet syndrome.

Venous TOS (VTOS)

This is the second commonest presentation and patients may present acutely with cyanosis and arm swelling. If established there may be prominent veins seen in the upper arm or chest. Thrombosis of the subclavian vein develops at the site of compression as the vein passes over the first rib, and it often occurs after strenuous activity to the upper limb and is referred to as effort thrombosis or Paget–Schroetter syndrome. It is also found in younger patients who are athletes, such as swimmers. It is thought that repeated extrinsic compression of the subclavian vein may cause fibrosis, stenosis and eventually thrombosis of the subclavian vein. It may also be due to a sudden hyper-abduction injury causing intimal damage and thrombosis of the subclavian vein.

Arterial TOS (ATOS)

This is the rarest presentation (1%). Constriction and repetitive trauma of the subclavian artery can lead to stenosis, aneurysm formation or complete occlusion. Poststenotic dilatation of the second part of the subclavian artery may lead to aneurysm formation, which can present with thromboembolic complications, such as acute ischaemia of the arm or a digit (Figure 11.3). Patients might present with attacks of pallor, pain and paraesthesia, or display Raynaud's phenomenon. The radial pulse may be absent and provocative tests may cause the radial pulse to disappear although this is often found in normal subjects and is not diagnostic.

Investigations

Cervical spine film and chest radiograph can rule out cervical ribs, lung lesions or clavicular abnormalities. Magnetic resonance imaging and computed tomography (CT) scan of the cervicothoracic area can be helpful in detecting the non-bony anomalies (fibrous bands, muscular abnormality, tumours), and in excluding cervical spine lesions. Magnetic resonance imaging findings in patients in a provocative position (the shoulder is abducted by placing the hand behind the head) are also valuable [4].

Neurophysiologic testing is largely unhelpful and may show non-specific abnormalities although it can be useful to exclude other disorders. Recently a new nerve test has been shown to be abnormal in the majority of patients with neurogenic TOS. It is the determination of the response to medial antebrachial cutaneous nerve stimulation. Electromyography (EMG) may reveal abnormalities in the intrinsic muscles of the hand in late cases but is unreliable in early diagnosis. Anterior scalene nerve blocks provide temporary relief but these patients usually respond well to surgery.

Venous Duplex ultrasound, contrast venograms or magnetic resonance venography are useful to rule out venous obstruction or arterial involvement and these can also be performed with the shoulder in abduction.

Arterial Duplex ultrasound of the upper extremity is the first-line investigation in most cases. Arteriography or MRAs help to confirm the diagnosis and to plan reconstruction. Angiography can highlight subclavian stenosis, aneurysms or irregular filling defects consistent with mural thrombus and allow for dynamic views with the arms in abduction and adduction.

Treatment

Neurogenic TOS

Conservative measures to avoid repetitive overhead work, correct posture and strengthen the shoulder elevating muscles, such as the trapezius, are useful and have proven to be effective at reducing symptoms and improving function [5].

Selective botulinum chemodenervation of the scalene muscles can provide temporary relief in NTOS [6, 7]. This can be done under electrophysiological and fluoroscopic guidance and has proven to be more effective than injections with local anaesthetics and steroids.

Surgery is indicated in NTOS if the conservative treatment failed to improve symptoms, and in the case of severe symptoms that interfere with work or daily activities. This includes anterior scalenectomy with or without cervical rib resection, removal of fibrous bands and excision of the first rib. Various approaches to the first rib including transaxillary, supraclavicular and infraclavicular approaches have been described. Several combinations of surgery have been presented in large series and there is no consensus on the optimal approach.

Venous TOS

Therapeutic protocols now include thrombolysis and correction of the anatomical abnormalities contributing to the thrombosis by surgery or endovascular means. First rib resection is recommended as soon as possible after thrombolysis [8]. Without decompression of the thoracic outlet rethrombosis may occur and likewise without decompression there is almost universal failure of venous stenting due to external compression to the stent causing stent fracture or thrombosis.

Arterial TOS

Thrombectomy, followed by excision of the cervical or first rib is carried out. Arterial reconstruction may include repairing a subclavian aneurysm, which forms as a result of the post-stenotic dilatation or bypass grafting.

Symptomatic improvement after surgery is difficult to quantify and is largely subjective. It has been shown to vary from 43% to 88% [9].

Results have usually been classed as excellent, good and fair, based on patients' perceptions. Previous acute ischaemia, sensory or motor deficit and extended resection of the first rib have been shown to be poor predictors of outcome [10].

References

1. Thompson JF, Jannsen F. Thoracic outlet syndromes. *Br J Surg* 1996; **83**: 435–6.
2. Sanders RJ, Hammond SL, Rao NM. Diagnosis of thoracic outlet syndrome. *J Vasc Surg* 2007; **46**: 601–4.
3. Rayan GM, Jensen C. Thoracic outlet syndrome: provocative examination manoeuvres in a typical population. *J Shoulder Elbow Surg* 1995; **4**: 113–17.
4. Jordan SE, Machleder HI. Diagnosis of thoracic outlet syndrome using electrophysiologically guided anterior scalene blocks. *Ann Vasc Surg* 1998; **12**: 260–4.
5. Vanti C, Natalini L, Romeo A, Tosarelli D, Pillastrini P. Conservative treatment of thoracic outlet syndrome. A review of the literature. *Eura Medicophys* 2007; **43**: 55–70.
6. Jordan SE, Ahn SS, Gelabert HA. Combining ultrasonography and electromyography for botulinum chemodenervation treatment of thoracic outlet syndrome: comparison with fluoroscopy and electromyography guidance. *Pain Physician* 2007; **10**: 541–6.
7. Jordan SE, Ahn SS, Freischlag JA, Gelabert HA, Machleder HI. Selective botulinum chemodenervation of the scalene muscles for treatment of neurogenic thoracic outlet syndrome. *Ann Vasc Surg* 2000; **14**: 365–9.
8. Lee MC, Grassi CJ, Belkin M, Mannick JA, Whittemore AD, Donaldson MC. Early operative intervention after thrombolytic therapy for primary subclavian vein thrombosis: an effective treatment approach. *J Vasc Surg* 1998; **27**: 1101–7.
9. Bhattacharya V, Hansrani M, Wyatt MG, Lambert D, Jones NA. Outcome following surgery for thoracic outlet syndrome. *Eur J Vasc Endovasc Surg* 2003; **26**: 170–5.
10. Degeorges R, Reynaud C, Becquemin JP. Thoracic outlet syndrome surgery: long-term functional results. *Ann Vasc Surg* 2004; **18**: 558–65.

12 Diagnosis and management of hyperhidrosis

Hassan Badri and Vish Bhattacharya

Key points

- Postganglionic sympathetic C fibres supply the sweat glands
- Iontophoresis involves passing a small current into the skin using tap water
- Botox injections are useful for axillary, palmar or frontal hyperhidrosis but repeat injections are required
- Thoracoscopic sympathectomy of T2 and T3 ganglion for palmar and T2 T3 and T4 ganglia for axillary hyperhidrosis is very effective
- Patients should be warned of side effects such as compensatory hyperhidrosis, Horner's syndrome, pneumothorax and haemothorax
- Local surgical treatments include curettage, skin excision or liposuction

Introduction

Hyperhidrosis is the production of excessive quantities of sweat, and is caused by hyper-function of the exocrine sweat glands, which are controlled by the sympathetic nervous system via postsynaptic cholinergic fibres.

Nerves from the hypothalamic preoptic sweat centre synapse in the intermediolateral cell columns without crossing. The myelinated preganglionic fibres pass out in the anterior roots to the sympathetic chain. Unmyelinated postganglionic C fibres arising from the sympathetic ganglia join the peripheral nerves and pass out to the sweat glands.

Sweating can be induced by thermal stimuli and emotional stress. Emotional sweating can occur over the entire skin but is more prevalent in the palms, axillae and soles. This stops during sleep when thermal sweating can continue.

A dysfunction of the central sympathetic nervous system, possibly of the hypothalamic nucleus or prefrontal areas is suspected to be the cause of hyperhidrosis.

Hyperhidrosis may be primary or secondary; localized or generalized. Secondary hyperhidrosis may be due to hyperthyroidism or phaeochromcytoma.

Primary hyperhidrosis is not uncommon, affecting between 0.6% and 1% of the general population. The palms, soles and axillae are the most commonly affected sites. Patients are usually in their second or third decade of life, with a positive family history noted in 30% to 50% of cases [1, 2].

Postgraduate Vascular Surgery: The Candidate's Guide to the FRCS, eds. Vish Bhattacharya and Gerard Stansby. Published by Cambridge University Press. © Cambridge University Press 2010.

Symptoms

The only presentation is excessive sweating in a localized area of the patients' body, which restricts their private and professional lives. The condition itself might cause bromhidrosis, dermal mycoses, and gram-negative infections of the feet or palmar and plantar warts.

Diagnosis

The diagnosis of this condition is usually made on clinical grounds. However, Minor described a test in which a 2% iodine solution is applied to the affected area, followed by starch powder once the solution has dried. The hyperhidrotic skin then develops a blue-black colouration. Colorimetry is a similar procedure where colour changes, occurring on specially coated paper placed in contact with the sweat, are analysed.

Management

Topical therapy

Aluminium chloride hexahydrate in absolute anhydrous ethyl alcohol is the most effective antiperspirant for treating hyperhidrosis. The product is applied to the affected areas every night until symptoms are controlled and then weekly or fortnightly to maintain control of sweating. The drawbacks of topical treatment are that they are time consuming, and cannot be applied to irritated, broken or recently shaven skin. They also can cause irritation, hypersensitivity and staining. Boric acid, glutaraldehyde, formaldehyde, potassium permanganate and tannic acid have shown less satisfactory results.

Systemic therapy

Anticholinergic agents block sweat production at the level of the neuroglandular junction by competing with acetylcholine. Treatment with glycopyrollate, at a dose of 1–2 mg, has been tried with some success. This does not cross the blood–brain barrier and does not have any systemic side effects unlike atropine and probathaline bromide, which can cause dry mouth, blurred vision, mydriasis, urinary retention and constipation.

Iontophoresis

Iontophoresis involves passing a direct electrical current of about 15 mA through the skin, thereby reducing sweat excretion. The patients' hands or feet are placed on a metal plate and gauze in two trays containing tap water or anticholinergic agents such as glycopyrronium bromide solution. The mechanism of action is poorly understood but it is thought to act by either causing obstruction of sweat pores or impairment of the electrochemical gradient of sweat secretion [3]. A repeated course of treatment is usually required with maintenance to prevent relapse. Tap water has been shown to be more effective than saline. Adverse effects include initial aggravation of symptoms, sensory disturbances and skin eruptions. Iontophoresis is contraindicated in patients with pacemakers and in pregnancy. It is not as effective for axillary symptoms as for palmo-plantar hyperhidrosis but it is simple, effective and not associated with rebound compensatory hyperhidrosis [4]. The treated area may become dry, cracked or fissured.

Botulinum toxin

Botulinum toxin A is a neurotoxin produced by *Clostridium botulinum*, which is a gram positive, spore-producing, anaerobic bacteria. It acts at the acetylcholine presynaptic nerve endings at neuromuscular junctions and exocrine sweat glands. The toxin works over an area of approximately 1.2 cm and injections should therefore be spaced up to 2.5 cm apart. Injections are made in the intracutaneous rather than subepidermal layer. The effect however gradually wanes between 4–13 months and top-up injections may be needed [5].

Common side effects include transitory pain, intrinsic muscle wasting of the hand in patients undergoing palmar injections, haematoma and itching. Nerve blocks are the most effective way of combating pain around injection sites and have been found to be more effective than topical solutions of local anaesthetic.

It is both effective and well tolerated in axillary, palmar and frontal hyperhidrosis.

Surgical treatment

Sympathectomy

Sympathectomy is used to eliminate the sympathetic innervation of the sweat glands and consequently reduce the amount of sweating. Thoracoscopic sympathectomy has proved to be the most effective and durable treatment for patients suffering from moderate to severe hyperhidrosis. For palmar hyperhidrosis sympathectomy should be restricted to T2, T3 ganglions. For axillary hyperhidrosis, the T2, T3, T4 ganglia are denervated. In a large study with a 6-year follow up, Dumont et al. found satisfaction rates and improved quality of life of 93% and 100% after sympathectomy for palmar hyperhidrosis and 67% and 83% after sympathectomy for axillary hyperhidrosis [6]. A recent 10-year follow up showed that satisfaction rate were lower (47%) after a mean follow up of 12 years after surgery [7]. In the case of plantar hyperhidrosis, ablation of the L2, L3, L4 ganglia is required. Clipping of the sympathetic chain has also been advocated in patients who have severe compensatory hyperhidrosis as this would make the procedure reversible.

The commonest complication after sympathectomy is compensatory sweating with reported rates of 33–87% [8]. This affects previously unaffected areas such as trunk, chest, back, and lower limb. This can be avoided by limiting the extent of symapthectomy to T2 level only.

Other surgical complications included haemothorax (0.1%), pneumothorax (0.5%), segmental atelectasis (0.35%), and mild wound infections (0.1%). The recurrence rates for palmar and axillary hyperhidrosis 5 years after surgery have been reported to be 1.3% and 16.7%, respectively [9]. Transient Horner's syndrome has been reported in up to 0.8% of patients and permanently in 0.1% [10].

Local surgical treatments

Other surgical treatment options are local excision of sweat glands, curettage and liposuction. Excision requires identification using the starch-iodine test. While studies have shown this to be effective it can lead to ugly scars, haematoma, wound infection and reduced shoulder abduction. Recurrence rates can be as high as 20–25%. Subcutaneous curettage involves smaller incisions and a curette to remove all the subcutaneous fat within a demarcated area. This reduces keloid and poor scar formation but has a high failure and relapse rate. Liposuction enables the removal of sweat glands without comprising the overlying skin and has better cosmesis than excision and less bleeding than curettage. This may require more than one procedure and can be time consuming, with some authors proposing a trial of inotophoresis prior to liposuction

Chemical/thermo coagulation sympathectomy

Chemical sympathectomy is another method in which sympathetic ganglion blockade is achieved by injecting ethanol or phenol using a closed percutaneous needle technique. In addition to the risks of pneumothorax, intradural or intravascular injection, neuralgia and compensatory sweating have been reported. This technique has been greatly facilitated by use under CT-guidance.

Dorsal percutaneous stereotactic thermocoagulation sympathectomy is a newer alternative procedure. It involves the insertion of a thermocoagulation probe through the skin of the back under local anaesthetic. Recurrence rates are low and retreatment can easily be performed in an outpatient setting. However, complications such as Horner's syndrome and pneumothorax have been noted with this procedure as well.

References

1. Moran KT, Brady MP. Surgical management of primary hyperhidrosis. *Br J Surg* 1991; **78**: 279–83.
2. Mosek A, Korczyn A. Hyperhidrosis in the palms and soles. In: Korczyn A, ed. *Handbook of Autonomic System Dysfunction.* New York: Marcel Dekker, 1995; pp. 167–77.
3. Hill AC, Baker GF, Jansen GT. Mechanism of action of iontophoresis in the treatment of palmar hyperhidrosis. *Cutis* 1981; **28**: 69–70, 72.
4. Karakoc Y, Aydemir EH, Kalkan MT, Unal G. Safe control of palmoplantar hyperhidrosis with direct electrical current. *Int J Dermatol* 2002; **41**: 602–5.
5. Karamfilov T, Konrad H, Karte K et al. Lower relapse rate of botulinum toxin A therapy for axillary hyperhidrosis by dose increase. *Arch Dermatol* 2000; **136**: 487–90.
6. Dumont P, Denoyer A, Robin P. Long-term results of thoracoscopic sympathectomy for hyperhidrosis. *Ann Thorac Surg* 2004; **78**: 1801–7.
7. Walles T, Somuncuoglu G, Steger V, Veit S, Friedel G. Long-term efficiency of endoscopic thoracic sympathectomy: survey 10 years after surgery. *Interact Cardiovasc Thorac Surg* 2009; **8**(1): 54–7.
8. Kwong KF, Hobbs JL, Cooper LB, Burrows W, Gamliel Z, Krasna MJ. Stratified analysis of clinical outcomes in thoracoscopic sympathectotomy for hyperhidrosis. *Ann Thorac Surg* 2008; **85**: 390–4.
9. Lin TS, Kuo SJ, Chou MC. Uniportal endoscopic thoracic sympathectomy for treatment of palmar and axillary hyperhidrosis: analysis of 2000 cases. *Neurosurgery* 2002; **51**: 84–7.
10. Kestenholz PB, Weder W. Thoracic sympathectomy *Curr Probl Dermatol* 2002; **30**: 64–76.

Final FRCS vascular topics

Chronic mesenteric ischaemia

Mohamed Abdelhamid, Robert Davies and Rajiv Vohra

Key points

- Chronic mesenteric ischaemia (CMI) is a rare condition, accounting for less than 5% of all intestinal ischaemic events
- More than 90% of cases are due to atherosclerotic occlusion or severe stenosis
- Classic symptoms include postprandial abdominal pain, sitophobia and weight loss
- At least two of the three main splanchnic arteries must be significantly compromised to result in chronic mesenteric ischaemia
- Duplex ultrasonography is non-invasive and expedient but may miss up to 20% of vascular lesions in the coeliac trunk
- Computed tomography angiography (CTA) and magnetic resonance angiography (MRA) are equally excellent non-invasive modalities with highly accurate diagnosis of vascular disease in the coeliac axis (CA) and superior mesenteric artery (SMA) and replace conventional catheter angiography
- Conventional catheter angiography should be reserved for diagnosis of CMI only when other modalities have been unhelpful or if intervention such as percutaneous transluminal angioplasty (PTA) is planned
- Surgical vascular bypass is the traditional definitive therapy for CMI with an overall 5-year graft patency of 78%
- Endovascular therapy is optimal in short segment atherosclerotic lesions at the ostia of the SMA and CA. Stenting and PTA in short-term follow up have a clinical benefit with stent patency in more than 90% of cases

Background

CMI is an uncommon cause of abdominal pain. It accounts for 5% of all intestinal ischaemic events with acute ischaemia being much more common. Atherosclerotic occlusion, or severe stenosis of the mesenteric arteries, is the most common aetiology and the incidence of atherosclerotic lesions affecting the mesenteric arteries in a person >65 years is 17.5% [1]. Symptoms of CMI such as intestinal angina, weight loss and sitophobia (=fear of eating) usually only occur when at least two of the three main splanchnic arteries are affected. This is because the mesenteric arterial circulation is rich in collaterals. allowing for the gradual stenosis/occlusion of one or two main arteries without any symptoms.

Postgraduate Vascular Surgery: The Candidate's Guide to the FRCS, eds. Vish Bhattacharya and Gerard Stansby. Published by Cambridge University Press. © Cambridge University Press 2010.

Table 13.1 Aetiology and differential diagnosis of chronic mesenteric ischaemia

Aetiology	Differential diagnosis
• Atherosclerosis	• Gall bladder disease
• Median arcuate ligament syndrome	• Peptic ulcer
• Takayasu arteritis	• Abdominal malignancy
• Dysplastic lesions	• Chronic pancreatitis
• Thromboangiitis obliterans	• Spastic colon
• Radiation induced vascular injury	• Indigestion

Pathophysiology

The majority of those affected are elderly patients with generalized atherosclerosis. Atherosclerotic occlusion or severe stenosis of the mesenteric arteries accounts for more than 90% of causes of CMI [2]. Hyperlipidemia, diabetes and smoking contribute to the occurrence of CMI. Thrombotic occlusion or stenosis usually occurs at the origin of the artery adjacent to the ostium. Diffuse atherosclerosis of the whole vessel is seen in fewer patients. The CA and SMA are more commonly affected than the inferior mesenteric artery (IMA). In patients with peripheral arterial disease and renal artery stenosis a quarter of the individuals examined had greater than 50% stenosis in either the CA or SMA but only 3.4% had significant occlusion of both arteries [3]. Other causes of CMI include constriction of coeliac artery blood flow by diaphragmatic compression (median arcuate ligament syndrome, which is more predominant in women), Takayasu arteritis, dysplastic lesions, thromboangiitis obliterans and radiation-induced vascular injury (Table 13.1).

Clinical presentation

Relative ischaemia occurs after eating when there is an increased demand for flow within the mesenteric circulation while the arteries are unable to dilate due to the fixed occlusive lesions. This results in transient ischaemic pain, known as intestinal angina. Pain is dull in nature and typically postprandial, 30 min after eating, and occurs in the periumbilical region. It may last 1–4 hours and fades gradually. The patients develop fear from eating resulting in reduction of the size of meals in order to avoid the pain, which eventually leads to weight loss [2]. Chronic mesenteric ischaemia involving the coeliac artery may result in disorders such as gastroparesis, gastric ulceration and gall bladder dyskinesia. Physical examination is usually unremarkable except for abdominal pain that is out of proportion to examination. Sometimes, an epigastric bruit may be audible.

Diagnosis

Diagnosis requires careful history-taking and exclusion of other illnesses such as malignancy, chronic pancreatitis and gastric ulcer (Table 13.1). The traditional modality used to diagnose CMI is mesenteric angiography. Other modalities include visceral Duplex ultrasound, CTA and MRA.

Visceral Duplex ultrasound (VDU) evaluation of the mesenteric arteries is non-invasive. It has been used successfully to document occlusive disease in the proximal SMA and, to a lesser extent, in the CA. The IMA is rarely imaged by transabdominal ultrasound due to its anatomic location. Overall, VDU has a 90% accuracy in identifying significant proximal SMA stenosis and 80% accuracy for coeliac trunk lesions [4]. Turbulence and velocity of blood flow are the features of stenotic and occlusive lesions affecting the proximal portion of the arteries. Peak systolic velocity of greater than 200 cm s^{-1} and an end-diastolic velocity exceeding 55 cm s^{-1} have been shown to have high correlation with CA stenosis [2]. End-diastolic velocity greater than 45 cm s^{-1} is specific to lesions of the proximal SMA, together with peak systolic velocity greater than 275 cm s^{-1}. However, limitations of Duplex include effects of respiration, obesity, food ingestion, bowel gas, anatomic variations and operator. If screening ultrasonography detects vascular stenosis or occlusion, further detailed imaging is usually indicated.

Conventional interventional angiography is reserved until other more common disorders of chronic abdominal pain have been excluded. Selective arterial catheterisation of the branches of the CA or SMA is possible. It usually shows occlusion or near occlusion of the CA and/or SMA near their origins from the aorta. The IMA is usually occluded due to diffuse atherosclerosis and prominent collaterals are often present. Contraindications to arteriography include hypotension or hypovolemia as these may cause vasoconstriction and make the findings less accurate. Contrast-induced nephrotoxicity is another drawback. The overall rate of major complications from mesenteric angiography is 1.9–2.9% and may include external iliac artery dissection or deep venous thrombosis.

CTA is used increasingly with high sensitivity and specificity to identify significant splanchnic vascular stenosis. The availability of three-dimensional image reconstruction can diagnose significant atherosclerotic lesions of all the three major mesenteric arteries and many of their main branches. In addition to providing three-dimensional images, this modality has faster scanning time. Thinner collimation of 0.5–1.0 mm thickness facilitates better visualisation of small vessels and branches. This minimally invasive method is highly comparable to conventional angiography but with less cost and morbidity. In suspected intestinal angina, a negative CTA study of the mesenteric arteries makes the diagnosis of CMI virtually unlikely. Recently, it has been shown that using multiple radiographic criteria, CTA has a sensitivity of 96% and specificity of 94% for diagnosis of CMI [5].

In recent years MRA has become a valuable tool for diagnosing CMI, particularly since its cost and image acquisition times have substantially decreased. MRA images provide high-resolution mesenteric angiograms with sensitivity greater than 90% of SMA and CA lesions, 81–88% of portal vein disease, and 25% of lesions affecting the IMA vessels [6]. Contrast-enhanced MRA has 100% sensitivity and 95% specificity for stenosis of the CA and SMA when compared to conventional angiography. However, small peripheral arterial branches are less well visualised. Unlike Duplex ultrasonography, the detection of proximal CA and SMA stenosis by contrast-enhanced MRA is accurate with minimal interobserver variability.

The choice between these investigations depends on the availability of technology, allergy to contrast and renal function. It is therefore recommended that invasive angiography should be used when IMA occlusion is suspected or when endovascular therapy of stenotic or occlusive lesions is planned (Table 13.2)

Treatment

In most cases, the treatment of CMI is not considered urgent. However, the therapeutic goal in patients with CMI is to revascularize the mesenteric arterial circulation to prevent the

Table 13.2 Diagnostic methods of chronic mesenteric ischaemia

	Advantages	Disadvantages
Duplex ultrasound	Non-invasive, low cost, 90% and 80% sensitivity for SMA and CA, respectively	Operator dependent, not for IMA, limited by obesity, respiration, bowel gas and food ingestion
Angiography	100% sensitive for three arteries, angioplasty possible	Invasive, contrast allergy, renal impairment, complications
CTA	Non-invasive, 96% sensitive for CA and SMA, operator non-dependent,	Not for IMA, contrast allergy, renal impairment, cost
MRA	Non-invasive, 90% sensitive for CA and SMA, operator non-dependent	Low sensitivity for IMA, cost, claustrophobia

SMA, superior mesenteric artery; CA, coeliac axis; IMA, inferior mesenteric artery; CTA, computed tomography angiography; MRA, magnetic resonance angiography.

development of bowel infarction. Mesenteric vascular stenosis or occlusion usually requires open surgical repair or endovascular therapy.

Surgical repair

Surgical repair has been the standard treatment for CMI since the first successful repair reported by Shaw in 1958. The surgical options include:

1. Transaortic endarterectomy. This is indicated for osteal lesions of patent CA and SMA. This can be achieved by left medial visceral rotation to expose the aorta and its mesenteric branches. Initial success of trap-door transaortic endarterectomy was found to reach 93% with overall patency at 1 and 3 years of $85\pm10.0\%$ and $77\pm11.7\%$, respectively [6]. However, others reported high failure rates with recurrent thrombosis and symptoms using this method. Transaortic endarterectomy is also beneficial in patients with concomitant renal artery stenosis and CMI due to atherosclerosis. When significant lesions are located at the origin of both the renal artery and splanchnic arteries, transaortic endarterectomy can be effectively used to treat both conditions with minimal mortality.

2. Surgical bypass is indicated for occlusive lesions located 1–2 cm from the origin of the mesenteric arteries. Surgical bypass can be performed through either antegrade or retrograde reconstruction using either autogenous or prosthetic grafts. Single or multivessel reconstruction with outflow into the CA, SMA or rarely the IMA should be achieved. Isolated IMA revascularization has been used for CMI in selected cases when it is not possible to revascularize from either the CA or SMA.

Antegrade versus retrograde inflow reconstruction

In antegrade reconstruction, the arterial inflow arises from the thoracic or supracoeliac aorta, so the bypass is placed in the direction of normal blood flow to reduce anastomotic turbulence. This could be done through abdominal or thoracoabdominal incision. Apart from a slightly higher 30-day mortality with the antegrade approach, there is no statistic-ally significant difference between the antegrade and retrograde approaches concerning

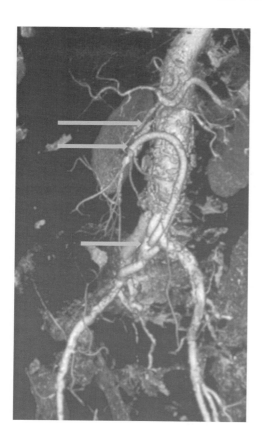

Figure 13.1 Retrograde bypass. (Top) Superior mensenteric (SMA) stenosis, (middle) proximal anastomosis from the right limb of the aorto-bi-iliac graft, (bottom) distal anastomosis to the distal SMA.

symptom free survival. In addition, an antegrade approach may lead to a higher incidence of postoperative ileus [7]. In retrograde reconstruction (Figure 13.1), inflow arises from the infrarenal aorta or the common iliac artery.

The drawbacks of retrograde revascularization include kinking of the graft and progression of atherosclerosis to the origin of the retrograde bypass graft from the infrarenal aorta or from the common iliac artery. Kinking of the vein grafts occurred immediately after surgery in the earlier series when short vein grafts were used. This problem has been avoided with the use of prosthetic grafts, especially when a long loop is constructed.

The retrograde approach is useful in high-risk patients requiring shorter surgical time, in patients with previous abdominal surgery and in those who have had a failed previous antegrade bypass [8].

Autogenous versus prosthetic grafts

Both autogenous and prosthetic vascular reconstructions have been used with satisfactory results. Both the long saphenous vein and and superficial femoral vein have been used with equally good results although polytetrafluoroethane (PTFE) and Dacron have more long-term durability. Surgical reconstruction has been associated with morbidity and mortality (5–30%) in most series [8]. This could be expected in this group as many are elderly with significant weight loss, malnutrition, and low albumin levels, which are all predictors of increased morbidity and mortality after any major surgery. Symptomatic recurrence requiring reintervention is required in about 10–40% of patients.

Percutaneous transluminal angioplasty and stenting (PTA/stent)

In the last two decades, endovascular therapy has become a more acceptable approach for stenotic or occlusive lesions in the mesenteric arteries. This consists of percutaneous transluminal angioplasty and stenting (PTA/stent) of the mesenteric arteries. Interest in this method arose from the potential for decreased morbidity and mortality in comparison to surgical bypass. However, reported series on percutaneous transluminal angioplasty and stenting (PTA/stent) have contained small numbers of patients. Short occlusive or stenotic lesions are ideal for this modality (Figure 13.2 and Figure 13.3).

An endovascular approach could also be used for graft angioplasty in the case of recurrent symptoms after surgical repair (Figure 13.4).

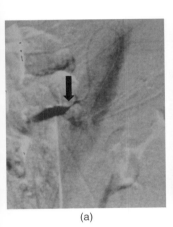

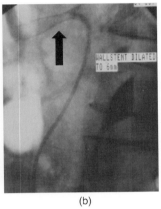

(a) (b)

Figure 13.2 (a) Tight stenosis at the origin of coeliac artery, (b) successful angioplasty and stent deployment.

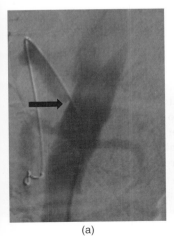

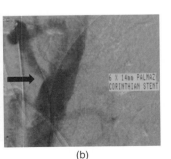

(a) (b)

Figure 13.3 (a) Tight stenosis at the origin of the superior mesenteric artery (SMA), (b) successful angioplasty and stent insertion.

Table 13.3 A comparison of surgical and endovascular repairs

	Surgical repair		Endovascular repair
	Endarterectomy	**Bypass**	
Suitable lesions	Osteal lesions	Lesions 1–2 cm from the origin	Stenotic or short occlusive lesions
Success rate	Initial success 93%	90–100% success	80–100% success
Suitable arteries	Suitable for CA, SMA and associated renal artery stenosis	Suitable for CA, SMA and IMA stenosis	Suitable for renal artery, CA, SMA, IMA and graft stenosis
Complications	30–60%		10–30%
Perioperative mortality	5–10%		0–5%
Primary patency	60–80%		60–90%
Recurrent symptoms	10–40%		10–50%
Re-intervention at 1 year	7–20%		8–20%

CA, coeliac axis; SMA, superior mesenteric artery; IMA inferior mesenteric artery.

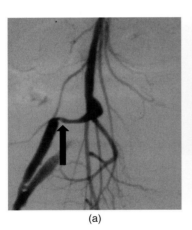
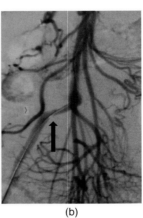

(a) (b)

Figure 13.4 (a) Tight stenosis in vein graft 18 months after surgery, (b) successful graft angioplasty.

Endovascular mesenteric revascularization has been associated with high immediate technical success of 91% ± 8% with immediate symptom relief in 79% ± 9%. Complications occurred in 18% of cases with a periprocedural mortality rate of 4%. Subjective long-term pain relief was found in 72% ± 10% with a radiographic patency of 70% ± 18% [9].

In a review of their practice during 14 years, the Mayo Clinic Group examined the results of 229 patients undergoing surgery or PTA/stent for CMI. They found that open repair was associated with higher morbidity and longer hospitalization. However, periprocedural mortality was not statistically significant (2.5% surgery versus 3.6% PTA). They reported that patients undergoing PTA/stent were five times more likely to develop restenosis, seven times more likely to have recurrent symptoms, and four times more likely to undergo reintervention. They concluded that surgical repair was the preferred first-line treatment in good-risk patients and that PTA/stent was reserved for those at increased risk from surgery (Table 13.3) [10].

Conclusion

Although uncommon, CMI remains an important cause of abdominal pain that may lead to serious consequences if misdiagnosed. The clinician has to have a high degree of suspicion for its early detection. Diagnosis requires good history taking, physical examination and diagnostic testing. Non-invasive investigations, CTA or MRA, are replacing the traditional angiography as the standard investigation with high levels of accuracy and less side effects. Whenever indicated, the minimally invasive endovascular approach should be attempted and if there is restenosis or recurrence of symptoms, standard open surgical repair is the definitive therapy.

References

1. Hansen KJ, Wilson DB, Craven TE et al. Mesenteric artery disease in the elderly. *J Vasc Surg* 2004; **40**: 45–52.
2. Van Bockel JH, Geelkerken RH, Wasser MN. Chronic splanchnic ischaemia. *Best Practice Res Clin Gastroenterol* 2001; **15**: 99–119.
3. Zwolak RM. Can duplex ultrasound replace arteriography in screening for mesenteric ischaemia? *Semin Vasc Surg* 1999; **12**: 252–60.
4. Kirkpatrick ID, Kroeker MA, Greenberg HM. Biphasic CT with mesenteric CT angiography in the valuation of acute mesenteric ischaemia: initial experience. *Radiology* 2003; **229**: 91–98.
5. Laissy JP, Trillaud H, Douek P. MR angiography: noninvasive vascular imaging of the abdomen. *Abdom Imaging* 2002; **27**: 488–506.
6. Lau H, Chew DK, Whittemore AD et al. Transaortic endarterectomy for primary mesenteric revascularization. *Vasc Endovasc Surg* 2002; **36**: 335–41.
7. Kansal N, Logerfo F, Belfield A et al. A comparison of antegrade and retrograde mesenteric bypass. *Ann Vasc Surg* 2002; **16**: 591–6.
8. Cho JS, Carr JA, Jacobsen G et al. Long-term outcome after mesenteric artery reconstruction: a 37-year experience. *J Vasc Surg* 2002; **35**: 453–60.
9. Kasirajan K, O'Hara PJ, Gray BH et al. Chronic mesenteric ischaemia: open surgery versus percutaneous angioplasty and stenting. *J Vasc Surg* 2001; **33**: 63–71.
10. Oderich GS, Bower TC, Misra S et al. Open versus endovascular revascularization for chronic mesenteric ischaemia: risk stratified outcomes. Society for Vascular Surgery Annual Meeting, Philadelphia, PA, 3 June 2006.

Final FRCS vascular topics

Acute ischaemic colitis

Vish Bhattacharya and Gerard Stansby

Key points

- Acute ischaemic colitis can be due to occlusive or non-occlusive causes
- A high index of suspicion should be present in elderly patients presenting with sudden abdominal pain and bloody diarrhoea
- Computed tomography (CT) scan may show a 'halo sign' and also rule out other abnormalities
- D-Lactate is more specific for intestinal ischaemia than L-Lactate
- Angiography and lysis may be considered in early cases with no sign of peritonitis
- In case of bowel resection primary anastomosis is best avoided and a re-look laparotomy recommended
- Postaneurysm repair colitis can be prevented by selective reimplantaion of the inferior mesenteric artery (IMA) in high risk cases

Introduction

Ischaemic colitis is the result of an event that leads to a reduction in colonic blood flow sufficient to cause ischaemia or infarction of the colonic wall but not sufficient to produce full thickness infarction and perforation.

The term ischaemic colitis was first introduced by Marston et al. [1] in 1966. It is commonly due to acute thrombosis or embolism of the superior mesenteric artery (SMA) or IMA, causing compromise of the colonic blood supply or due to hypotension causing hypoperfusion and ischaemia.

The term is often used for cases where full thickness infarction is present acutely but this usage is incorrect – not all ischaemic colons have ischaemic colitis, although the two may coexist if the involvement is patchy.

Pathophysiology

The following causes predispose the colon to ischaemia more readily than the small bowel:

1. The colon differs from the small bowel in having no villi and therefore no countercurrent mechanism.
2. The overall blood supplied per gram of tissue is lower in the colon compared to the small bowel.

Postgraduate Vascular Surgery: The Candidate's Guide to the FRCS, eds. Vish Bhattacharya and Gerard Stansby. Published by Cambridge University Press. © Cambridge University Press 2010.

3. The mucosa may be relatively hypoperfused in conditions of low cardiac output because it is at the end of the microvascular arcades supplying the colonic wall.
4. There is decreased capacity for autoregulation, especially when the perfusion pressure is lower than 50–60 mmHg [2].
5. In periods of physiological or surgical stress blood is shunted away from the splanchnic circulation as part of the physiological responses to shock and vasoconstrictors.

The ischaemic colonic mucosa loses its barrier function rapidly allowing invasion by luminal bacteria and absorption of endotoxins. In less severe cases inflammatory cytokine release may contribute to multiple organ failure with renal and respiratory impairment. The mucosa may also slough in a patchy fashion and this can result in increased peristalsis and diarrhoea mixed with blood. In the more severe forms of the condition, bacterial invasion leads to portal pyaemia and death.

The gut mucosa is rich in the enzyme xanthine dehyrogenase, which results in the production of reactive oxygen species and free radicals, such as superoxide. This causes oxidative tissue damage, which is actually most severe when reperfusion follows a period of ischaemia.

This reperfusion injury also results in the activation of polymorphonuclear leucocytes, which then result in systemic events, which may potentially lead to tissue injury and systemic inflammatory response syndrome (SIRS). In addition endothelin 1 (ET-1), a potent vasoconstrictor, is released following ischaemia and reperfusion and may lead to splanchnic vasoconstriction, thus further exacerbating the situation.

Aetiology

The following causes lead to ischaemic colitis:

1. Occlusive vascular disease of the major vessels due to embolism, thrombosis, trauma or surgical ligation.
2. Low perfusion states with low cardiac output, e.g. in cardiogenic or septic shock.
3. Mesenteric venous occlusive disease, where increased venous resistance leads to impaired microcirculatory arterial perfusion, e.g. in portal hypertension, mesenteric venous thrombosis or sequestration of red cells in sickle cell disease.
4. Drug induced ischaemic colitis due to cocaine, catecholamines, oral contraceptives [3], phenobarital and sumitriptan.
5. Hypercoagulability states caused by dehydration and physiological shunting, e.g. in marathon runners [4].
6. Small vessel disease, e.g. in acute pancreatitis, polyarteritis nodosa, systemic lupus erythematosus, Wegener's granulomatosis.

Anatomical factors

The colon is normally supplied by the SMA and IMA, with some contributions from the internal iliac arteries via the superior haemorrhoidal vessels. This anatomical arrangement usually allows for free collateralisation between the coeliac, SMA and IMA territories, such that occlusion of individual vessels does not necessarily result in ischaemia.

Important in the collateral pathways between SMA and IMA territories is the marginal artery of Drummond, which runs along the splenic flexure and the Arc of Riolan forming a collateral between the left colic artery and the SMA (meandering mesenteric artery). These collaterals may not always be adequate, either because of congenital variations or previous surgery. In acute conditions, for example after surgery or myocardial infarction, there may be no time for collaterals to form.

The internal iliac arteries provide an important collateral supply to the IMA territory of the rectum and descending colon via the middle and inferior haemorrhoidal vessels.

The watershed between the areas of the colon supplied by the SMA and IMA is usually described to be between the proximal two thirds and distal third of the transverse colon, based on the embryological division between the mid- and hind-gut. This anatomical arrangement explains the vulnerability of the splenic flexure to ischaemia. However in the arteriopath with an occluded inferior mesenteric artery the watershed point will be shifted distally towards the rectum.

In up to 50% of people the marginal artery of the colon may be poorly developed and this may result in right-sided ischaemic colitis. Right colonic involvement appears to be associated with severe forms of ischaemic colitis and occurs frequently in patients with chronic cardiac disease, such as aortic stenosis and in patients with chronic renal failure requiring haemodialysis.

Clinical features

The typical presentation is of an elderly man with a history of vascular disease complaining of abdominal pain and tenderness with bloody diarrhoea.

Mild degrees of ischaemic colitis may in fact be subclinical and never diagnosed. Clinically evident ischaemic colitis appears to affect 1–2% of patients after aortic surgery but it is found more frequently if colonoscopy or biopsy evidence is sought. In a study by Welch et al. [5] where colonoscopy and biopsies were performed post-aortic surgery a surprisingly high 30% were found to have features of ischaemic colitis on biopsy, although virtually all of these were asymptomatic. If only the submucosa and mucosa are involved then the presentation is more likely to be mild. If the muscularis is involved then symptoms are likely to be worse and the colitis may fail to resolve or cause subsequent stricture formation.

Full thickness infarction of the muscularis can lead to perforation and peritonitis. This situation should not be classified as true ischaemic colitis, but most series do include 10–20% of such cases, presumably reflecting the fact that full thickness infarcts and true ischaemic colitis can coexist in a patchy fashion.

Differential diagnosis

This includes infective colitis, pseudomembranous colitis due to *Clostridium difficile* toxin, inflammatory bowel disease, an acute diverticulitis and radiation colitis.

Perhaps the most common diagnostic dilemma is between *C. difficile* colitis and ischaemic colitis in the postoperative patient where *C. difficile* is probably more common.

C. difficile can be tested by detecting the toxin A and/or B in a fresh or frozen stool sample. Biopsy specimens may show diffuse pseudomembranes in *C. difficile*. Hyalization and haemorrhage in the lamina propria along and atrophic micro crypts and a diffuse microscopic distribution of pseudomembranes are more commonly seen in ischaemic colitis [6]. Full-thickness mucosal necrosis is also significantly more common in ischaemia than *C. difficile*.

Escherichia coli 0157 may cause a haemorrhagic colitis resembling ischaemic colitis. In addition it may also be a cause of ischaemic colitis by causing thrombosis in the colonic vessels as a secondary event.

Investigations

The diagnosis of ischaemic colitis requires a high index of clinical suspicion and confirmation by further investigations.

Plain X-ray

Plain X-ray of the abdomen may show fluid levels in the colon, toxic colonic dilatation, intramural gas, or free gas if a perforation has occurred. In severe cases intraportal air may be seen, a finding that suggests an outcome with a high mortality. In the postoperative patient it may help to exclude mechanical obstruction or indicate the need for laparotomy.

Stool culture

Stool samples should be sent for microscopy for ova cysts and parasites, culture and sensitivity and for analysis for *C. difficile* toxin.

Endoscopic examination

Sigmoidoscopy may reveal blood in the lumen but the mucosa may appear normal at this point if the 'watershed zone' is higher up. If the mucosa appears macroscopically normal but ischaemic colitis is suspected, mucosal biopsies should be taken.

Colonoscopy will determine the extent of ischaemia and may need to be undertaken in an unprepared bowel if the patient is unwell. Examination will determine the extent of the ischaemia. In mild disease the mucosa has a pale appearance with petechiae. In more severe disease the mucosa may be blue or black with slough and ulceration. Colonoscopy can help diagnose ischaemic colitis, but cannot separate transmural from mucosal ischaemia.

Barium enema

An instant enema may reveal thumb printing due to mucosal oedema. However, endoscopy with biopsy is preferable as a means of investigation, if available.

Computed tomography (CT)/magnetic resonance imaging (MRI) scanning

These may be normal in the early stages of ischaemic colitis or show non-specific thickening or oedema with a 'double halo' or 'target' appearance. CT can be used to confirm the clinical suspicion of ischaemic colitis and to diagnose complications. In ischaemic colitis, CT typically demonstrates circumferential, symmetric wall thickening with fold enlargement. CT may also demonstrate a thrombus in the mesenteric vessel, toxic megacolon or gas in the colonic wall. Modern spiral CT may also allow assessment of patency of visceral vessels as may gadolinium-enhanced magnetic resonance angiography (MRA).

Blood gases

In severe intestinal infarction the patient will develop a metabolic acidosis with a large base excess and low pH. However, these metabolic changes are usually signs of advanced full thickness infarction rather than ischaemic colitis.

L-lactate is produced by all cells as a product of glycolysis and is produced in excess during conditions of hypoxia. Raised levels of L-lactate are therefore related to inadequate tissue perfusion. However since L-lactate from the intestine is mostly removed by the liver it is not usually helpful in the diagnosis of ischaemic colitis, although it may be raised in colonic infarction. D-Lactate is produced by intestinal bacteria and may be more predictive of colonic ischaemia after aortic surgery than L-lactate, although there has been no prospective study.

Angiography/Duplex scanning

Angiography and Duplex scanning of mesenteric vessels are rarely helpful or diagnostic for ischaemic colitis in the acute situation.

Management

Conservative

Conservative management is appropriate in most patients if they are clinically stable and there are no signs of full thickness involvement or peritonitis. Patients should be given intravenous fluids and antibiotics and be carefully monitored. If there are conditions predisposing to intestinal ischaemia, such as hypercoagulability, they should be treated.

Pharmacological

A number of pharmacological treatments have been shown experimentally to improve intestinal blood flow, such as glucagon and prostanoid infusions, but are not widely used clinically. Early colonoscopy should be carried out to confirm the diagnosis. The question of angiography and other investigations remains controversial. In the case of a patient who appears to be settling and who is systemically well, intervention is probably best avoided.

Surgical

In a patient who continues with significant bowel disturbance or systemic symptoms angiography may be considered in order to assess the visceral circulation. If there is a significant stenosis or occlusion of visceral arteries then thrombolysis followed by angioplasty may be considered. Thrombolytic therapy should be undertaken within 8 hours of onset of symptoms and only if there is no sign of peritonitis or bowel necrosis. Angioplasty may be considered if there is any stenosis of the SMA. Heparin should be given concomitantly, provided there is no bowel necrosis.

In cases with embolic acute myocardial infarction (AMI), where lysis is not indicated, surgical embolectomy can be carried out. A transverse arteriotomy is made and the clot removed. If the embolectomy fails, an aorto bi-iliac graft can be inserted.

Patients who have peritonitis or who deteriorate should have a laparotomy with resection of the ischaemic segment and both ends of the bowel should be brought out as stomas. A primary anastomosis is probably always best avoided when the colon is involved. If attempted then the anastomosis certainly should be covered by a defunctioning stoma. Re-look laparotomy the following day should also be considered. Although there is a high-associated mortality, in patients who survive it is often possible to reverse the stoma at a later date [7].

Mortality rates in patients requiring emergency surgery for peritonitis and resection of ischaemic bowel may be as high as 50%. This is due to the associated comorbid medical conditions including peripheral vascular disease, ischaemic heart disease and cerebrovascular disease. If the original surgery has involved aortic grafting then there is also a high risk of subsequent graft infection.

Colonic stricture may develop as a late complication of ischaemic colitis, especially where the muscularis has been involved. Clinically these patients will typically present with features of subacute obstruction. Bowel resection and anastamosis for these strictures may lead to anastomotic dehiscence in cases where there has been an occlusive aetiology.

As postaortic ischaemic colitis is commonly seen this will be discussed in detail below.

Ischaemic colitis after aortic surgery

The single commonest cause of ischaemic colitis is postaortic surgery where a combination of inferior mesenteric occlusion, postoperative hypoxia or hypotension and a vulnerable, elderly patient are predisposing factors.

Incidence

The incidence of this condition is of the order of 1–2% in most series. In ruptured aortic aneurysm repair, however, the incidence is much higher, up to 30%. Studies with colonoscopy or sigmoidoscopy have, however, shown an even higher incidence: 7–35% of elective cases and up to 60% of survivors of ruptured aneurysm repair.

Fanti et al. [8] reported a series of 105 patients who underwent rectosigmoidoscopy within 72 hours of aortic surgery. Colonic ischaemia was found in 12 patients but 7 were asymptomatic and all were managed conservatively.

Welch et al. studied a group of patients undergoing elective aortic surgery with pre- and postoperative colonoscopy with biopsy in order to assess the true incidence of the condition [5]. They studied 28 patients each in two groups having aneurysm repair and reconstruction for occlusive aortoiliac disease, respectively. Postoperative colonoscopy and biopsy was carried out at one week. All patients had normal appearances and biopsies before surgery. Postoperatively, however, 30% had features of ischaemic colitis upon biopsy. Interestingly there was no difference in the incidence of this finding between those with occlusive and those with aneurysmal disease.

It has also been described following aortic stent grafting.

Risk factors

Renal disease, emergency surgery, age, type of hospital, aortobifemoral graft, operating time, cross-clamping time and ligation of one or both internal iliac arteries are independent risk factors for developing ischaemic colitis. Duration of hypotension, temperature less than $35°C$, pH <7.3, fluid requirement of >5 l and packed red cells >6 units have been found to be predictive of ischaemic colonic complications following ruptured aortic aneurysm repair.

Ischaemic colitis after aortic surgery may be due to interruption to colonic blood supply due to division of the IMA, hypotension and hypoxia in the perioperative period and stenosis of other visceral vessels due to the underlying atherosclerotic disease process. Inferior mesenteric artery ligation is probably the most important factor in the majority of cases. Other possible factors include embolisation into the IMA territory during dissection of the aneurysm, injury to mesenteric vessels by retractors and mesenteric compression by haematoma.

Prevention

As postoperative ischaemic colitis occurs in an unpredictable fashion there are no clear guidelines as to how surgeons may avoid its development. The normal IMA is not well demonstrated at routine angiography and preoperative angiography may demonstrate only the occasional at-risk patient with enlarged collaterals. Routine angiography can therefore not be justified in all patients undergoing aortic surgery.

Various suggestions have been made to either reimplant the patent IMA routinely, or selectively based on stump pressure, Doppler and intraoperative inspection.

Seeger et al. [9] reimplanted all patent IMAs routinely in 151 aortic reconstructions. None of the patients developed colonic infarction compared with 2.7% of patients in the previous series of 186 patients where reimplantation was done based on stump pressure, Doppler and inspection.

Killen et al. [10] used IMA stump pressure of less than 50 mmHg as an indicator for implantation of the IMA. However this did not improve the incidence of ischaemic colitis in his series.

Routine reimplantation of IMAs may increase the risk of bleeding from the anastomosis, is technically demanding and takes extra time. However this is recommended in patients whose preoperative angiography has shown occlusion or stenosis of the SMA. This is also recommended if neither of the internal iliacs is reconstructed and the colon appears ischaemic at the end of the operation.

In summary the following steps can prevent this complication after aneurysm repair:

1. At least one internal iliac artery should be revascularised whenever possible.
2. Blood pressure and oxygen levels should be maintained as any fall may be critical in patients with an already compromised colonic mucosal perfusion.
3. Inspection of the colon after surgery is important, although confounding factors such as hypovolemia, hypotension and the use of inotropes can make this unreliable.
4. Selective reimplantation of the IMA in high-risk patients as mentioned above.

Conclusion

Acute mesenteric ischemia is a serious condition associated with a 60–80% mortality. The SMA is the main vessel usually involved in 85% of cases. CT angiography with three-dimensional reconstruction is the diagnostic tool of choice. Conventional angiography is only useful if this is associated with thrombolysis and or stenting.

The elderly are most commonly affected due to their higher incidence of underlying systemic pathology, most notably atherosclerotic cardiovascular disease. A high index of suspicion should be present, especially in the elderly arteriopath presenting with abdominal pain. Early recognition and an aggressive therapeutic approach are essential if the usually poor outcome is to be improved. Blood pressure support typically involves careful, but often massive, fluid resuscitation and pharmacologic support. Thrombolysis and stenting have a limited role and only in the early hours of diagnosis. A second look laparoscopy or laparotomy is indicated in the case of bowel resection.

References

1. Marston A, Pheils MT, Thomas ML, Morson BC. Ischaemic colitis. *Gut* 1966; 7: 1–15.
2. Kvietys PR, Granger DN. Physiology, pharmacology and pathology of the colonic circulation. In: Shepherd AP, Granger DN, eds. *Physiology of the Intestinal Circulation*. New York: Raven Press, 1984.
3. Mann DE Jr, Kessel ER, Mullins DL, Lottenberg R. Ischemic colitis and acquired resistance to activated protein C in a

woman using oral contraceptives. *Am J Gastroenterol* 1998; **93**: 1960–2.

4. Lucas W, Schroy PC 3rd. Reversible ischaemic colitis in a high endurance athlete. *Am J Gastroenterol.* 1998; **93**: 2231–4.

5. Welch M, Baguneid MS, McMahon RF et al. Histological study of colonic ischaemia after aortic surgery. *Br J Surg* 1998; **85**: 1095–8.

6. Dignan CR, Greenson JK. Can ischaemic colitis be differentiated from *C difficile* colitis in biopsy specimens? *Am J Surg Pathol* 1997; **21**: 706–10.

7. Longo WE, Ward D, Vernava AM 3rd, Kaminski DL. Outcome of patients with total colonic ischaemia. *Dis Colon Rectum* 1997; **40**: 1448–54.

8. Fanti L, Masci E, Mariani A et al. Is endoscopy useful for early diagnosis of ischaemic colitis after aortic surgery? Results of a prospective trial. *Ital J Gastroenterol Hepatol* 1997; **29**: 357–60.

9. Seeger JM, Coe DA, Kaelin LD, Flynn TC. Routine reimplantation of patent inferior mesenteric arteries limits colon infarction after aortic reconstruction. *J Vasc Surg* 1992; **15**: 635–41.

10. Killen DA, Reed WA, Gorton ME et al. Is routine postaneurysmectomy hemodynamic assessment of the inferior mesenteric artery circulation helpful? *Ann Vasc Surg* 1999; **13**: 533–8.

Final FRCS vascular topics

Vascular trauma

Robbie George and Paul Blair

Key points

- Remember the whole patient, do not just focus on the vascular injury
- Time is of the essence, avoid delay
- Do not attempt to mobilise large veins, use local pressure
- Consider temporary intravascular shunts in complex limb injuries
- Consider damage limitation surgery in patients developing hypothermia or acidosis

Trauma is a leading cause of mortality in the first four decades of life. Vascular surgeons are often involved in the management of a multiply-injured patient who may have limb- and/or life-threatening vascular injuries. In addition the extended range of procedures carried out by open and minimally invasive surgical and radiological techniques has created its own unique set of vascular injuries. It is beyond the scope of this short chapter to deal with specific vascular injuries in detail, however, general principles will be discussed with specific details given in the more common sites of injury.

General considerations

Vascular trauma can occur as a result of a variety of mechanisms including penetrating, blunt, crush, irradiation and a variety of iatrogenic injuries. The majority of penetrating injuries in civilian life in the UK are caused by knives or low-velocity handguns. Penetrating injuries in military and terrorist theatres are more often associated with high-velocity weapons, bombs and missiles, the latter can cause extensive tissue damage due to a combination of blast and shrapnel injuries.

Blunt vascular trauma is usually seen following road traffic accidents, falls, building collapses, major disasters, etc.

Time is of the essence when dealing with vascular trauma and the need for early control of haemorrhage and restoration of blood flow must be balanced with potential delay caused by over investigation. Patients should be managed along the principles of the Advanced Trauma Life Support (ATLS) system as is it important not to miss occult torso injuries. Rapid exsanguinating local haemorrhage is best controlled with local pressure. The use of vascular clamps should be avoided in the emergency department. A small but significant number of trauma patients may benefit from immediate transfer to the operating room without further investigation (see Table 15.1).

Postgraduate Vascular Surgery: The Candidate's Guide to the FRCS, eds. Vish Bhattacharya and Gerard Stansby. Published by Cambridge University Press. © Cambridge University Press 2010.

Table 15.1 Indications for immediate transfer to the operating room

Cardiopulmonary resuscitation (CPR) in progress and penetrating torso injury
Systolic blood pressure <90 after 2 l of fluid
Major amputation of hip/shoulder
Major complex wounds and hypotension

Limb trauma

Pathophysiology

Distal ischaemia can result from a wide range of arterial injury, including complete transection or laceration of vessels, contusions and haematomas, dissections, thromboses, occlusion by haematoma from adjacent injury, false aneurysms and delayed presentation of arteriovenous fistula.

Arterial injury affects distal flow and results in ischaemia and tissue hypoxia. Striated muscle will likely undergo irreversible damage if warm ischaemia time exceeds 6–8 hours and may result in multi-organ dysfunction as well. Limb ischaemia is associated with oedema; tight fascial compartments can cause a further fall in perfusion pressure with worsening of ischaemia resulting in compartment syndrome. Revascularisation of ischaemic limbs can result in significant ischaemia reperfusion injury and rapidly destabilize an already unwell patient as toxic metabolites are washed out. Although the upper limb will tolerate a prolonged period of warm ischaemia, >6 hours ischaemia is poorly tolerated in the lower limb. Revascularisation of a non-viable limb is futile and hazardous for the patient.

Initial assessment and management

Clinical signs of limb vascular injuries can be classified into hard and soft signs. See Table 15.2. The majority of patients with a single-level penetrating injury and one hard sign should be transferred immediately to the operating theatre, without further imaging, for immediate exploration. Exceptions to this rule include:

- proximal upper limb injuries with suspected subclavian or axillary artery involvement;
- extensive bone or soft tissue injury;
- close range shotgun injuries or multiple entry wounds;
- elderly patients with co-existing peripheral vascular disease (PVD).

Other issues to be considered:

- Is there any neurological deficit associated with the trauma?
- Is the limb salvageable? Various scores such as the Mangled Extremity Severity Score (MESS) are in use. They are good predictors of likely limb salvage but not of likely limb loss [1].
- Duration since injury, i.e. warm ischaemia time.
- Any features of compartment syndrome – is the arm/calf soft.

Investigations [2]

It can be difficult to assess distal limb perfusion in a hypothermic, hypovolaemic, multiply-injured patient. Hand-held Doppler can be helpful but should be used with caution. Accuracy

Table 15.2 Clinical signs of vascular injury in a limb

Hard signs	Soft signs
Absent pulses	Pulses present but decreased (compare with opposite limb and/or measure ankle brachial pressure index)
Arterial thrill or bruit over or near the artery	History of haemorrhage at the scene
Observed pulsatile bleeding	Unexplained hypotension
Signs of distal ischaemia	Peripheral nerve deficit
Haematoma (large or expanding)	

is improved significantly when formal ankle brachial pressure index (ABPI) measurements are performed. An ABPI of <0.9 should raise the suspicion of an upstream vascular compromise. Stable patients with hard signs of vascular trauma, not falling into the urgent category (Table 15.1), or those patients with single-level penetrating injury and hard sign of vascular trauma, may be investigated in a more timely fashion.

Computed tomography (CT) is widely available and can provide superb contrast resolution with the additional visualisation of non-vascular structures, particularly useful in the investigation of a trauma patient. Multi-slice technology has further expanded the image quality of run-off vessels, although images can be sub-optimal. Catheter-directed angiography remains the gold standard, particularly if therapeutic interventional procedures are required. The development of endovascular surgery has improved the quality of digital subtraction angiography (DSA) available in the operating theatre.

The investigation of patients with soft signs of vascular trauma is more controversial. The majority of publications, in the literature, concerning investigation of such patients, are often produced from high volume North American or South African trauma centres and are, therefore, not always applicable to the UK where the incidence of vascular trauma is relatively low. While it is not appropriate to over-investigate patients, once the suspicion of a vascular injury is raised it should be excluded by appropriate imaging. There is a high incidence of occult arterial injury with posterior knee dislocations and investigations should be utilised freely in this situation. Over-investigation of penetrating proximity injury, with 'soft signs', should be balanced with the risk of late sequelae of missed injuries such as false aneurysms and arteriovenous fistulae.

General principles of arterial repair

Prior to exploring any vascular injury, proximal and distal control must be attempted, with the use of additional axial incisions if required. Major bleeds from the femoral vessels in the groin are best controlled by direct pressure until proximal control of the external iliac vessels is obtained via an extraperitoneal approach in the iliac fossa. The contralateral limb should be prepped in case great saphenous vein (GSV) harvest is required and the abdomen should also be prepped in case iliac control is required. Axillary artery injuries may require proximal control of the subclavian artery in the supraclavicular space while the axillary artery itself is approached through an incision just below the clavicle with division/separation of pectoralis fibres. Axillary and subclavian artery injuries should be approached with care due to the close association of the brachial plexus. Embolectomy catheters may be employed to gain temporary proximal control.

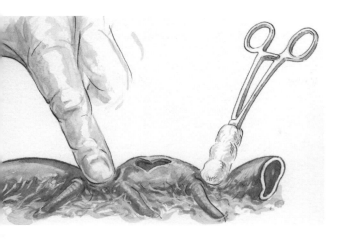

Figure 15.1 Proximal and distal compression using fingers and swabs in venous injury.

In complex limb injury, or delayed management of simple arterial injury, the use of a temporary intravascular shunt should be considered [3, 4]. This allows early restoration of tissue perfusion prior to a planned arterial repair with appropriate soft tissue cover. It is important to have a healthy vessel exposed proximally and distally, particularly in crush injury, and a gentle distal embolectomy should be performed to remove distal thrombus prior to shunt insertion. Temporary intraluminal shunts may also be employed in venous injury although this is rarely required. Once the shunt is in place, associated damage to bone, nerve, muscles and skin can be fully assessed and may require the presence of an orthopaedic and plastic surgeon. If there is an associated fracture, bony stability via internal or external fixation can be achieved with the shunt in place. This allows stability prior to definitive arterial and/or venous repair. Intravenous heparin may be employed although is best avoided in unstable hypovolaemic trauma patients.

Arterial repair can be in the form of lateral suture, patch angioplasty or some form of arterial graft. Patch angioplasty can be difficult in a young patient, due to spasm, and if in doubt a short segment GSV graft is the operation of choice. It is the authors' opinion that resection of a damaged vessel with end-to-end anastomosis is rarely possible and an interposition graft is preferable. In the majority of cases GSV should be harvested from the contralateral limb in case of deep vein damage in the traumatised limb. The majority of venous injuries require lateral suturing or occasionally ligation. Venous repair is rarely required in the upper limb but may be required in the lower limb at popliteal level. Complex venous repair employing panel or spiral grafts is best avoided in the majority of trauma patients.

Limb distal vessel injury

Isolated distal radial or ulnar artery injuries can be ligated if collateral circulation, as assessed by Allen's test, is adequate. However, they frequently need exploration because of the risk of associated nerve injury. Isolated lower limb crural vessel injury rarely requires repair and may be ligated in the majority of cases. If both anterior and posterior tibial vessels have been transected in a young patient, attempts should be made to repair at least one of them, preferably the posterior tibial artery. Achieving tissue cover for the vascular repair is critical to success. Use of soft tissue flaps and involvement of the plastic surgeons is very helpful. In extensive soft tissue loss extra-anatomic bypasses may be utilised.

Fasciotomies should be used liberally as compartmental hypertension from a combina tion of ischaemic damage, direct trauma, haematomas and third space losses associated with trauma can all compromise blood flow.

Strong indications for fasciotomy include an ischaemia time greater than 6 hours major artery and vein injury, significant soft tissue injury or evidence of muscle damage proximal half of below-knee vascular tree injury or compartment pressures of greater than 40 mmHg.

Vascular injuries of the chest [5, 6]

Thoracic vascular injuries may occur in road traffic accidents associated with rapid decelera tion. They may also result from penetrating and gunshot wounds.

Diagnosis and assessment

Penetrating thoracic vascular injuries may be obvious while major vascular injury in the setting of blunt trauma is typically one component of polytrauma and must always be sus pected. Following a major deceleration injury or gunshot wound a combination of severe interscapular pain, decreased air entry and dullness in the chest, with reduced or diminished pulses, is highly suggestive of free aortic rupture.

Hypotension and other major signs of significant blood loss may not be seen in a patient with a contained rupture. Dissection or partial laceration of the aortic wall may be contained by spasm and surrounding mediastinal tissues. This, however, is a very temporary situation and it is imperative to detect and treat the injury as soon as possible. The clinical triad of grossly widened mediastinum on chest X-ray, haemothorax and transient hemodynamic instability is highly indicative of aortic injury. Aortic injuries can be associated with a 2–3% incidence of paraplegia resulting from spinal cord ischaemia.

Investigations

Chest X-ray should be part of the adjuncts to primary survey in the management of al trauma patients and the signs of aortic injury include a widened mediastinum, loss of aortic knuckle, apical cap, depression of left main bronchus and deviation of the trachea/nasogas tric tube to the right.

If a vascular injury is suspected the next investigation should be contrast enhanced helical CT. Transoesophageal echocardiography and arch aortography are other useful modalities. The choice of investigation is dictated by the hemodynamic state, other injuries, local avail ability and expertise.

Management

A rapid rise in blood pressure in these patients may convert a contained rupture into a free rupture, resulting in rapid exsanguinations and death. A regime of permissive hypotension, where the aim is to maintain cerebral perfusion rather than a normal blood pressure, is followed. In the conscious patient this is easy to implement, in unconscious or intubated patients a systolic pressure of 70–80 mmHg is probably acceptable.

Injuries presenting with features of free bleeding need minimum investigations and should quickly proceed to resuscitative surgery. In more contained situations the airway and cervical spine should be secured and cardiac tamponade and tension pneumothorax relieved prior to transfer to a trauma centre. No attempt should be made to drain a haemothorax unless there is respiratory compromise.

Operative management

In penetrating trauma, surgical intervention is required in the presence of cardiac arrest, significant or sustained haemorrhage from the chest, mediastinal traversing injury, major vascular injury, sucking chest wound, persistent massive air leak or diaphragmatic rupture. In a minority of patients this might necessitate emergency room thoracotomy, however this is a procedure best carried out in the operating theatre.

Contained thoracic aortic rupture due to blunt trauma is managed by blood pressure control and treatment of other life threatening injuries with repair of the thoracic aorta on a semi-urgent basis. β-blockers are the drug of choice in this situation.

A recent meta-analysis of retrospective cohort studies indicates that endovascular treatment of descending thoracic aortic trauma is an alternative to open repair and is associated with lower postoperative mortality and ischaemic spinal cord complication rates [7].

Vascular injuries of the neck [8, 9]

Carotid artery injury accounts for approximately 10% of all vascular trauma with penetrating trauma responsible for 90% of cases. The carotid artery is most commonly involved in penetrating trauma with the vertebral artery more commonly damaged by blunt trauma. Mortality remains around 10–30% and in survivors permanent neurological sequelae are present in approximately 40%.

Diagnosis and assessment of penetrating neck vascular injuries

If a penetrating injury has breached the platysma, surgical exploration or arterial imaging is essential. Besides active bleeding, a cervical bruit or thrill or a rapidly expanding haematoma and an absent carotid pulse are diagnostic of carotid artery injury. It is essential to look for evidence of neurological deficits, which may be the result of vessel occlusion (contralateral deficits) or direct cranial nerve injuries (IX–XII). Associated head injuries, psychotropic substance or systemic hypotension and hypothermia may make neurological assessment difficult.

Investigations and management

Penetrating carotid injuries

Carotid artery injuries are classified into three zones and management is dependent on the zone of injury.

Zone 1 – injuries from clavicle to cricoid cartilage.
Zone 2 – injuries from cricoid to angle of mandible.
Zone 3 – injuries above the angle of mandible.

Surgical access in zone 1 and 3 injuries is problematic and, therefore, imaging is essential. The gold standard imaging modality is catheter angiography although CT angiography and occasionally Duplex may be employed. Catheter-directed angiography has the additional benefit of offering therapeutic endovascular interventions. Most patients, unless unstable will need further investigation to rule out concomitant aero-digestive tract injury.

Injuries with active bleeding, expanding cervical haematomas or airway compromise should undergo immediate surgical exploration. In such patients early control of the airway by intubation must be considered.

Management

Patients with minor angiography abnormalities, such as small pseudoaneurysms, small intimal defects and non-obstructive downstream intimal plaques may be managed non operatively with close follow up.

Patients with carotid artery occlusion on angiography and a dense neurological deficit due to brain infarct have a poor outcome, regardless of operative management.

Those with an occluded vessel but no neurological deficit should be managed with anti coagulation to prevent thrombus extension. High zone 3 injuries and those involving the vertebral artery may be best managed by endovascular methods, such as the use of embolisa tion and covered stents. Most other injuries seen on angiography are likely to need surgical intervention.

Operative management

The carotid artery is approached by an incision along the anterior border of the sternomas toid with the chest being prepped for access if needed. If possible proximal and distal control should be obtained prior to entering a haematoma although this may not always be possible. Digital pressure may be used prior to vessel control, but care should be taken to avoid dam aging the vagus, hypoglossal and recurrent laryngeal nerves. Repair is undertaken by suture patch or interposition or transposition grafting as required. Occasionally a thrombosed occluded vessel may be ligated to reduce the risk of embolic stroke. Thorough exploration of the aerodigestive tract is essential to ensure that no other injuries are missed.

Blunt carotid artery injury in the neck

Blunt injury may cause dissection and thrombosis of the carotid or, more commonly, ver tebral arteries. These injuries can be extremely difficult to diagnose and may be missed in up to two-thirds of patients. High-risk criteria for associated blunt cerebrovascular injuries include severe hyperextension, rotation or flexion of the neck, a significant anterior triangle haematoma or soft tissue injury, transient ischaemic attack (TIA) or stroke, cervical spine fracture (vertebral artery), seat belt around the neck, bruit or thrill and a basilar fracture involving the petrous bone (carotid artery). Occasionally patients develop transient neuro logical signs at the time of injury. There may be a classic history of a neurologically intact road traffic victim later developing hemiparesis or other lateralising neurological signs. Some patients may present with Horner's syndrome.

Catheter angiography is the diagnostic gold standard, though there is also a role for CT angiography and perhaps Duplex sonography. Imaging of the brain and spine is also essential.

The keystones of management are to optimise haemodynamics and anticoagulation. Hypotension must be avoided to prevent thromboses. Hypertension risks the development of an intimal flap and dissection. Systemic anticoagulation is the preferred treatment for most patients. Heparin or combinations of antiplatelets have both been utilised, with no clear benefit for either. Endovascular placements of stents may have a role in the management of pseudoaneurysms but their role in the management of dissections remains unclear. These patients need to be followed up with MRI to detect late onset false aneurysm formation.

Vertebral artery injuries

The majority of vertebral artery injuries are silent due to the vertebral artery's capacity for collateral flow. However in 2–3% of patients the contralateral artery may be hypoplastic, precipitating the development of neurological signs. Injuries occur rarely in the setting of penetrating trauma and are more commonly associated with cervical spine injuries.

Catheter angiography is usually required for diagnosis and, where possible, endovascular interventions are the treatment of choice, as surgical access can be very difficult.

Abdominal vascular trauma

Patients with significant abdominal vascular trauma are usually haemodynamically unstable with obvious signs of haemorrhage. A small group of patients, however, may present late with relatively subtle signs. Abdominal vascular trauma can present as hypovolaemia, limb ischaemia, anuria or obvious intraoperative haemorrhage. Most patients, unless extremely unstable, will have a contrast enhanced CT of the abdomen and pelvis. Resuscitation and diagnosis usually takes place simultaneously and unstable patients should proceed, without delay, to the operating room as stated in Table 15.1.

Stable patients, who have sustained blunt trauma following CT evaluation, may have attempted embolisation of arterial bleeding points i.e. those associated with pelvic fractures, distal renal artery injury and lumbar vessels. It is important, however, to exclude non-vascular injuries in these patients, e.g. occult bowel perforation.

Operative management

A standard mid-line laparotomy is performed with the patient prepped for additional thoracotomy if required. Initial assessment requires four quadrant packing and careful evaluation of injuries. If faced with uncontrollable haemorrhage, from multiple sites, control of the aorta at the diaphragmatic hiatus may be a useful manoeuvre. Mobilisation of the left lobe of liver is required and care must be taken to avoid damaging the oesophagus (more easily identified if a nasogastric [NG] tube has been inserted). Finger dissection of the diaphragmatic crus in a vertical plane is required before the aorta can be visualised and clamped in a vertical fashion. Formal vascular repair, in the abdomen, depends on the location of the injury and also the general condition of the patient. In the extremely unstable patient, principles of damage control surgery should be applied. The presence of metabolic acidosis, hypothermia and coagulopathy may preclude formal vascular repair. In such patients, packing the abdomen and pelvis, followed by a period of resuscitation in intensive care, may be entirely appropriate prior to second-look laparotomy.

Management of retroperitoneal haematomas

The decision to explore a retro-peritoneal haematoma depends on the mechanism of injury, stability of the patient and the appearance of the haematoma. Exploration of a retro-peritoneal haematoma can be challenging for an experienced vascular surgeon and it may be best to simply pack the area and wait for additional help to arrive. Retro-peritoneal haematomas, caused by penetrating trauma, require mandatory exploration, while a more selective policy may be employed for those caused by blunt trauma. They are classified into three zones - central, lateral and pelvic.

Central haematomas (zone 1) are always explored as the likely source of bleed is the great vessels, pancreas or duodenum. For suprarenal haematomas proximal control of the aorta is obtained at the diaphragmatic hiatus. The lesser sac is then opened to isolate the injury. If that fails left or right visceral rotation is carried out to expose the aorta or inferior vena cava (IVC), respectively. Infrarenal haematomas or those at the base of the mesentery are approached after infrarenal aortic control. Special care must be taken to avoid injury to the extremely delicate IVC, renal and iliac veins.

Lateral (zone 2) haematomas are likely of renal pedicle origin and should be explored if expanding or pulsatile or if there is radiological evidence of serious injury. Renal vessels should be controlled prior to opening the haematoma. Avulsed or lacerated renal arteries are best treated by using a saphenous graft although outcomes are often poor.

Pelvic fracture associated injuries (zone 3) can be due to torn pelvic veins or injury to the iliac vessels. In case of a pelvic fracture, fixation of the same is essential to reduce the pelvic volume and therefore blood loss. If the patient is reasonably stable following pelvic fracture fixation, investigation via catheter guided angiography may be particularly useful in achieving embolisation of arterial bleeders.

The retro-peritoneum often provides tamponade for zone 3 haematomas and if this is entered catastrophic blood loss may occur. When faced with uncontrollable venous haemorrhage in this situation damage limitation surgery and packing should be considered. If the haematoma is actively bleeding or expanding and pulsatile, especially with a missing pulse in the groin, it should be explored. Some of these injuries can be managed by endovascular means.

Mesenteric vessel injuries [10]

The superior mesenteric artery (SMA) proximal to the trunk of the middle colic should be repaired if at all possible or a saphenous graft taken off the aorta. Segmental branches to the small bowel can be ligated and in between injuries should be repaired or ligated, dependent on the patient's condition.

- Coeliac artery injuries will tolerate ligation but should be repaired if possible.
- IVC injuries are best controlled by direct pressure and suture repair where possible. For major uncontrollable haemorrhage IVC ligation is the best option and is well tolerated. Retrohepatic IVC injuries have over an 80% mortality. Patients may need a median sternotomy and atriocaval shunt or total occlusion of the portal system to achieve control and repair.
- Portal vein injuries are also associated with extremely high mortality. Where possible they should be repaired by direct suture or interposition grafting. Failing that ligation would be the best option.
- Renal vein injuries on the right side need repair as the right kidney does not tolerate ligation. On the left the vein can be ligated, providing drainage through collaterals to the gonadal and adrenal vein are preserved.
- Iliac vein injuries are treated by packing if associated with pelvic fractures. Where possible common or external iliac vein injuries should be repaired but ligation is a feasible option as well.

Delayed presentation abdominal vascular injury

Patients may present with a pulsatile mass suggestive of a pseudoaneurysm. GI haemorrhage may result from haemobilia secondary to liver injury or from false aneurysms eroding into the rectum, colon and duodenum. Aortocaval fistula can present with lower limb oedema and an arteriovenous bruit in the abdomen. They may present late with congestive heart failure and venous hypertension. The main investigation in this patient group is an angiogram and investigations of the involved organ.

Iatrogenic injuries

A wide scope of iatrogenic vascular injuries may occur as surgical advances continue.

Injuries of arterial or venous catheterisation and endovascular procedures

Arterial catheterisation and puncture may cause bleeding, stenosis or occlusion as a result of laceration, thromboembolism, dissection or foreign body occlusion. If recognised at the time of intervention numerous endovascular interventions in the form of angioplasty, covered stents etc. are available.

Major haemorrhage can occur especially if the back wall of the artery is perforated and a concealed bleed into the retroperitoneum occurs. If suspected after a groin puncture, and time allows, a quick CT scan will confirm the diagnosis. Most such injuries in the femoral artery can be explored and controlled from the groin.

Thromboembolic occlusion or dissection will require surgical exploration.

Pseudoaneurysms formed as a result of arterial catheterisation should proceed to surgical repair if there are any signs of active bleed or impending rupture. In stable patients Duplex sonography can confirm the diagnosis. Pseudoaneurysms < 2 cm in maximum diameter will likely respond to thrombin injection and compression.

Central venous line insertion can inadvertently puncture the subclavian artery or carotid artery. If the catheter is withdrawn, especially after a dilator has been used, significant bleeding can occur. A bleed from the carotid artery can rapidly cause airway compromise. If the carotid artery is punctured and dilated, it will need formal exploration and repair and the dilator should be left in place until control has been achieved. Surgical access to the subclavian artery can be especially difficult and endovascular solutions should be considered.

Endovascular procedures with catheters and balloons can also cause vascular trauma in the form of perforation and rupture of vessels distant from the site of puncture.

Immediate control can usually be achieved by balloon tamponade followed by surgical exploration.

Specific injuries of open surgery

Lumbar disc surgery, especially at L4/L5 level, can cause vascular injury to the aorta, IVC or iliac vessels. Significant intraoperative bleeding may necessitate an immediate laparotomy and repair. Patients can also present late with arteriovenous fistulae, which are ordinarily best dealt with by endovascular means.

Hip and knee surgery beside fracture fixation have all been associated with injury to major lower limb vascular structures. Vascular injuries after hip/knee arthroplasty/replacement are rare but have been known to result in amputations.

Varicose vein surgery has resulted in femoral vein injuries, ranging from laceration to stripping of the vein. Redo groin surgery and attempts to pass a vein stripper from distal to proximal are significant causative factors. Blind attempts at applying haemostats can make a bad situation worse. Compression will control bleeding until help is available. Repair may be by simple lateral suture, patch or interposition grafting.

Accidental injection of sclerosant into arteries can produce significant tissue damage. If that is suspected and the needle is still *in situ*, heparinised saline and an α-blocker should be injected through it.

Laparoscopic surgery and especially the creation of a pneumoperitoneum have been reported to cause major vascular trauma, which will require rapid recognition and treatment if a successful outcome is to be achieved.

Hepatic artery injury during cholecystectomy is often best dealt with by ligation, rather than attempts at repair. Significant hepatic damage is unlikely to occur because of the dual blood supply of the liver.

A variety of other vascular injuries have been reported in association with abdominal surgery, hernia repairs and gynaecological surgery among others. The application of the general principles and approaches to vessels should allow control of such injuries.

References

1. Ly TV, Travison TG, Castillo RC, Bosse MJ, MacKenzie EJ. LEAP Study Group. Ability of lower-extremity injury severity scores to predict functional outcome after limb salvage. *J Bone Joint Surg Am* 2008; **90**: 1738–43.

2. Fishman EK, Horton KM, Johnson PT. Multidetector CT and three-dimensional CT angiography for suspected vascular trauma of the extremities. *Radiographics* 2008; **28**: 653–65.

3. Barros D' Sa AA, Harkin DW, Blair PH, Hood JM, McIlrath E. The Belfast approach to managing complex lower limb vascular injuries. *Eur J Vasc Endovasc Surg* 2006; **32**: 246–56.

4. Taller J, Kamdar JP, Greene JA et al. Temporary vascular shunts as initial treatment of proximal extremity vascular injuries during combat operations: the new standard of care at Echelon II facilities? *J Trauma* 2008; **65**: 595–603.

5. Neschis D, Scalea T, Flinn W, Griffith B. Blunt aortic injury current concepts. *New Engl J Med* 2008; **359**: 1708–16.

6. Arthurs ZM, Sohn VY, Starnes BW. Vascular trauma: endovascular management and techniques. *Surg Clin N Am* 2007; **87**: 1179–92.

7. Xenos ES, Abedi NN, Davenport DL et al. Meta-analysis of endovascular vs open repair for traumatic descending thoracic aortic rupture. *J Vasc Surg* 2008; **48**: 1343–51.

8. Rathlev NK, Medzon R, Bracken ME. Evaluation and management of neck trauma. *Emerg Med Clin N Am* 2007; **25**: 679–94.

9. Newton EJ. Acute complications of extremity trauma. *Emerg Med Clin N Am* 2007; **25**: 751–61.

10. Asensio JA, Forno W, Roldán G et al. Visceral vascular injuries. *Surg Clin North Am* 2002; **82**: 1–20, xix.

16

Indications and management of lower limb amputation

Mark Kay and Colette Marshall

Key points

Peripheral vascular disease is the leading cause of amputation in the Western world

Diabetics are 8–12 times more likely to suffer amputation

Mortality and subsequent loss of the contralateral limb following amputation is high

The level of amputation requires careful consideration of the rehabilitative potential of the patient, level and pattern of vascular disease and likely healing

Careful preoperative assessment and periopertive care using the multidiscliplinary team is essential for successful outcomes

Epidural analgesia provides the best perioperative analgesia but does not prevent subsequent phantom pain

The general principles of amputation surgery apply to all sites of amputation

Rehabilitation of the patient should start immediately postoperatively

Postamputation pain is the commonest postoperative complication, is multifactorial and requires thorough assessment and possible onwards referral to a multidisciplinary pain team for management

Phantom limb pain is common and effective treatments remain elusive

History of amputation

Amputation, derived from the latin *amputare*, 'to cut away', is one of the oldest surgical operations. The first recorded amputation appears in the book of the Vedas, written in Sanskrit in India, dated between 3500 and 1800 BC. It records that the leg of Queen Vishpla was amputated in battle, and after healing, an iron leg was fitted to enable the Queen to return to the battlefield [1, 2].

The early descriptions of amputation by Hippocrates and Celsus focused on amputation for the treatment of gangrene. Hippocrates, in the latter half of the fifth century BC, recommended amputation for gangrene of the joint below the 'boundaries of blackening' as soon as it is 'fairly dead and lost its sensibility.' Celsus described the use of ligatures to control bleeding, although the use of cautery was more commonly used. By AD 100, Archigenes and Heliodorus described amputation for the management of ulcer, tumour, injuries and deformity.

Postgraduate Vascular Surgery: The Candidate's Guide to the FRCS, eds. Vish Bhattacharya and Gerard Stansby. Published by Cambridge University Press. © Cambridge University Press 2010.

War served as the impetus for surgical developments in amputation. The mid-fourteenth century saw the arrival of gunpowder into the wars of Europe, and with it came a new era of injury that required control of major haemorrhage and limb fracture.

Amboise Paré, surgeon to the colonel general of the French infantry, is most famous for re-introducing the use of the ligature to control bleeding. Paré first employed the ligature in amputation of the leg at the siege of Danvier in 1552, and published his technique in 1564. Paré is also known for his work on prosthetics, having designed an artificial hand and above knee prosthesis with a knee joint. The introduction of the tourniquet in 1674, by the French barber surgeon Morell, further advanced surgical practice of haemorrhage control during amputation.

During the Napoleonic wars, Dominique Larrey, Napoleon's chief of surgery, advocated the use of amputation 'on-site' rather than waiting for transfer to conventional hospital settings. This practice was continued in the American civil war with immediate transfer to adjacent field surgical sites, where some 50 000 amputations were carried out.

The introduction of ether anaesthetic by Morton and Warren in 1846 and the antiseptic technique by Lord Lister in 1867 reduced mortality from amputation and allowed better healing of wounds. Prior to antisepsis, mortality following limb amputation due to sepsis was approximately 60%. However, as medical advances have developed, so too have weapons of increasing destruction. The First World War saw somewhere between 300 000 and 500 000 amputations carried out.

Epidemiology of amputation

In the Western world, peripheral vascular disease is the dominant cause of lower limb amputation. Implicit to this is an increased prevalence of diabetes, currently over 1.7 million in the UK, obesity, together with an ageing population. Amputation carries with it a significant economic burden, and a high mortality rate, approaching 50% in diabetics at 2 years. A 1.6% annual incidence of major limb amputation is reported in patients with intermittent claudication [3].

The incidence of amputation is reported to be 8–12 times higher in diabetics than non diabetics [4]. The mortality rate in both groups increases with age, the level of amputation and is twice as high in men compared to women. A half of all diabetics who have a major amputation will lose their contralateral leg within 5 years [5].

The UK National Amputee Statistical Data Base reported a total of 5000 new amputee referrals in 2005–2006. Seventy-two per cent of these were due to dysvascularity, 9% trauma, 7% infection and 2% neoplasia (10% other or not specified). More than two-thirds of lower limb amputees referred were male (70%).

In the USA an estimated 134 000 amputations occur annually, such that there are approximately 1.7 million amputees in the USA. Dysvascularity accounts for 82% of amputations with the highest incidence among males.

Rates of trauma- and cancer-related amputations have both declined by approximately half over the past 20 years. However, unlike the UK, the risk of traumatic amputations in the USA has increased steadily with age, reaching its highest level among people age 85 or older.

There is evidence that focused management can reduce the incidence of amputation. Regional UK studies have shown significant reduction of lower limb amputation rates in diabetics of 70–80%, following the introduction of diabetic foot care monitoring [6].

These improvements are unlikely to be due to any single factor. Dedicated diabetic foot care services with a multidisciplinary approach, advances in radiology such as the use of subintimal angioplasty, and tighter control of risk factors with statins, antihypertensives and antiplatelet agents are all important developments.

Aetiology of amputation

- Critical limb ischaemia
- Sepsis
- Trauma
- Neoplasm
- Congenital

Critical limb ischaemia warrants revascularisation by angioplasty or bypass, to relieve rest pain or for the management of tissue loss/gangrene, in order to avoid major amputation. Amputation may become necessary after unsuccessful attempts at revascularisation or it may be considered as a primary option to control symptoms. Some patients choose primary amputation over potentially complex and lengthy surgery, or it may be recommended if they have significant comorbidities. The aims of amputation are to improve patient function and quality of life.

Sepsis, with or without, gangrene is most commonly seen in the diabetic foot, but can result from systemic infections such as meningitis. The diabetic foot is subject to a combination of neuropathy, ischaemia and biomechanical changes that result in abnormal weight bearing. Pressure ulceration ensues and ischaemia impairs healing, allowing superimposed infection. Minor infection may be treated with antibiotic treatment, but diabetic foot sepsis can progress rapidly and have devastating consequences if not managed appropriately. The diabetic patient with foot sepsis and palpable pedal pulses has a good prognosis with early surgical intervention. Digital gangrene is treated by amputation of the digit and metatarsal head with the wound left open. However the extent of underlying infection is often more extensive than is apparent externally, necessitating a higher and more major level of amputation. This should be borne in mind when consenting such patients. In diabetics with absent pulses attempts at revascularistion should be made at the earliest opportunity, ideally prior to surgery but this may not be practical until after.

Trauma was a common reason for amputation during wartime but in the UK is now more commonly performed following traumatic injury sustained in road traffic or machinery accidents. Thermal injury by severe burns or extreme cold exposure may also necessitate amputation.

Bone or soft tissue tumours (e.g. osteosarcoma, fibrosarcoma) may require limb amputation as their management. Finally, congenital deformities such as polydactyly may require amputation to improve patient function.

Preoperative assessment

Preoperative assessment of the patient includes consideration of the level of amputation. Decision on the level of amputation should include the likely rehabilitative potential of the patient. Patients with peripheral vascular disease often have concomitant disease that will limit ambulation due to the energy expenditure required for more proximal

Table 16.1 Key considerations in decision making about the level of major lower limb amputation

Level of amputation	Energy expenditure above normal (%)	Ambulation rate (%)	Advantages	Disadvantages
Below-knee amputation long stump	10	>80	Best chance of restoring ambulation	Flaps require well-perfused tissues, up to 10% conversion rate to above-knee amputation. Not suitable for bed-bound patients who are unlikely to ambulate due to stump contracture and pressure ulceration
Below-knee amputation short stump	40	80	May excise poorly perfused tissues	If stump is too short a prosthesis cannot be successfully used
Through-knee amputation	71.5	31	Useful if orthopaedic metalware present in femur. Provides long stump for balance in a wheelchair	Unpredictable healing of skin flaps. Poor cosmesis from prosthesis with leg appearing to dangle further than the normal side
Above-knee amputation	63	38–50 (less in vascular patients)	Excellent healing rates	Vascular or elderly patients unlikely to become ambulant, poor balance due to short stump

amputations. A summary of the key considerations for major amputations are given in Table 16.1.

Preoperative assessment should involve a multidisciplinary approach with input from physiotherapists, occupational therapists, prosthetists, rehabilitation medicine specialists, psychologists, nursing staff, and the surgical and anaesthetic teams. As well as the rehabilitative considerations a decision on the level of amputation should also include an assessment of the likelihood of the flaps healing. This should take into account the degree of tissue loss and ulceration, pattern and severity of vascular occlusion and the viability of tissues in the area of the proposed flaps. Toe pressures measured by Doppler should be >40 mmHg for successful healing of toe amputations. Several adjunctive tests exist to aid decision making, e.g. laser Doppler flowmetry, transcutaneous oxygen measurement or isotopic measurement of skin blood flow. However, the role of these tests is currently unclear and usually decision making is based on clinician judgement.

A checklist of the other preoperative tests and assessments routinely required are given in Table 16.2. Additional, more detailed tests and referral on to the appropriate subspecialty may be required for individual patients based on clinical findings. Amputation patients are

Table 16.2 Preoperative checklist of tests and assessments required routinely prior to major lower limb amputation

Test/assessment required	Reason	Action required
Full blood count	Patients often anaemic from chronic ulceration or other causes	Tranfuse if haemoglobin less than $10\,g\,dl^{-1}$
	Raised white cell count may indicate ongoing infection	Preoperative antibiotic treatment may be required if clinical supporting evidence of infection
Urea and electrolytes	Vascular patients often have associated renal disease and often are on medications that may disturb electrolyte balance	Perioperative intravenous rehydration whilst patient is fasted
		Treatment of individual disturbances
		Involve renal team if necessary
Clotting screen	Vascular patients may often be on a variety of anticoagulants or may have disturbed clotting function secondary to sepsis	Stop anticoagulants perioperatively to bring INR < 1.5. Patients at high risk of cardiac thromboembolism may need perioperative intravenous heparin or treatment dose low molecular weight heparin – consult local protocols
		Correct clotting disorders in discussion with a haematologist
Crossmatch (usually two units)	Transfusion frequently required perioperatively due to high blood losses. Concomitant disease such as ischaemic heart disease dictates maintaining relatively high haemoglobin levels	Monitor haemoglobin postoperatively
Blood glucose	Many amputation patients are diabetic, good perioperative diabetic control is associated with better outcomes	Monitor blood glucose perioperatively, prescribe insulin sliding scale or glucose/potassium/ insulin infusion for insulin dependent diabetics depending on local protocols
		Put diabetic patients first on the operating list
Electrocardiogram	Patients often have concomitant ishaemic heart disease	Referral to cardiology if necessary based on clinical findings
Chest X-ray	Only if clinically indicated for suspected acute or new chest problems	Delay surgery if possible until active problems treated
Thromboprophylaxis risk assessment	Major amputation puts patients at high risk of thromboembolic disease	Prescription of low molecular weight heparin
		Avoid TED stocking in patients with known peripheral arterial disease.

Table 16.2 (*cont.*)

Test/assessment required	Reason	Action required
MRSA screening/ microbiological screen	Guides use of perioperative antibiotics Allows isolation of MRSA-positive patients	Routine prescription of intravenous broad spectrum antibiotics at induction of anaesthesia. Modify according to swab results
Anaesthetic assessment	To assess and plan analgesic requirements To plan safe anaesthesia To plan level of critical care facilities required	Instigate preoperative epidural analgesia if possible Book bed at appropriate level of care (levels 1, 2 or 3)
Careful history and examination	To detect unexpected conditions that may impact on surgery e.g. previous orthopaedic metalware or vascular prostheses	Inform operating surgeon and other team members
Consent	Some patients undergoing amputation may be unable to give consent Life-changing procedure that requires careful counselling Surgery high risk with associated high mortality and morbidity rates	In-depth discussion with patient and family about procedure, its risks and impact on quality of life Two doctor consent form may need to be signed if necessary

INR, international normalized ratio; TED thromboembolic deterrent; MRSA, methicillin-resistant Staphylococcus aureus.

often very sick, frail and elderly. Careful attention to detail with delivery of optimal perioperative care is essential for successful outcomes.

Principles of amputation surgery

The underlying general principles of amputation surgery apply to all surgical sites:

- Avoid undermining or devitalizing skin flaps.
- Use a tourniquet to control haemorrhage – a recent randomized trial has shown that this reduces blood loss but does not compromise healing [7].
- Ligate vessels as they are encountered.
- Divide nerves cleanly and away from bone ends to avoid neuroma formation.
- Presence of muscle that does not bleed or contract in response to diathermy stimulation indicates devitalisation and that a higher level should be selected for amputation.
- Guillotine amputation of highly-infected tissue with later stage completion of amputation is indicated for severe sepsis and may reduce revision rates.
- Avoid unnecessary tension on the flaps and unnecessary bulk in the stump when closing.
- Use a suction drain/s for major amputation.
- Avoid stump bandaging, which can cause skin breakdown.

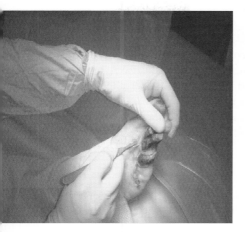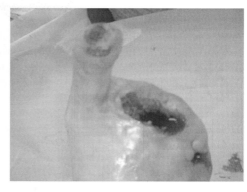

Figure 16.1 Toe amputation: amputation of diabetic gangrenous toes.

Lower limb amputation

Toe amputation

An evaluation of the vascular supply must be performed prior to toe amputation. Fishmouth or circular incisions are used to excise the affected toe. Amputation should not be performed through a joint as the avascular cartilage that is exposed prevents healing. Therefore toe amputations are usually performed through the proximal phalanx (Figure 16.1).

Ray amputation

This involves removal of a toe through the metatarsal bone. A tennis racquet-shaped incision is used to expose the distal part of the metatarsal bone and amputation is performed through the neck. Dissection must be kept close to the bone to avoid damaging the blood supply to neighbouring toes. Tendon remnants need to be excised as far proximally as possible. Ray amputation usually involves subsequent near normal ambulation but amputation of the hallux or fifth toe can sometimes cause ulceration of the plantar skin due to tendon imbalances and abnormal weight bearing.

Transmetatarsal amputation

This involves amputation of all the toes through the mid-metatarsal bones. A plantar flap is fashioned to cover the end of the foot. Excellent ambulation results from a well-healed amputation.

Mid-foot amputation

For more proximal foot disease amputation can be carried out proximal to the metatarsal bones. Named amputations include the Chopart amputation – a disarticulation of the talonavicular and cacaneocuboid joints or the Lisfranc amputation between the metarsal and tarsal bones. Other unnamed amputations at this level can also be successful. Healing rates at his level may be unpredictable and ambulation limited by the development of equinus varus deformity due to sacrifice of tendons. Mid-foot amputation should only be considered in patients without or with corrected ischaemia.

Ankle-level amputation

The Syme and Pirogoff amputations at ankle level are seldom performed in vascular surgical practice. The Syme amputation occurs through the ankle joint with the distal tibia and fibula cut in line with the joint. The Pirogoff modification conserves a piece of posterior calcaneum, which is screwed onto the distal tibia. Problems associated with these amputations include difficulty fitting a prosthesis, posterior migration of the heel pad and sloughing of the skin. The failure rate in dysvascular patients is approximately 41%. Usually below-knee amputation is preferable and allows a more reliable stump to be fashioned.

Below-knee amputation (BKA)

The most common technique for BKA is the long posterior flap technique first described by Burgess and Romano in 1967. The preferred site for section of the tibia is 14 cm below the knee joint or 10–12 cm below the tibial tuberosity. The absolute minimum required for successful limb-fitting is a length of 7.5 cm below the joint line. The flaps are marked out accurately using the rule of thirds (Figure 16.2). The tibia is divided 1 cm proximal to the skin wound and bevelled smoothly. The fibula is divided 2 cm proximally. The posterior flap is fashioned by excluding soleus from the wound to provide suitable coverage for the bone end that is not too bulky. An alternative technique uses skew flaps. This technique is useful when a long posterior flap is unsuitable due to tissue loss or non-viability extending onto the proposed site of the posterior flap. A systematic review has demonstrated comparability of the two techniques [8].

Through-knee amputation

Through-knee amputation may be useful when a BKA is contraindicated due to tissue nonviability. The through-knee amputation provides a long lever and an end-bearing stump. The patella may be preserved and wired onto the end of the femur (Gritti–Stokes

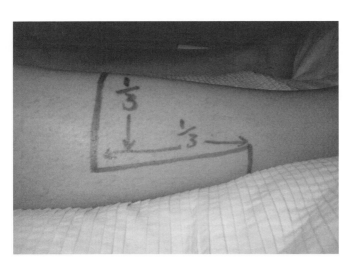

Figure 16.2 Marking the amputation flaps of a below-knee amputation using the rule of thirds.

amputation) or may be sacrificed. Problems with through-knee amputation include unpredictable healing of tissues and a stump that cosmetically is bulbous with unequal levels of the knee when fitted with a prosthesis. However, when successful it can provide good ambulation with less energy demands than a more proximal amputation. For the non-ambulant patient the long stump provides good leverage for transfer and good balance for sitting.

Above-knee amputation (AKA)

The preferred site of AKA is at the mid-femoral level at least 15 cm above the tibial plateau. The aim is to achieve a stump long enough to act as a lever arm for locomotion whilst allowing adequate clearance at the knee for a jointed prosthesis. The shortest stump recommended is 8 cm below the inferior pubic ramus. The flaps are fashioned using fishmouth incisions to achieve equal anterior and posterior myoplastic flaps.

Hip disarticulation and hindquarter amputation

These may occasionally be required in cases of severe ischaemia extending proximally, usually due to occlusion of aorto-iliac inflow. Mortality is high and successful ambulation exceedingly low.

Upper limb amputation

Upper limb amputation is rare in vascular surgical practice and may result from trauma, failed or delayed revascularization or infection. Amputations for congenital causes or malignancy may be undertaken by other specialties. The general principle considerations for amputations apply to amputations of the upper limb.

Postoperative complications

Early complications

- Deep vein thrombosis
- Flap necrosis
- Wound infection
- Post-amputation pain
- Stump haematoma
- Flexion contractures
- Psychological problems

Late complications

- Excess bulbosity of the stump
- Bone erosion through the skin
- Neuroma formation
- Ischaemia
- Osteomyelitis
- Adherent scar tissue
- Ulceration

Table 16.3 Causes of post-amputation pain

Type of pain	Definition	Treatment strategies
Immediate postoperative pain	Pain occurring in the immediate postoperative period due to the trauma of surgery	Opiate analgesia Epidural analgesia
Phantom limb sensation	Any sensory phenomenon (except pain) felt in the amputated limb	Reassurance
Phantom pain	Pain felt in the amputated limb or a portion of the absent limb	Referral to a multidisciplinary pain team. Useful approaches may include: simple analgesia, opiates, amitriptyline, gabapentin or pregabalin, ketamine, biofeedback, transcutaneous nerve stimulation, psychological techniques, spinal cord stimulation, use of metallic stump liners and application of hot or cold to stump. No treatment has been conclusively proven in robust randomized trials to be effective
Residual limb pain		
Internal pain:		
• Neuroma formation	Overgrowth of nerve-ending in stump – may cause spontaneous or mechanically induced pain	Nerve injections, amitriptyline, gabapentin or pregabalin Surgical exision/revision of nerve
• Bony overgrowth	New bony formation may produce spurs that cause local pain	Revision of stump
• Ischaemic pain	Coldness, blueness and pain associated with elevation in the stump +/– ulceration	Revascularisation using inflow procedure, amputation at higher level
• Sympathetically mediated pain	Rare type of pain maintained by the sympathetic nervous system and similar to complex regional pain syndrome. Associated with coldness, blueness, increased sweating and allodynia (pain associated with a stimulus that is not usually painful)	Referral to multidisciplinary pain team
• Neuropathic pain	Neuropathic pain usually associated with diabetes may affect a stump	Amitryptilline, gabapentin, pregabalin
External pain:		
• Mechanical causes from ill-fitting prosthesis	Ill-fitting prosthesis	Adjustment of prosthesis
Myofascial pain	Pain occurring at the supporting joint usually from an ill-	Physiotherapy, adjustment of prosthesis

Post-amputation pain

Because post-amputation pain is so common and challenging to treat it deserves special mention. Post-amputation pain occurs in about 80% of patients following amputation. There are several different causes, which are categorized in Table 16.3. A careful history and examination is the key to identifying the cause of the pain and a treatment plan can then be tailored to the underlying cause. Phantom limb pain occurs in about 70% of patients. Despite the wide variety of treatments described none has been conclusively proven to be of benefit in preventing or treating phantom limb pain. Pre-emptive epidural analgesia does not prevent phantom pain in the long term but does provide superior perioperative analgesia [9]. For cases recalcitrant to treatment with first-line oral agents referral to a multidisciplinary pain team is recommended.

Rehabilitation and prosthetics

Rehabilitation of the amputee should start as soon as possible postoperatively. Physiotherapy in the early period is important to prevent flexion contractures and to commence practice in transferring, sitting in bed, etc. Once the stump is healed, elasticated graduated compression stump socks are used to shrink the stump to an acceptable shape for fitting of a prosthesis. Early walking aids allow the patient to stand and start walking early. The Pneumatic Post Amputation Mobility Aid uses a maximal pressure of 40 mmHg to attach a pneumatic aid to the stump to achieve early walking in the physiotherapy gym.

Limb fitting is usually delayed until about 6 weeks postoperatively when oedema in the stump has subsided and it has shrunk to an acceptable size. A prosthesis is a device that is designed to replace, as much as possible, the function or appearance of a missing limb or body part. Advances in prosthetic technology have developed very sophisticated artificial limbs that use microchip technology to anticipate and respond to movements. These can be useful for young athletic patients to maintain prior levels of activity. However, for elderly dysvascular patients simpler and lighter modular components are recommended. Modern materials such as silicone or thermoplastic materials are used for stump liners and sockets to achieve a good fit with the stump [10].

References

1. Ellis H. *The Cambridge Illustrated History of Surgery*. Cambridge: Cambridge University Press, 2009; 127–8.
2. Stansbury LG, Branstetter JG, Lalliss SJ. Amputation in military surgery. *Trauma* 2007; 63: 940–4.
3. Dormandy JA, Murray GD. The fate of the claudicant. *Eur J Vasc Surg* 1991; 5: 131–3.
4. Johannesson A, Larsson GU, Ramstrand N et al. Incidences of lower limb amputation in the diabetic and nondiabetic general population. *Diabetes Care* 2009; 32: 275–80.
5. Nathan DM. Long-term complications of diabetes mellitus. *N Engl J Med* 1993; 328: 1676–85.
6. Canavan RJ, Unwin NC, Kelly WF, Connolly VM. Diabetes- and nondiabetes-related lower extremity amputation incidence before and after the introduction of better organized diabetes foot care: continuous longitudinal monitoring using a standard method. *Diabetes Care* 2008; 31: 459–63.
7. Choksey PA, Chong PL, Smith C, Ireland M, Beard J. A randomized

controlled trial of the use of a tourniquet to reduce blood loss during transtibial amputation for peripheral arterial disease. *Eur J Vasc Endovasc Surg* 2006; **31**: 646–50.

8. Tisi PV, Callam J. Type of incision for below knee amputation. *Cochrane Database of Systematic Reviews* 2004, Issue 1. Article no. CD003749.

9. Halbert J, Crotty M, Cameron ID. Evidence for the optimal management of acute and chronic phantom pain: a systematic review. *Clin J Pain* 2002; **18**: 84–92.

10. Tang PCY, Ravji K, Key JJ, Mahler DB, Blume PA, Sumpio B. Let them walk! Current prosthesis options for leg and foot amputees. *J Am Coll Surg* 2008; **206**: 548–60.

Leg swelling and lymphoedema

Arun Balakrishnan and Tim Lees

Key points

- The commonest cause of lymphoedema worldwide is filariasis
- In the Western world the commonest cause is malignancy and its treatment
- Oedema is initially pitting, but becomes non-pitting due to fibrosis of subcutaneous tissues
- Diagnosis is confirmed by isotope lymphangioscintigraphy
- Satisfactory treatment can usually be achieved by conservative measures that include manual drainage, compression hosiery, complex decongestive therapy and prevention of infection

There are various conditions that cause chronic lower limb swelling (Table 17.1). The two most common are chronic venous insufficiency and lymphoedema. Lymphoedema is a debilitating condition that has no cure. Several million people are affected worldwide.

Definition

Lymphoedema can be defined as the accumulation of fluid rich in protein in the skin and sub-cutaneous tissues due to a defect in the lymphatic system resulting in swelling of the limb.

Classification

Lymphoedema can be primary or secondary.

Primary

Primary lymphoedema can be classified based on the age of onset (Table 17.2). Women are more likely to be affected than men. The lower limbs are more frequently affected than the upper limbs.

- Congenital lymphoedema is present at birth and can be autosomally inherited (Milroy's disease). Oedema is present at birth and two-thirds of affected patients have bilateral lymphoedema. It accounts for 25% of all cases.
- Lymphoedema praecox presents up to the age of 35 years, usually during adolescence. It is the commonest form of congenital lymphoedema. Most patients have unilateral limb involvement.
- Lymphoedema tarda presents after the age of 35 years. This is the least common form and accounts for about 10% of cases.

Postgraduate Vascular Surgery: The Candidate's Guide to the FRCS, eds. Vish Bhattacharya and Gerard Stansby. Published by Cambridge University Press. © Cambridge University Press 2010.

Table 17.1 Differential diagnosis of chronic leg swelling

Venous disease
- Primary varicose veins
- Primary deep venous incompetence
- Post-thrombotic syndrome
- Arteriovenous malformations

Lymphoedema
- Primary
- Secondary

General disease
- Lipoedema
- Congestive cardiac failure
- Pretibial myxoedema
- Nephrotic syndrome
- Hepatic failure

Tumours
- Pelvic tumours causing extrinsic compression

Drugs

Dependency

All forms of primary lymphoedema are likely to arise from an abnormality present at birth that may manifest at birth or later in life. It is likely that these three groups represent different parts of the same spectrum of disease, which has been attributed to aplasia, hypoplasia or hyperplasia of the lymph vessels during development.

Secondary

Secondary lymphoedema occurs when the lymphatic vessels become occluded by an acquired pathology. The lymphatic channels distal to the obstruction become dilated and the valves secondarily incompetent. Worldwide the commonest cause is an infection caused by the parasite *Wuchereria bancrofti*, resulting in filariasis.

In the Western world the commonest cause is neoplasia and its treatment, resulting in damage or removal of lymph nodes, for example post-mastectomy lymphoedema of the upper limb. This is particularly common in patients who undergo radiotherapy following axillary lymph node removal.

The causes of secondary lymphoedema are listed in Table 17.2.

Pathophysiology

Interstitial fluid is composed of proteins, lipids and water. It is formed by the high hydrostatic pressure in the capillaries that forces fluid into the interstitial space. This results in an increase in the oncotic pressure, which attracts more water. Normally functioning lymphatics return interstitial fluid to the intravascular space. High molecular weight proteins and associated water pass through the lymphatics and eventually into the venous system.

Table 17.2 Causes of lymphoedema

Primary

- Congenital (age <1 year)
- Familial (Milroy's disease)
- Non-familial
- Praecox (age <35 years)
- Familial
- Non-familial
- Tarda (age >35 years)

Secondary

- Malignant disease
- Surgery
- Radical mastectomy
- Radical groin dissection
- Radiotherapy
- Infection
- Parasitic (filariasis)
- Pyogenic (β-haemolytic streptococci, *Staphylococcus aureus*)
- Tuberculosis
- Arterial surgery
- Venous disease and venous surgery

If a disease process has caused obstruction of the lymphatics, the above transport system is overwhelmed. There is a stagnation of protein-rich fluid in the interstitial space and high concentrations of protein result in accumulation of more water. The lymphatic vessels dilate and this results in secondary valvular incompetence.

Limbs may swell due to other local or systemic conditions. Chronic venous insufficiency results in a rise in venous pressure. This pressure is transmitted to the capillary bed, resulting in structural changes in the endothelium, causing an increase in capillary permeability. This results in an increase in interstitial fluid volume, causing oedema. Systemic conditions such as congestive cardiac failure, hypoproteinemia and nephrotic syndrome result in a state of retention of salt and water, causing oedema. This may compound the situation in the presence of diseased lymphatics or overwhelm a normally functioning lymphatic system.

Initially the oedema is pitting. The accumulation of protein and fluid in the interstitial space results in an inflammatory reaction. This, in time, leads to fibrosis of subcutaneous tissues and the oedema becomes non-pitting.

Presentation

Patients initially present with peripheral oedema. Lymphoedema can be differentiated from other causes of limb swelling by history and examination. A detailed history and examination of the patient may help to differentiate primary from secondary lymphoedema.

History

The initial presentation is swelling of the limb of varying degrees. As the swelling progresses the patient may have difficulty fitting into clothes and footwear. As the oedema progresses skin complications develop. Bacterial and fungal infections are common. Patients may have discomfort related to the size of the limb, cosmetic concerns, difficulty mobilizing and impairment of activities of daily living. Primary lymphoedema occurs predominantly in females in their early teens. Patients with secondary lymphoedema will commonly have a history of previous surgery, neoplastic disease or radiotherapy.

Examination

The patient may have unilateral or bilateral limb swelling. Initially the oedema is pitting but with time the swelling becomes non-pitting due to fibrotic changes in the skin and subcutaneous tissues. The swelling is uniform and as it progresses the leg appears like a tree trunk. The skin gradually thickens and becomes less elastic. The dorsum of the foot (Figure 17.1) is usually involved, producing the characteristic 'buffalo hump' appearance. The skin becomes thickened and has a typical peau d'orange appearance. There are thick deposits of keratin on the epidermis.

Investigation

The diagnosis of lymphoedema can usually be made clinically. Investigation is needed when the diagnosis is uncertain, to confirm diagnosis, when considering surgery, to plan treatment and to exclude pelvic masses as the cause for lower limb lymphoedema. Oedema associated with generalized disorders such as hypoproteinemia, congestive cardiac failure and nephrotic syndrome are excluded or diagnosed by examination, biochemical analysis and urinalysis.

Duplex ultrasonography

This is useful to exclude chronic venous insufficiency. Chronic venous insufficiency is the commonest differential diagnosis for lymphoedema. Deep venous thrombosis may cause unilateral lower limb swelling.

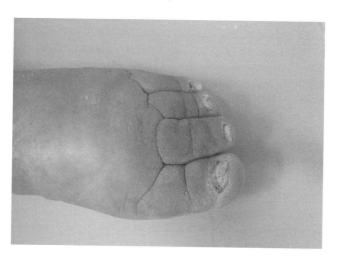

Figure 17.1 Chronic lymphoedema of the foot.

Lymphangioscintigraphy (isotope lymphangiography)

This is the most commonly performed investigation (Figure 17.2). It defines anatomy, evaluates dynamics and determines the severity of obstruction [1]. A radiolabelled (usually technetium) colloid is injected into the interdigital space and gamma-camera pictures are taken at 5-min intervals to assess transit through the lymph channels. If the time taken for the tracer to appear in the regional lymph node is greater than 60 min then this would suggest delayed lymphatic transport. A negative scintigram effectively excludes the diagnosis of lymphoedema. Primary and secondary lymphoedema are frequently associated with similar scintigraphic appearances, including delayed transit, the presence of collaterals, dermal backflow, and reduced uptake in one or more groups of lymph nodes. It can be used to distinguish between a venous and lymphatic cause of limb swelling [2]. The test cannot differentiate primary from secondary lymphoedema.

Computed tomography

The primary role of computed tomography (CT) is in the diagnosis of primary and secondary malignancy as a cause for lymphoedema. The common findings on computed tomography are skin thickening, thickening of subcutaneous fat and thickening of the perimuscular aponeurosis. It will also provide evidence of lymphoedema by the presence of a honeycomb appearance of fluid in the subcutaneous tissues [3] and has been used to monitor the response to compression therapy. Patients with a previous history of pelvic or abdominal malignancy

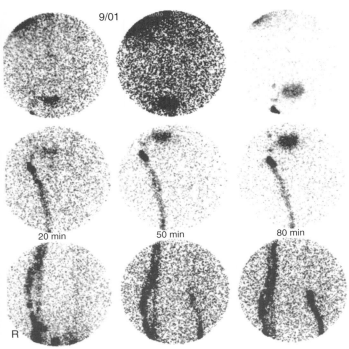

Figure 17.2
Lymphangioscintigram.

should be scanned for recurrent disease in order to diagnose enlarged lymph nodes or pelvic masses that may be compressing the lymphatic channels.

Magnetic resonance (MR) imaging

The MR features of lymphoedema include circumferential oedema, increased volume of tissues, honeycomb pattern of subcutaneous tissues and thickening of the dermis. Nodal architecture can be demonstrated. It can distinguish between lymphatic and venous swelling but is not good at separating primary and secondary causes of lymphoedema.

Contrast lymphangiography

Lymphangiography used to be the gold standard test for evaluating lymphatic disorders. It is an invasive test and can cause an inflammatory reaction in the lymphatics. This investigation is now rarely used in the diagnosis of lymphoedema and has been largely replaced by scintigraphy.

Treatment

The aim of treatment is to reduce limb swelling, reduce the risk of infection and improve function. Treatment can be surgical or non surgical. If management begins early in the disease process, before irreversible fibrotic changes occur, then conservative measures should be successful. Once achieved the improvement must be maintained. Surgery is indicated only in a small proportion of patients, and is palliative and not curative.

General measures

There is no cure for lymphoedema. The nature of the condition and its management should be clearly explained to the patient. General measures are of benefit and should be followed religiously throughout life to obtain maximum benefit. These include the following:

- skin care is essential to maintain healthy skin and reduce risk of infection;
- elevation of the limb at rest;
- regular exercise to encourage flow of lymph;
- weight reduction;
- high protein and low sodium diet;
- avoiding pressure, tight footwear and constrictive clothing;
- simple lymphatic drainage, which involves gentle massage of the affected area by patients or their carers [4].

Manual lymphatic drainage

This is performed by specially trained therapists. Beginning with the proximal portion of the affected limb, the limb is massaged over short segments in a distal to proximal manner. Massage stimulates the flow of lymph via superficial lymphatics from an affected area to an adjacent normal area.

Compression therapy

Compression can be achieved by multilayer bandaging during the intensive treatment phase. Multi Layer Lymphoedema Bandaging (MLLB) involves the use of several layers of bandages to achieve compression [4]. The pressure is more uniformly distributed. Compression stockings need to exert a pressure of approximately 40–50 mmHg at the level of the ankle and are generally used during the maintenance phase. The compression should be graduated from distal to proximal. Support garments are essential to maintain limb size in the treatment of lymphoedema.

Intermittent sequential pneumatic compression therapy

Intermittent pneumatic compression is a means of reducing the size of a limb in lymphoedema. They can be used at home or in an outpatient setting. They work best if used before subcutaneous fibrosis sets in. The affected limb is placed in a sleeve or cuff that is alternately inflated and deflated, creating a pressure gradient that moves fluid out of the affected limb. These devices may have a single sleeve of uniform pressure or may consist of several chambers that can be inflated in sequence. The direction of inflation should be graduated from distal to proximal. Compression hosiery should be used between treatments.

Thermal treatment

Hyperthermia of the leg is produced by immersing the limb in hot water or by microwave heating. The reason behind its efficacy is not clear. It is presumed to mobilize fluid and soften tissues.

Complex decongestive therapy

Complex decongestive physiotherapy generally involves an intensive treatment programme over 4 weeks. The first phase (intensive therapy) involves skin care, exercise, multilayer bandages and manual lymphatic drainage. Phase 2 (maintenance phase) aims to conserve and optimize the results obtained in Phase 1. It involves the regular use of support garments, continued exercise, skin care and massage therapy. Reduction in limb volume can be achieved and maintained. There is a reduction in the incidence of infection. Worldwide, people have achieved good results but this process is resource intensive and compliance can be poor.

Prevention of infection

Macrophages and lymphocytes are activated by inflammatory processes and carried through the lymphatics to regional lymph nodes. Antigens are presented and an immune response is mounted. Stagnation of lymph prevents this and increases the risk and severity of infection. The common pathogens are β-haemolytic streptococci and staphylococcus aureus. With each episode of infection there is further destruction of the lymph channels, making the oedema worse. Well-fitting comfortable shoes prevent small cracks in the skin that may act as a portal of entry. The affected limb should be washed daily with a mild soap and the feet must be dry before putting on shoes. The patient must keep a very careful eye on the foot and any early signs of infection must be treated aggressively with antibiotics. Recurrent infection can be managed by long-term, prophylactic, low-dose antibiotics such as amoxicillin, flucloxacillin or a cephalosporin.

A Consensus Document on the Management of Cellulitis in Lymphoedema has been published by the British Lymphology Society and the Lymphoedema Support Network [6].

This document makes recommendations about the use of antibiotics for cellulitis in patients with lymphoedema, and advises when admission to hospital is indicated. Prompt treatment is essential to avoid further damage to the affected part, which in turn may predispose to repeated attacks.

Drugs

Drug therapy for lymphoedema is limited. Diuretics can be used in the early stages but have no value in long-term treatment. Underlying filarial infection should be treated with diethylcarbamazine. Benzopyrenes have been advocated by some. They induce phagocytosis of proteins and proteolysis. The resulting fragments are more readily removed.

Surgical treatment

Surgery is indicated only in a very small proportion of patients as symptoms are usually controlled adequately by conservative measures. Surgery is indicated if conservative measures have failed and there is severe disability, gross deformity or lymphorrhagia. These can be divided into debulking operations and bypass procedures. Obliterative causes are best treated by debulking procedures, whereas in lymphatic obstruction surgical bypass is recommended.

Debulking operations

These procedures, which involve removal of variable amounts of the excess skin and subcutaneous tissue from the affected limb, are indicated when there is gross oedema:

- Homan's operation involves making an incision along the length of the limb. Anterior and posterior skin flaps are fashioned and raised. Excess subcutaneous tissue is excised. Tissue is removed down to the level of the deep fascia. The skin flaps are then fashioned appropriately and closed primarily. The skin should be reasonably healthy to carry out this procedure.
- Charles' procedure involves excision of skin, subcutaneous tissues and deep fascia. The resulting defect is closed with a split skin graft. The cosmetic results of this procedure are poor and the procedure can be complicated by hyperkeratotic scars.
- Liposuction has been used to reduce the size of a lymphoedematous limb. It is generally more effective in patients with minimal pitting oedema. Post-procedure, patients are required to wear compression garments for life. The National Institute for Health and Clinical Excellence (NICE) has issued guidance regarding treating chronic lymphoedema by liposuction. NICE has said that if a doctor wants to use liposuction to treat chronic lymphoedema, they should make sure that extra steps are taken to explain the uncertainty about how well it works in the long term, as well as the potential risks of the procedure. The patient should be told that they will need to wear compression garments indefinitely after the procedure. This should happen before the patient agrees (or does not agree) to the procedure. The patient should be given this leaflet (Treating chronic lymphoedema by liposuction, Interventional procedure guidance 251) and other written information as part of the discussion. There should also be special arrangements for monitoring what happens to the patient after the procedure [6].

Table 17.3 Bypass procedures for lymphoedema

- Skin and muscle flaps
- Omental bridges
- Enteromesenteric bridges
- Lymphatico-lymphatic anastomosis
- Lymphatico-venous anastomosis

Bypass procedures

Several procedures have been described (Table 17.3). Only a small number of patients show long-term improvement.

Patients with proximal obstruction of lymphatics in the pelvis and patent distal lymphatics can have a bypass procedure. Of note are lymphovenous anastomosis and lympholymphatic anastomosis. They are physiological methods for correcting lymphoedema. Multiple lymphatics are anastomosed to subdermal venules using micro-surgical techniques to produce an improvement in signs and symptoms. Autologus lymphatic vessels harvested from the contra lateral normal limb can be used to bypass obstruction by performing lympholymphatic anastomosis. For the procedures to succeed the patients should have patent distal lymphatics and mild-to-moderate oedema. In patients with distal obliterative disease reconstruction is not an option. The techniques of omental and enteromesenteric bridges have been described to help improve lymphatic drainage.

Lipeodema

This condition is often diagnosed as lymphoedema. It is characterized by symmetrical enlargement of the lower limbs, excluding the feet. The age of onset is early and the condition almost exclusively affects women. There is no cure for the condition. Treatment is multimodal and mainly involves the use of exercise and compression hosiery. Liposuction has been used with some effect. Patients require adequate support.

References

1. Mortimer PS. Evaluation of lymphatic function: abnormal lymph drainage in venous disease. *Int Angiol* 1995; **14**: 32–5.
2. Brautigam P, Vanscheidt W, Foldi E, Krause T, Moser E. The importance of the subfascial lymphatics in the diagnosis of lower limb edema: investigations with semi quantitative lymphoscintigraphy. *Angiology* 1993; **44**: 464–70.
3. Hadjis NS, Carr DH, Banks L, Pflug JJ. The role of CT in the diagnosis of primary lymphoedema of the lower limb. *AJR Am J Roentgenol* 1985; **144**: 361–4.
4. Lymphoedema Support Network. What is lymphoedema? 2004. www.lymphoedema.org (accessed 13 June 2009).
5. British Lymphology Society. Cellulitis Management Consensus 2007. www.thebls.com (accessed 13 June 2009).
6. National Institute for Health and Clinical Excellence. Treating chronic lymphoedema by liposuction. 2008. www.nice.org.uk/IPG251 (accessed 13 June 2009).

Varicose veins and chronic venous insufficiency

Marcus Cleanthis and Tim Lees

Key points

- Truncal varices are common with an age-adjusted prevalence of 40% in men and 32% in women
- Varicosities may be primary or secondary due to previous deep vein thrombosis (DVT), pelvic obstruction or deep venous reflux
- Patients present with discomfort, swelling, pain, pruritis, bleeding, thrombophlebitis and skin changes
- Hand held Doppler has replaced the tourniquet test as a 'bedside examination' for evaluating incompetence of valves
- Current treatments for varicose veins include conventional surgery, radiofrequency ablation, laser ablation and injection sclerotherapy (liquid or foam)
- Surgery to the great saphenous vein involves high tie and stripping and has a recurrence rate of 15%–20%
- Surgery to the small saphenous vein involves saphenopopliteal ligation, stripping and phlebectomy
- Foam sclerotherapy and catheter ablation techniques using laser or radiofrequency can be used under local anaesthesia, but less is known about their long-term outcome
- Chronic venous insufficiency affects between 7% and 9% of the adult population and is due to venous reflux, obstruction or calf pump failure
- Clinical signs include swelling, venous eczema, pigmentation lipodermatosclerosis and ulceration
- Multilayered compression is the gold standard used to heal venous ulceration
- The Effect of Surgery and Compression on Healing and Recurrence (ESCHAR) trial showed a reduced ulcer recurrence rate with combined surgery and compression
- Venous reconstruction is rarely performed and usually reserved for severe disease, resistant to other forms of treatment

Varicose veins

Epidemiology

Data from the Edinburgh Vein Study suggest a slightly greater prevalence of varicose veins in males compared to females (4 : 3.2) [1]. The age-adjusted prevalence of truncal varices

Postgraduate Vascular Surgery: The Candidate's Guide to the FRCS, eds. Vish Bhattacharya and Gerard Stansby. Published by Cambridge University Press. © Cambridge University Press 2010.

was found to be 40% in men and 32% in women. Mild varices (hyphenweb and reticular varices) were identified in 80% of the population aged 18–64 years.

Asymptomatic disease detected with duplex scanning and defined as significant venous reflux greater than or equal to 0.5 s is estimated to occur in 35% of the population between the ages of 18 and 64 years. The prevalence of varicose veins increases with age and affects approximately 15% of the population aged between 25 and 34 years and 50–60% of the population aged 55–64 years [1].

Aetiology

Primary varicose veins

Primary varicose veins occur in the absence of any known underlying cause. Risk factors for developing primary varicose veins include age, parity, weight, posture and bowel habit.

- Pregnancy: it is not uncommon for female patients to relate the onset of their varicose veins to pregnancy and childbirth. The question as to whether these individuals have underlying predisposition to venous disease or whether the pregnancy causes it remains unanswered. Venous tone is affected by changes in female sex hormones and increased blood volume. Interestingly most varices appear in the first trimester when uterine size is unlikely to cause obstruction to venous return. Multiparity is also a risk factor for venous disease with a 20–30% increased risk associated with two or more pregnancies.
- Weight: increased weight is a risk factor for varicose veins and the evidence for this is stronger in women. The association with elevated body mass index (BMI) has been shown in numerous studies. However, although the risk of developing varicose veins has been shown to increase with increasing BMI there is no defined BMI level at which this risk is greatest.
- Posture: it has been suggested that prolonged standing may exacerbate varicose veins. Prolonged sitting has also been linked in some studies. The mechanism may be related to prolonged, increased hydrostatic pressure making the veins more susceptible to other factors.
- Diet: the effect of diet is suggested by the geographical variation in venous disease. Varicose veins are more common in Western societies with low fibre diets. Western diets result in straining during defacation associated with raised intra-abdominal pressures. This pressure may be applied hydrostatically to leg veins.
- Genetics: patients frequently describe the occurrence of varicose veins in other family members suggesting an inherited component to the occurrence. Although this is plausible, the evidence for genetic factors is limited. The prevalence of venous disease is so high that it is of no surprise that other family members are afflicted.

Secondary varicose veins

Secondary varicose veins occur as a consequence of another condition (post deep venous thrombosis [DVT], pelvic tumours, congenital malformations, deep venous reflux and out-flow obstruction). In these situations the superficial veins act as a collateral venous return.

Clinical features (Table 18.1)

Asymptomatic varicose veins

The majority of patients with varicose veins are asymptomatic. Many seek medical attention for cosmetic reasons. This may have psychological implications altering a patient's

Table 18.1 Clinical features of varicose veins

Symptoms	Types of varices	Chronic skin changes	Acute complications
Pain	Corona phlebectatica	Eczema Lipodermatosclerosis	Haemorrhage
Swelling Heaviness	Hyphenweb varices	Pigmentation	Superficial thrombophlebitis
Pruritis	Reticular varices	Ulceration	
Burning Restlessness	Truncal varices	Atrophie blanche	
Cramps			

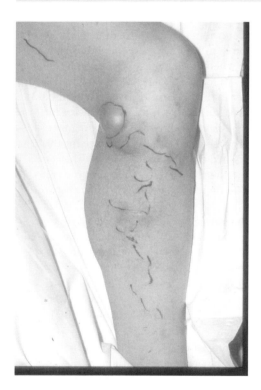

Figure 18.1 Typical features of thrombophlebitis are displayed. This patient presented with inflammation affecting varicosities arising from the long saphenous system.
MIMS Cardiovascular Journal 2007; 2 No. 3.
Reproduced with permission.

confidence. Such concerns should be identified and discussed prior to any intervention to ensure that the expectations of any treatment are realistic.

Some patients have concerns about the risk of future complications. Many have a fear of developing ulceration and some are concerned about the risk of deep venous thrombosis. Other patients are concerned about the risk of developing a DVT during flying. These patients should be offered reassurance as not all patients develop skin changes. If a patient is likely to be travelling on a long-haul flight they should take the same precautions as a person without varicose veins. Many of the available treatments have an underlying risk of DVT and hence treatment of varicose veins should not be offered as a form of DVT prophylaxis.

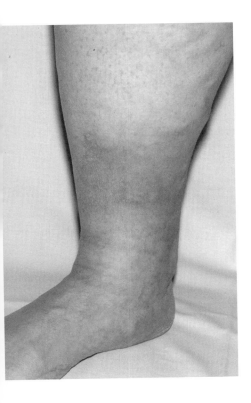

Figure 18.2 Clinical features of chronic venous insufficiency include swelling, pigmentation, eczema, lipodermatosclerosis (shown above) and ulceration. *MIMS Cardiovascular Journal* 2007; 2 No. 3. Reproduced with permission.

Symptomatic varicose veins

Symptoms can be variable and may include pain, swelling, heaviness, pruritis, burning, restlessness and cramps. These symptoms may be exacerbated by ambulation and alleviated by lower limb elevation. Consequently symptoms may be more troublesome during the day or in the evening after prolonged standing or sitting and less problematic in the morning after the legs have been elevated overnight.

Presentation with acute complications of varicose veins is not uncommon. The acute complications are haemorrhage and thrombophlebitis (Figure 18.1).

Haemorrhage can be torrential, occasionally life threatening and frequently associated with trauma (often trivial). Bleeding is initially managed with compression and elevation. However after a single episode patients frequently seek definitive treatment to avoid further haemorrhage. It can be very distressing and subsequent treatment is indicated to prevent further episodes. Superficial thrombophlebitis is a consequence of thrombosis and subsequent inflammation of the vein. The clinical presentation is that of an inflamed swollen tender vein. The early phase is managed with analgesics and anti-inflammatory agents. It is not uncommon for patients to receive a course of antibiotics in the community, although the process is that of a sterile inflammation. Subsequent fibrosis can result in a thickened nodule with subsequent skin pigmentation. As recurrence is common many surgeons would regard this as an indication for surgery after the acute phase has been controlled. Chronic complications (pigmentation, eczema, lipodermatosclerosis (Figure 18.2) and ulceration) are more commonly seen with chronic venous insufficiency (CVI) although they can occur with isolated superficial venous reflux.

Clinical signs

Varicose veins show features of tortuosity, elongation and dilatation. They are described as hyphenweb varices, reticular or truncal varicosties.

- Hyphenweb varices are also referred to as telengiectasia, thread veins, spider veins and venous flare. They are intradermal dilated venules occurring in isolation or associated with truncal or reticular varices.
- Reticular varices are subcuticular varices that do not belong to the main trunk or its tributaries. They frequently appear as a bluish reticular pattern of veins beneath the skin and can occur physiologically.
- Truncal varices arise from the long or short saphenous veins or their major tributaries (first and second order tributaries).
- Chronic venous skin changes include eczema, lipodermatosclerosis and ulceration.
- Eczema results in dry, scaly, itchy skin. Scratching can result in bleeding, infection and subsequent ulceration.
- Lipodermatosclerosis is the term given to the pigmented skin associated with thickened/inflamed subcuticular and cutaneous tissue. The mechanism is unclear but it is believed that elevated venous pressure facilitates extravasation of cells and fluid, leading to inflammation.
- Pigmentation/skin staining is a consequence of haemosiderin deposits.
- Chronic venous ulceration is most commonly (but not exclusively) seen in the gaiter area above the medial malleolus. It commonly occurs in an area of pre-existing lipodermatosclerosis following trauma. Long-standing ulcers are at risk of malignant conversion to squamous cell carcinoma (Marjolin's ulcer) and this should be considered in long-standing ulceration and those that fail to heal.
- Other skin changes seen include malleolar flare/corona phlebectatica (intradermal or subdermal collection of dilated veins at the medial malleolus) and atrophie blanche (scar tissue at a site of previous ulceration).

Investigations for venous disease

Hand held Doppler

Hand held Doppler has replaced the tourniquet test in assessing the source of incompetence. It is now the initial choice of investigation at the bedside. The test is performed with the patient standing. The probe is placed at the junction suspected of being incompetent and the calf muscle squeezed. This produces a characteristic venous signal. On releasing the muscle the presence of an audible signal suggests reflux. The great saphenous vein, saphenofemoral junction and saphenopopliteal junction can all be assessed although false positives are more commonly seen at the saphenopopliteal junction. Hence reflux at this site should always be confirmed with a duplex scan.

Duplex

Duplex combines B-mode ultrasound and Doppler. This allows identification of individual vessels and can generate information on the direction of flow in a vessel. Hence both anatomical and functional information can be obtained. As well as defining the communication points between the deep and superficial venous systems (perforators, saphenofemoral and saphenopopliteal junctions) the direction of blood flow through these junctions and within the veins themselves can be assessed and hence venous reflux confirmed. Duplex is non-invasive, quick and cheap. It is the first-line imaging technique for venous disease and frequently the only imaging ever required.

There is controversy regarding the use of duplex scanning for all patients with varicose veins. Some centres reserve duplex for recurrent disease, small saphenous disease, deep venous disease and equivocal hand held Doppler examination of the long saphenous system. Surgery may be offered on positive hand held Doppler examination of primary long saphenous varicose veins. There is evidence to support the use of duplex scanning for all patients presenting with varicose veins. Reliance on clinical examination alone can result in inappropriate surgical procedures being performed [2, 3]. The increasing availability of affordable portable scanners allows quick and convenient scanning in the outpatient environment, reduces diagnostic error and decreases clinic follow-up requirements prior to surgery.

Venography

Prior to duplex scanning investigation of the venous system was an invasive technique requiring direct injection of contrast into the venous system. Duplex scanning has almost abolished the need for this investigation. Occasionally more detailed imaging is required and venography can be performed using magnetic resonance venography (MRV) and computed tomography venograpy (CTV). These techniques have almost abolished the need for contrast venography described below.

Magnetic resonance venography (MRV)

MRV is useful for imaging the venous system, especially within the main body cavities (thorax, abdomen and pelvis) where duplex imaging may be limited (especially in the obese). It can be used to diagnose deep venous occlusions, stenosis, thrombosis and malformations. Various techniques exist including non-contrast imaging, which utilises time of flight techniques and contrast enhanced MRV. The contrast-enhanced techniques have the advantage of being quicker and less susceptible to flow artefact in parallel vessels. It is also able to differentiate between acute and chronic DVT and is less invasive than conventional venography. The greatest limitation with MRV is its cost compared to other forms of venography and duplex. Magnetic resonance venography has largely replaced conventional venography.

Computed tomography venograpy (CTV)

CTV, like MRV, may provide better imaging of the iliac and caval venous system than duplex scanning. Extrinsic compression of the iliac veins or vena cava (inferior and superior) can also be identified and pelvic/abdominal masses can be visualised. Computed tomography venography has become the investigation of choice for pulmonary embolism.

Contrast venography

Varicography requires the injection of the contrast into a superficial varicosity. It was previously used to identify perforators and localise the saphenopopliteal junction. This is now performed with duplex scanning although varicography may still have a role in defining ovarian reflux (e.g. patients with vulval varices) and in the investigation of venous malformations. Ascending venography requires cannulation of a pedal dorsal vein. Contrast is encouraged into the deep venous system via occlusion of the superficial system using a tourniquet above the ankle. This technique was traditionally used to define deep occlusions, stenosis, thrombosis and perforator vein incompetence. In addition iliac and inferior vena caval imaging can be obtained. Deep venous incompetence cannot be diagnosed using ascending venog raphy. Prior to duplex the diagnosis of valvular incompetence required descending venog raphy. This requires injection of contrast directly into the common femoral vein. Contrast venography is usually reserved for investigation of the deep venous system when duplex and MRV are equivocal.

Functional calf measurements

Plethysmography

Overall lower limb venous function is influenced by valvular function, venous outflow and calf muscle activity. All of these will affect venous filling, which subsequently influences calf volume. The change in calf volume can be quantified using plethysmography. Photoplethysmography utilises infrared light absorption to quantify the change in blood flow within cutaneous veins. This is correlated with ambulatory venous pressure refilling time. Air plethysmography involves enclosing the leg in a bag and measuring changes in the pressure within the bag fol lowing ankle exercise. From these measurements, changes in calf volume can be measured. A similar principle is used in foot volumetry where patients stand in water filled boots. Change in foot volume are detected by measuring the volume of water expelled.

Ambulatory venous pressure (AVP)

This is an invasive technique requiring the cannulation of a dorsal foot vein and direct meas urement of the superficial venous pressure by connection to a pressure transducer, ampli fier and a computer. It remains the gold standard method for measuring venous pressure. Patients are asked to tip-toe ten times and the pressure changes are recorded. Although AVP can provide detailed information its use is now largely confined to research of venous disease.

Treatment

Reassurance

Many patients require no treatment other than reassurance. Patients with asymptomatic varicose veins who have no cosmetic concerns can be discharged after the benign nature of the disease has been explained. Patients who are due to fly on long-haul flights should be advised to wear anti-DVT flight socks and exercise their calves as for patients without varicose veins. The risk of developing DVT with varicose veins is not significant enough to justify intervention and patients should be reassured of this, especially as intervention itself is associated with a risk of DVT.

Compression stockings

These can provide symptomatic relief in patients with varicose veins and should be offered to those who do not want any form of invasive intervention. They have an important role in the management of chronic venous insufficiency and reduce ulcer recurrence after healing with compression dressings. They create a graduated pressure on the leg, aiding the action of the venous calf pump and improving deep venous blood flow, which in turn reduces reflux into the superficial system. Compression stockings are classified (and should be pre scribed) according to the pressure applied at the ankle. These stockings may be described as class I to IV but this classification should be avoided as significant differences exist between the British and European standard pressure classification (Table 18.2). The most commonly

Table 18.2 Classification of compression stockings

Indication	Support	European standard class pressure	British standard class pressure
Mild varices, deep vein thrombosis, prophylaxis	Light	I 18–21 mmHg	I 14–17 mmHg
Marked varices, oedema, chronic venous insufficiency	Medium	II 23–32 mmHg	II 18–24 mmHg
Chronic venous insufficiency, lymphoedema, prevention of venous ulcers	Strong	III 34–46 mmHg	III 25–35 mmHg
Severe lymphoedema, chronic venous insufficiency	Heavy	IV >49 mmHg	

used stockings are those that produce a pressure ranging between 25 and 35 mmHg at the ankle. Before prescribing compression stockings it is vital to exclude co-existing occlusive arterial disease. They should be used with caution in diabetic patients. Stockings can result in ulceration in these groups of patients and hence close monitoring is required.

Foam sclerotherapy

Foam sclerotherapy is an advancement on a technique used for many years to treat varicose veins. The original use of sclerosing agents for varicosities became less popular after the recurrence rate was shown to be significantly higher compared to surgery. However, the efficacy of sclerosing agents was found to be improved by mixing with air and administering the agent as foam. This facilitated the displacement of blood from the vein and improved contact with the vein wall.

Today, foam sclerotherapy injection is achieved under ultrasound guidance. The most common agents used are sodium tetradecyl sulphate (1–3%) and polidocanol (0.5–3%). These agents are converted to foam by mixing with air using two syringes and a 3-way tap. Using ultrasound the great saphenous or small saphenous vein is cannulated with a venflon and the foam administered in 1 ml aliquots. Smaller tributaries are cannulated with butterfly needles and treated with lower concentrations of foam. While the foam is administered, the leg is elevated and the patient encouraged to dorsiflex the ankle. This latter manoeuvre encourages blood flow in the deep veins, reducing the risk of deep venous thrombosis. After treatment, compression bandaging is applied for one or two weeks. The more common complications include thrombophlebitis, haemosiderin skin staining and ulceration from extravasation of sclerosant (Table 18.3). Less common complications include deep venous thrombosis, transient visual disturbance and stroke (three cases reported worldwide). Foam sclerotherapy can be offered as an outpatient treatment and is also suitable for recurrent varicosities. It is the first-line treatment for patients unfit for general anaesthetic. Long-term studies are required to compare recurrence rates of foam with conventional surgery.

Catheter ablation

Catheter ablation is a technique used to generate heat resulting in transmural injury to the vein wall. There are two techniques in common use: radiofrequency ablation (RFA) and endovenous laser treatment (EVLT). One trial comparing RFA with surgery has shown that

RFA is associated with less postoperative pain and faster recovery compared to surgery [4] Early results have shown that both are effective in eliminating reflux. Endovenous laser treatment has been shown to produce less postoperative bruising and swelling compared to surgery [5]. One trial has shown RFA to be superior to EVLT in postoperative pain and quality of life parameters [6].

Radiofrequency ablation (RFA)

Radiofrequency energy is used to provide the thermal insult required to destroy the vein. Using a Seldinger technique the vein (e.g. great saphenous vein) is cannulated under ultrasound guidance and the RFA catheter inserted and guided to a position just distal to the saphenofemoral junction. Bipolar electrodes on the end of the catheter are exposed and an alternating electrical current passes between the electrodes and the vein wall. The cells of the vein wall offer resistance to the passage of the alternating current and as a result of this resistance the cells become heated and the vein ablated. Temperatures of 120°C are generated. Complications include nerve injury (resulting in paraesthesia) and skin burns (Table 18.3). The risk is reduced or prevented by using tumescence anaesthesia (ultrasound guided injection of anaesthetic solution into the facial envelope surrounding the vein). The solution injected usually consists of a vasoconstrictor such as adrenalin and local anaesthetic diluted in saline solution. This type of anaesthesia protects the surrounding tissue from thermal insult, anaesthetises and vaso-constricts the vein compressing it against the catheter/electrode within the lumen. The latter effect drains blood from within the vein and facilitates contact of the catheter with the wall of the vein lumen. This is aided further by manual compression. Successful long saphenous vein ablation is seen in approximately 85% of patients at 2 years [7].

Endovenous laser treatment (EVLT)

The main difference between EVLT and RFA is with the use of a laser diode to generate the thermal insult required for ablation of the vein. The technique of vein cannulation (ultrasound guidance, Seldinger technique) and tumescence anaesthesia is comparable to that of RFA. The catheter contains a laser diode that generates a laser (usually of 810 nm wavelength). This heats blood around the laser tip, generating steam, which heats the vein wall. The risks are the same as RFA, although the temperatures generated are higher and the results probably comparable. Both RFA and EVLT avoid the complications associated with groin incisions and thigh haematomas, and have improved postoperative recovery with less postoperative pain. Both techniques are dependent on causing cell death in the vein wall whilst avoiding perforation and luminal thrombus. Although there are few randomised controlled trials comparing recurrence after EVLT with surgery, published case series indicate successful early ablation rates of 80–90% with EVLT [8, 9].

Surgery

Saphenofemoral junction ligation and great saphenous vein stripping

Surgical treatment of varicosities arising from an incompetent saphenofemoral junction and/or its tributaries is one of the most common procedures performed by the vascular surgeon. Flush ligation of the saphenofemoral junction, division of its tributaries and stripping of the great saphenous vein (ideally to a level of approximately one hand breadth below the knee) has become the gold standard surgical procedure. Stripping of the long saphenous vein to this level reduces the risk of reoccurrence, disconnects the vein from the more proximal cal-

perforator (Boyd's perforator) and minimises the risk of damage to the saphenous nerve. Saphenous neuralgia and chronic pain was a complication associated with full length long saphenous vein stripping. The technique of full length stripping has now been abandoned because of this complication.

Saphenopopliteal junction ligation

Varicosities associated with reflux of the saphenopopliteal junction are treated by ligation of the saphenopopliteal junction. Preoperative diagnosis of saphenopopliteal reflux requires duplex confirmation, and prior to surgery all patients should have the saphenopopliteal junction marked with the aid of duplex ultrasonography. This is because there is considerable anatomical variation in the location of the saphenopopliteal junction location. Significant variation exists in the techniques for small saphenous vein surgery. Approximately 15% of UK surgeons strip the proximal third and there is evidence to suggest this reduces the risk of reoccurrence [10, 11]. Stripping of the small saphenous vein is not carried out routinely by all surgeons due to the risk of sural nerve damage. However, the sural nerve joins the vein in the distal two thirds of the calf. Many surgeons will excise a segment of the small saphenous vein, in the popliteal fossa.

Multiple stab avulsions (phlebectomies)

The cosmetic part of the procedure takes the form of phlebectomies performed through tiny stab incisions using a special vein hook. These should be sufficiently small enough to be closed with small steri-strip adhesive dressings.

Perforator surgery

Opinion remains divided regarding the relevance of perforator surgery. Open surgical ligation of venous perforators may be complicated by poor wound healing and recurrence. A number of perforators identified as being incompetent on duplex scan later become competent after treatment. Some ulceration associated with perforator incompetence together with incompetence in either the long or short saphenous system improves with treatment of the long/short system only. Hence the majority of surgeons would not treat perforators in primary varicose veins without skin changes or ulceration. Some would reserve perforator surgery for resistant venous ulceration not responding to treatment of either the long or short systems. As well as the technique of open ligation, perforator surgery may also be performed using the minimally invasive technique of subfascial endoscopic perforator surgery (SEPS). This involves endoscopic dissection of the sub-fascial plane, identification of the perforator veins and subsequent division. The port site is positioned away from the diseased skin. However, despite this advancement, there remains a lack of evidence to support the use of perforator surgery and randomised controlled trials are needed.

Recurrent varicose veins

There exist a number of reasons for developing recurrence. After excluding persistent varicosities (present but not treated at the time of original surgery) recurrent varicose veins may develop for a number of reasons. Neovascularisation is the development of a new connection between the deep and the superficial vein at a previously divided junction. The mechanism is not fully understood but is believed to be either the consequence of new vessel growth at a site of a previous junction or the dilatation of pre-exisiting tributaries.

Table 18.3 Complications of treatment

Catheter ablation (RFA/EVLT)	Surgery	Foam sclerotherapy
Bruising	Bleeding/bruising	Hyperpigmentation
Thrombophlebitis	Groin infection/abscess	Visual disturbance
Skin burns	Nerve injury	Skin necrosis
Nerve injury	Sensory loss	Deep vein thrombosis
Sensory loss	Motor loss	Thrombophlebitis
Neuralgia	Neuralgia	Stroke
Perforation of deep veins	Deep vein thrombosis	Recurrence
Erythema	Venous flare	
Deep vein thrombosis	Residual varicosities	
Recurrence	Arterial/venous injury	
	Recurrence	

RFA, radiofrequency ablation; EVLT. Endovenous laser treatment.

This is the commonest cause of recurrence at the saphenofemoral junction. Other causes of recurrence include the development of incompetent perforators and the development of varicosities in a second saphenous system.

Approximately one in five patients treated for varicose veins are likely to develop recurrent varicosities. Surgery for recurrent varicose veins can be hazardous with a greater risk of injuring the deep veins, wound complications such as bleeding, infections, lymphatic leakage and seromas. In addition there is a greater risk of nerve injury especially at the saphenopopliteal juction. The need for re-exploration of the groin or saphenopopliteal junction has diminished with the expansion of techniques available to treat varicose veins. Foam scleroterhpy, RFA and EVLT can all be used and hence reduce the need for complicated groin and popliteal re-explorations.

Complications of treatment (Table 18.3)

When consenting patients for surgery, potential complications need to be discussed. General complications include bleeding, infection (more common with groin surgery), recurrence, nerve injury (paraesthesia, chronic pain), DVT, residual varicosities, venous 'flare', haematoma, arterial and deep venous injury (common femoral vein, popliteal vein). Great saphenous vein stripping is associated with significant bruising to the thigh and patients should be warned of this. Saphenopopliteal ligation may be associated with injury to the common peroneal nerve and the risk of foot drop should be mentioned. The nerve can be affected by local anaethesia and any foot drop that persists beyond the duration of the local anaesthetic should be referred for immediate investigation and treatment (nerve conduction studies, exploration, nerve repair/grafting or tendon transfer). Other nerve injuries can occur as a consequence of the phlebectomies. These can result in numbness or chronic neuralgia. Nerves at risk include the common peroneal, saphenous, sural and tibial nerves. The latter two are especially at risk when avulsing behind the malleoli. Neuropraxia has also been seen following application of compression dressings and staff should be advised to release

Table 18.4 Aetiology of chronic venous insufficiency

Aetiology	Example
Superficial venous reflux	Great saphenous/small saphenous varicosities
Deep venous insufficiency	Valvular damage e.g. post DVT
Venous outflow obstruction	Stenosis/occlusion e.g. post DVT, venous cannulation
Calf muscle pump failure	Immobility, obesity, prolonged sitting

DVT, deep vein thrombosis.

ressings should the patient complain of significant pain and numbness in the postoperative recovery room. Any concern about perfusion to the foot following the application of dressings should be treated in the same way.

Chronic venous insufficiency

Epidemiology

As with varicose veins, the prevalence of chronic venous insufficiency (CVI) is marginally greater in men (9% of the population aged between 18–64 years) compared to women (7% of the female population aged between 18–64 years) [1]. The prevalence increases with age. It is a major cause of ulceration and has significant economic implications both in lost working days and cost to the NHS.

Aetiology

This condition results from impaired venous return and causes elevated ambulatory venous pressure within the lower limbs. As a consequence of this elevated venous pressure, skin changes occur in the form of eczema, pigentation, lipodermatosclerosis and ulceration. It is associated with lower limb oedema, varicose veins and chronic pain. There are a number of causes including venous reflux, venous obstruction and 'pump' failure of the calf muscle (Table 18.4).

The combination of normal venous anatomy and calf muscle contraction during exercise is responsible for reducing venous pressure in the lower leg and encouraging venous return. These mechanisms are impaired by venous reflux (affecting either the superficial, deep or perforating venous systems), venous occlusions (e.g. DVT) or abnormal calf pump action. Numerous causes exist for impaired calf muscle function and these range from neurological causes to reduced mobility associated with morbid obesity. The relevance of perforator reflux remains a topic of debate. Perforator reflux frequently occurs in association with superficial or deep reflux. Surgical treatment of the superficial system alone may be associated with a reversal of reflux in the perforator system. Ambulatory pressures have been shown to normalise after superficial venous surgery but not after perforator surgery. Studies of perforator surgery (open and SEPS) for chronic venous ulceration have been associated with a high incidence of ulcer recurrence. It is for this reason that primary surgical treatment should be directed at the superficial system and correction of perforator reflux only considered in resistant cases.

The mechanism by which raised ambulatory venous pressure generates skin changes is not fully understood. Numerous mechanisms have been suggested including the fibrin cuff hypothesis and white cell trapping hypothesis. The fibrin cuff hypothesis suggests tha elevated pressure associated with chronic venous insufficiency results in capillary damag leading to the deposition of fibrinogen. This subsequently forms fibrin and is allowed t accumulate due to an impaired fibrinolytic system. Subsequently oxygen transfer is impaire and the resulting local ischaemia results in ulceration. The white cell trapping hypothesi suggests that the elevated venous pressure slows and halts the passage of large white cell through the capillaries. These become 'plugged' with white cells. These cells are activate and release proteolytic enzymes and free radicals causing local tissue damage. A series events results in the release of factors, which favour increased vascular permeability facili tating the formation of the fibrin cuff. The latter and the trapped white cells cause loca ischaemia and facilitate the formation of ulcers.

Clinical features

Patients complain of a variety of symptoms including swelling, itching, ache and heaviness The symptoms tend to be exacerbated by prolonged standing and relieved by elevatior Initially, oedema is pitting but with chronicity becomes non-pitting. The venous eczem causes pruritis, which stimulates scratching and subsequent skin trauma. This can be th precipitating event leading to ulceration. The most common site of ulceration is the dista medial calf. Pigmentation results from haemosiderin deposition and when accompanied b fibrosis results in lipodermatosclerosis. Varicose veins may be present and superficial reflu should always be excluded. A previous history of deep venous thrombosis is not uncom mon and symptoms of venous claudication (pain and swelling exacerbated with exercise requiring rest and elevation for relief of symptoms) suggest significant venous occlusio (ilio-femoral veins).

Management

Non operative treatment

Certain co-morbidities are known to be associated with the development of chronic venou insufficiency and these should be treated. Obesity and immobility should be improved. Le elevation can reduce ankle venous pressure to 15 mmHg and should be encouraged. Be rest and elevation above the level of the heart may be required for patients with ulceratio resistant to other forms of treatment.

Most patients with chronic venous insufficiency are treated with either compression stock ings or dressings. These apply a graduated compression that decreases proximally. The com pression improves venous blood flow in the deep venous system. Multilayered compression i the gold standard and used to heal venous ulceration. Stockings are used to prevent reoccur rence. Below knee compression stockings of 25–35 mmHg are sufficient for most patients.

Operative treatment

Superficial venous surgery

The role of superficial surgery (e.g. ligation of saphenopopliteal junction, ligation saphenofemoral junction and long saphenous vein stripping) in ulcer healing has been pre viously studied [12]. The ESCHAR trial was a randomised trial involving 500 leg ulcers asso ciated with isolated superficial incompetence and showed the 1-year reccurrence rate of le ulceration to be reduced with combined superficial venous surgery and elastic compressio

9% recurrence) compared to compression alone (38% recurrence) [12]. The initial healing rate was not affected. Superficial surgery is recommended in patients with isolated superficial reflux and a previous history of ulceration.

Perforator surgery

The role of perforator surgery has already been discussed. There remains a debate regarding its benefits as correction of superficial reflux is frequently associated with improvement in perforator reflux. The use of minimally invasive perforator surgery (SEPS) is associated with less morbidity but usually reserved for resistant ulceration.

Venous reconstruction

Venous reconstruction is usually reserved for patients with severe ulceration, venous claudication and limb swelling that has not responded to compression and superficial/perforator surgery. The reconstruction may be either in the form of a venous bypass or, less commonly, valvular reconstruction. A variety of valvular reconstructive procedures have been described and include valvuloplasty, valve transplant, valve transposition, vein wall plication and external banding with a Dacron or polytetrafluoroethane (PTFE) cuff.

If the deep venous system is obstructed then bypass is the reconstructive procedure of choice. The most common cause for deep venous obstruction is deep venous thrombosis. A number of patients will undergo recanalisation and others will develop collaterals allowing for some improvement in symptoms. Venous bypass is usually reserved for patients who are severely symptomatic despite allowing sufficient time (at least 12 months) for collateral development. Other causes of deep venous obstruction include malignant disease, retroperitoneal fibrosis and May–Thurner syndrome. Iliac vein obstruction can be treated with Palma operation. Using the contra-lateral long saphenous vein a bypass is completed by anastomosing the distal end to the common femoral or profunda veins in the affected limb. In the absence of a suitable long saphenous vein a prosthetic conduit may be considered. Deep thigh vein occlusion can be treated with a sapheno-popliteal vein bypass (May–Husni operation). Again the long saphenous vein is the conduit of choice. This procedure is very rarely performed. Reconstructive surgery is contra-indicated in early DVT, arterial disease and thrombophilias.

Endovascular treatment

The techniques of endovenous catheter ablation (RFA and EVLT) and foam sclerotherapy described to treat the superficial system in varicose veins can also be used for treatment of the superficial venous system in chronic venous insufficiency. These are an alternative to surgery. Endo-luminal angioplasty and stenting can be used for treatment of the deep system. Long-term patency results are not known and have not been compared directly with surgery.

Management of leg ulcers

Venous ulceration accounts for approximately 80% of chronic ulceration. A significant number of ulcers are of mixed arterial and venous aetiology. Significant arterial disease should be treated especially if compression is to be considered. Neoplastic disease can be a cause of chronic ulceration and may occur in long standing ulcers (squamous cell carcinoma, Marjolin's ulcers). Biopsy needs to be considered.

In addition to management of the underlying venous disease, consideration should be given to appropriate skin dressings, emollients and nutritional supplements (vitamins and trace elements). Adjunctive surgical techniques that may facilitate wound healing should be considered e.g. wound debridement and skin grafts. Various techniques to facilitate debridement exist and range from topical applications to surgical debridement. Skin grafting may be considered to accelerate the healing. The graft is usually a split skin graft or pinch grafts.

Post-phlebitic syndrome

After a DVT a number of patients will develop chronic venous insufficiency. This is frequently referred to as post-phlebitic or post-thrombotic syndrome. Mild disease is seen in up to one-third of patients whilst severe disease may affect one in ten patients. The risk is increased with more proximal venous thrombosis. The underlying mechanism is of elevated ambulatory venous pressure. As a consequence of valvular destruction, outflow obstruction and calf muscle dysfunction ambulatory venous pressure fails to undergo the normal physiological reduction seen during walking. A normal pressure drop of 50% can be seen during ambulation compared to standing. In chronic venous insufficiency these pressures may actually rise and can result in venous claudication. The early management of DVT is aimed at preventing propagation of the thrombosis by anticoagulation. Elevation and compression stockings are encouraged to minimise swelling. If detected early, preferably within 14 days proximal/ileo-femoral DVTs may be treated with thrombolysis with the aim of restoring venous patency and minimising the loss of venous function. Long-term treatment includes compression stockings and all patients are encouraged to preserve calf muscle function with regular exercise.

References

1. Evans CJ, Fowkes FG, Ruckley CV, Lee AJ. Prevalence of varicose veins and chronic venous insufficiency in men and women in the general population: Edinburgh Vein Study. *J Epidemiol Community Health* 1999; 53: 149–53.
2. London NJM. Duplex ultrasonograpy and varicose veins. *Br J Surgery* 2007; 94: 521–2.
3. Makris SA, Karkos CD, Awad S, London NJM. An 'all comers' venous duplex scan policy for patients with lower limb varicose veins attending a one stop vascular clinic: is it justified? *Eur J Vasc Endovasc Surg* 2002; 32: 718–24.
4. Rautio T, Ohinmaa A, Perälä J et al. Endovenous obliteration versus conventional stripping operation in the treatment of primary varicose veins: a randomized controlled trial with comparison of the costs. *J Vasc Surg* 2002; 35: 958–65.
5. de Medeiros CA, Luccas GC. Comparison of endovenous treatment with an 810 nm laser versus conventional stripping of the great saphenous vein in patients with primary varicose veins. *Dermatol Surg* 2005; 31: 1685–94.
6. Almeida JI, Kaufman J, Göckeritz O et al. Radiofrequency endovenous ClosureFAST versus laser ablation for the treatment of great saphenous reflux: a multicenter, single-blinded, randomized study (RECOVERY study). J Vasc Interv Radiol 2009; 20: 752–9.
7. Suramonia S, Lees TA, Wyatt MG, Oates C. Radiofrequency ablation in the treatment of varicose veins. In: Wyatt WA, ed. *Endovascular Interventions.* Shrewsbury: TMF Publishing Ltd, 2004; 271–6.

8. Disselhoff BC, der Kinderen DJ, Moll FL. Is there recanalization of the great saphenous vein 2 years after endovenous laser treatment? *J Endovasc Ther* 2005; **12**: 731–8.

9. Sharif MA, Soong CV, Lau LL, Corvan R, Lee B, Hannon RJ. Endovenous laser treatment for long saphenous vein incompetence. *Br J Surg* 2006; **93**: 831–5.

10. Winterborn RJ, Campbell WB, Heather BP, Earnshaw JJ. The management of short saphenous varicose veins: a survey of the members of the vascular surgical society of Great Britain and Ireland. *Eur J Vasc Endovasc Surg* 2004; **28**: 400–3.

11. O'Hare JL, Vandenbroeck CP, Whitman B et al., Joint Vascular Research Group. A prospective evaluation of the outcome after small saphenous varicose vein surgery with one-year follow-up. *J Vasc Surg* 2008; **48**: 669–73.

12. Gohel MS, Barwell JR, Taylor M et al. Long term results of compression therapy alone versus compression plus surgery in chronic venous ulceration (ESCHAR): randomised controlled trial. *BMJ* 2007; **335**: 83.

19 Management of deep vein thrombosis

Dharmendra Garg and Vish Bhattacharya

Key points

- Deep vein thrombosis (DVT) and pulmonary embolism (PE) are the leading causes of preventable in-patient mortality following surgery
- Virchow's triad (stasis, hypercoagulable state, vessel wall injury) forms the basis for DVT formation
- Many DVTs are asymptomatic
- Heparin prevents propagation by its action on antithrombin III
- D-dimer level measurements are useful screening tests
- Heparin must be overlapped with warfarin because of the transient hypercoagulable state induced by warfarin
- Outpatient treatment is carried out with low molecular weight heparin (LMWH) and warfarin
- Newer anticoagulants such as rivoraxaban and dabigatran are now being used for prophylaxis
- Inferior vena cava filters can be used when anticoagulation is contraindicated

Background

DVT and its sequela, PE, are the leading causes of preventable in-hospital mortality [1, 2]. In 1846, Virchow recognized the association between venous thrombosis in the legs and PE. Heparin was only introduced to clinical practice in 1937. Over the last 25 years, considerable progress has been made in understanding the pathophysiology, diagnosis, treatment and prevention of venous thromboembolism (VTE). Many DVTs are asymptomatic and almost half of all fatal cases of PE are associated with asymptomatic DVTs.

Pathophysiology

DVT is multifactorial with interaction between hereditary and acquired risk factors. The Virchow triad (i.e. venous stasis, hypercoagulable state, vessel wall injury), continues to serve as the unifying concept in the pathogenesis of DVT. However the significance of interplay between the elements of Virchow's triad and environmental or

Postgraduate Vascular Surgery: The Candidate's Guide to the FRCS, eds. Vish Bhattacharya and Gerard Stansby. Published by Cambridge University Press. © Cambridge University Press 2010.

acquired risk factors is also important. The formation, propagation and dissolution of venous thrombi represent a balance between thrombogenesis and the body's protective mechanisms, specifically the circulating inhibitors of coagulation and the fibrinolytic system. Several risk factors in combination are needed for thrombosis to develop and the risk is cumulative.

Inherent hypercoagulable states include thrombophilias, which can be primary or secondary [3]. Whilst important they only account for <5% of VTE events and are not routinely screened for. Congenital thrombophilias include conditions such as AT III (antithrombin III) deficiency, protein C and protein S deficiency. Antiphospholipid syndrome is the most common cause of acquired thrombophilia. It is characterized by the combination of antiphospholipid antibodies, such as lupus anticoagulant or anticardiolipin antibodies. This syndrome is usually secondary to cancer or an autoimmune condition such as systemic lupus erythematosus (SLE) [3].

Clinical features

Traditional clinical features, such as swollen tender calf, venous swelling, are present in less than one-half the patients. Homan's sign, which is pain or dorsiflexion of foot, is rarely present. Phlegmesia alba dolens (phlegmasia = inflammation, alba = white, dolens = painful) was originally used to describe massive iliofemoral venous thrombosis and associated arterial spasm. The affected extremity is often pale with poor or even absent distal pulses. The physical findings may suggest acute arterial occlusion, but the presence of swelling, petechiae, and distended superficial veins point to a DVT.

In rare cases, the leg is cyanotic from extensive DVT where thrombosis extends into the collateral circulation, resulting in venous congestion. This ischaemic form of venous occlusion was originally described as phlegmasia cerulea dolens or painful blue inflammation. The leg is usually markedly oedematous, painful and cyanotic. Petechiae are often present and the viability of the limb may be threatened.

Calf vein thrombi are usually benign unless there is propagation into the proximal veins. Thrombi in the proximal veins can result in pulmonary emboli in 40–50% of cases and isolated calf vein DVTs cause pulmonary emboli in about 15% of cases.

Assessment of risks

Surgical patients are at increased risk of VTE if they meet one of the following criteria (NICE guidelines January 2010) [1].

- Surgical procedure with a total anaesthetic and surgical time of more than 90 minutes or 60 minutes if the surgery involves the pelvis or lower limb
- Acute surgical admission with inflammatory or intraabdominal condition
- Expected significant reduction in mobility
- One or more of the risk factors noted in Table 19.1.

The Wells clinical prediction guide incorporates risk factors, clinical signs, and the presence or absence of alternative diagnoses (Table 19.2). This clinical prediction guide quantifies the pre-test probability of DVT [4]. The model enables physicians to reliably stratify their patients into high-, moderate- or low-risk categories. Combining this with the results of objective testing greatly simplifies the clinical work up of patients with suspected DVT.

Table 19.1 Patient-related risk factors for venous thromboembolism (VTE) [1]

- Active cancer or cancer treatment
- Age over 60
- Critical care admission
- Dehydration
- Known thrombophilia
- Obesity with a BMI over 30 kg m^{-2}
- One or more significant medical comorbidities (e.g. heart, metabolic, endocrine or respiratory pathology)
- Personal history or first degree relative with a history of VTE
- Use of hormone replacement therapy
- Varicose veins with phlebitis

Table 19.2 Wells clinical score for deep vein thrombosis (DVT)

Clinical parameter score	Score
Active cancer (treatment ongoing, or within 6 months or palliative)	+1
Paralysis or recent plaster immobilization of the lower extremities	+1
Recently bedridden for >3 days or major surgery <4 weeks	+1
Localized tenderness along the distribution of the deep venous system	+1
Entire leg swelling	+1
Calf swelling >3 cm compared to the asymptomatic leg	+1
Pitting oedema (greater in the symptomatic leg)	+1
Previous DVT documented	+1
Collateral superficial veins (nonvaricose)	+1
Alternative diagnosis (as likely or greater than that of DVT)	−2
Total of above score	
High probability	≥3
Moderate probability	1 or 2
Low probability	≤0

Diagnostic evaluation

Because of the inherent inaccuracy of clinical diagnosis, the history, physical examination and assessment of risk factors should be used to determine who requires further objective diagnostic testing.

Objective diagnostic testing for acute DVT has changed considerably over the past two decades. Invasive tests such as venous angiography or fibrinogen uptake test have now been replaced by duplex ultrasound. In the fibrinogen uptake test, iodine labelled fibrinogen is injected intravenously and gets taken up by the developing thrombus. This test has a high sensitivity and detects many small DVTs that would normally resolve spontaneously. In addition this test is inaccurate in detecting the more serious clots in the pelvis and thigh. Duplex is 100% sensitive in detecting proximal thrombus but is less so for calf vein thrombi.

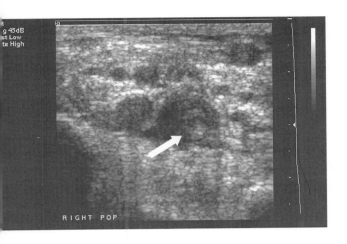

Figure 19.1 Right popliteal vein showing deep vein thrombosis.

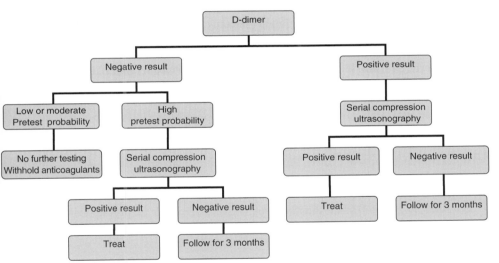

Figure 19.2 Systematic approach to the diagnosis of deep vein thrombosis using clinical prediction models, D-dimer assays, and ultrasound.

D-dimer testing is commonly indicated to rule out VTE in low risk patients. D-dimer is a degradation product of cross-linked fibrin with a high sensitivity in patients with clotting activity. It is measured using ELISA (enzyme linked immunosorbent assay) [5]. A negative D-dimer ELISA test effectively rules out VTE and the need for unnecessary ultrasound scans is therefore reduced. An algorithm combining the use of a clinical prediction score and a D-dimer assay is shown in Figure 19.2.

Information and assessment

- All surgical patients should be assessed to identify their risk factors for VTE (Table 19.1), ideally before admission.
- They should be given verbal and written information, before surgery, about the risks of DVT and the effectiveness of prophylaxis.

- They should be informed that the immobility associated with prolonged travel in the 4 weeks before or after surgery may increase the risk of DVT.
- Oestrogen containing oral contraceptive should be stopped 4 weeks before elective surgery although there is no added risk with progesterone only pills, implants or injections.
- Patients should be given verbal and written information on the signs and symptoms of DVT and PE and the correct use of prophylaxis at home as part of their discharge plan if extended prophylaxis is required [1].

Prophylaxis against DVT [1]

Several options for prophylaxis are available (Table 19.3).

- VTE prophylaxis for patients undergoing gastrointestinal, gynaecological or thoracic surgery and who are assessed to be at increased risk of VTE should be started on mechanical prophylaxis at admission with anti-embolism stockings, foot impulse devices or intermittent pneumatic compression devices.
- The stocking compression profile should be equivalent to the Sigel profile and approximately 18 mmHg at the ankle, 14 mmHg at the mid-calf and 8 mmHg at the upper thigh. These figures are based on Sigel's work in 1975 when he showed that optimal compression for elastic stockings to be used by hospitalized patients confined to bed should be 18 to 8 mmHg (ankle to mid thigh). At this compression, average femoral vein blood flow velocity is increased significantly. Graduated compression produced a greater femoral vein flow velocity than uniform compression of the lower limb.
- Pharmacological VTE prophylaxis for patients who have a low risk of major bleeding should include fondaparinux sodium, low molecular weight heparin (LMWH) or unfractionated heparin (UFH). This should be continued until the patient no longer has significant reduced mobility, generally for 5–7 days.
- NICE guidelines advise that in elective hip and knee replacement surgery and hip fractures, in addition to mechanical prophylaxis as above, VTE prophylaxis can be carried out with newer anticoagulants e.g. dabigatran etexilate and rivaroxaban, or fondaparinux sodium, LMWH or UFH.
- Dabigatran is started 1–4 hours after surgery, fondaparinux 6 hours after surgical closure and LMWH 6–12 hours after surgery. Rivaroxaban and UFH are started 6–12 hours after surgery.
- Patients who are already on antiplatelet agents and who are at increased risk of VTE should have pharmacological prophylaxis if the risk of VTE outweighs the risk of bleeding. Conversely, if the risk of bleeding is higher then mechanical prophylaxis should be used.
- If patients are on vitamin K antagonists and are within therapeutic range no prophylaxis is required provided anticoagulant therapy is continued.

Treatment of DVT

Unfractionated heparin

The primary objectives of the treatment of DVT are to prevent PE, reduce morbidity and prevent or minimize the risk of developing postphlebitic syndrome. Because of the risk of

Table 19.3 Methods of venous thromboembolism (VTE) prophylaxis

- General measures
Early mobilization
Leg exercises
Hydration
- Mechanical methods
Antiembolism stockings (thigh or knee length)
Foot impulse devices
Intermittent pneumatic compression devices (thigh or knee length)
- Pharmacological methods
Heparin
(i) unfractionated
(ii) low molecular weight
Direct thrombin inhibitors
(i) dabigatran
(ii) rivaroxaban
Synthetic pentasaccharides
(i) fondaparinux
Anticoagulants e.g. warfarin
Antiplatelet agents e.g. aspirin, clopidogrel (not usually used alone for VTE prophylaxis)
- Vena cava filters

proximal propagation with the potential risk of pulmonary embolism or post-thrombotic syndrome most authors believe that calf DVTs should be treated.

Anticoagulation remains the mainstay of initial treatment for DVT. Regular unfractionated heparin was the standard of care until the introduction of LMWH. Heparin prevents extension of the thrombus and has been shown to significantly reduce, but not eliminate, the incidence of fatal and nonfatal PE, as well as recurrent thrombosis [6]. The primary reason for this is that heparin has no effect on preexisting nonadherent thrombus. It does not affect the size of existing thrombus and has no intrinsic thrombolytic activity. Heparin is a heterogeneous mixture of polysaccharide fragments with varying molecular weights. The key unit is a pentasaccharide sequence that is responsible for binding to antithrombin III (AT III) to inhibit thrombin. Heparin also activates the plasma protein heparin cofactor II, which inactivates thrombin. At higher concentrations it also binds to factor IXa, resulting in the modulation of factor Xa generation.

The optimal regimen for the treatment of DVT is anticoagulation with heparin or LMWH followed by full anticoagulation with oral warfarin for 3–6 months. Warfarin therapy is overlapped with heparin for 4–5 days until the international normalized ratio (INR) is therapeutically elevated to 2–3. Heparin must be overlapped with oral warfarin because of the initial transient hypercoagulable state induced by warfarin. This effect is related to the differential half-lives of protein C, protein S and the vitamin K-dependent clotting factors II, VII, IX and X.

Long-term anticoagulation is definitely indicated for patients with recurrent venous thrombosis and/or persistent or irreversible risk factors. When IV UFH is initiated for DVT, the goal is to achieve and maintain an elevated activated partial thromboplastin time (aPTT) of at least 1.5 times control. After an initial bolus of 80 U kg^{-1}, a constant maintenance infusion of 18 U kg^{-1} is initiated. The aPTT is checked 6 hours after the bolus and adjusted accordingly. The aPTT is checked every 6 hours until two successive aPTTs are therapeutic. Thereafter, the aPTT, the haematocrit level and platelet count are monitored every 24 hours.

Heparin-induced thrombocytopenia (HIT) is a serious but uncommon side effect. Type I HIT occurs in 10% and Type II in 5% of patients on heparin. Type I is due to a mild lowering of the platelet count due to platelet clumping and occurs in the first 24 hours of therapy. Type II HIT results from the binding of heparin to platelets and subsequent generation of immune complexes consisting of immunoglobulin G and heparin platelet factor 4. This occurs five or more days after starting therapy and can cause thrombosis. Unfortunately, the subset of patients who develop thrombosis is unpredictable. Heparin can rarely cause hyperlipidaemia, hyperkalaemia, osteoporosis, skin necrosis and hypersensitivity reactions.

Low molecular weight heparin

LMWH is prepared by selectively treating UFH to isolate the low-molecular-weight (<9000 Da) fragments. Its activity is measured in units of factor X inactivation, and monitoring of the aPTT is not required. The dose is weight adjusted. LMWH is administered subcutaneously (SC), and its half-life permits single- or twice-daily dosing. Its use in the outpatient treatment of DVT and PE has been evaluated in a number of studies.

Indirect factor Xa inhibitors

A recent further refinement of the heparin molecule is fondaparinux, a synthetic form of the pentasaccharide sequence of heparin that binds to antithrombin. It acts as a selective potent, indirect antithrombin-dependent inhibitor of factor Xa. It is administered once a day via subcutaneous injection and does not require laboratory monitoring. Despite its advantages, it is not recommended for patients with renal failure and has limited use due to its parenteral route of administration and lack of an antidote.

Direct factor Xa inhibitors

Factor Xa inhibitors include rivaroxaban and apiaxaban. Rivaroxaban is well tolerated, has high bioavailability and predictable pharmacokinetics and is orally available. It does not require dose adjustments and laboratory monitoring. The RECORD trials (four multicentre double blind trials compared the efficacy of rivaroxaban compared to enoxaparin for the prevention of VTE following hip and knee replacement) showed significant reduction in primary efficacy end points (DVT, PE or death from all causes). Major bleeding was noted to be slightly higher in the rivaroxaban group although this was not statistically significant.

Direct thrombin inhibitors

Dabigatran and ximelagatran are a new class of drugs that act by binding directly to thrombin. There is no need for routine monitoring and drug interaction is rare. Clinical trials with dabigatran in patients undergoing hip and knee replacement surgery showed significantly less VTEs as compared to enoxaparin although bleeding risks were higher.

Other strategies

Inferior vena cava (IVC) filters [7]

IVC filters should be considered for surgical inpatients with recent (within 1 month) or existing DVT and in whom anticoagulation is contraindicated. They may be indicated in patients requiring abdominal surgery when anticoagulation is contraindicated or in trauma patients. Other indications include recurrent PE while being adequately anticoagulated or if there is a complication with the anticoagulation therapy requiring its termination. Designs of filters have improved since Greenfield first described his filter in 1973. Temporary and retrievable filters are also available. Most of these can now be placed via 6–12 French sheaths using a percutaneous route under fluoroscopic or ultrasound guidance. They are usually inserted via the jugular vein route. Complications include thrombosis of the filter and migration of the filter through the walls of the IVC.

Thrombolysis [8]

The indications for thrombolysis in acute DVT remain controversial and Level 1 evidence is missing for its long-term benefit. Thrombolysis can be performed for acute (<10 days) ileofemoral DVT when there is no contraindication to use of anticoagulants or recent bleeding episodes, trauma or recent surgery. It is usually reserved for patients with major ileofemoral thrombosis with significant acute swelling and symptoms. Techniques vary considerably and are rapidly developing [9]. Venous catheterization can be performed via the internal jugular, femoral or popliteal vein, depending on the site of thrombus and treatment aims. Infusion of thrombolytic agents such as r-tPA is performed via a multiple side hole catheter embedded into the thrombus. A Cochrane review has shown that complete clot lysis and improved patency is more often seen with thrombolysis than conservative treatment with anticoagulation [8]. Venous function is significantly improved and there is less post-thrombotic syndrome. Usually a temporary caval filter is used in addition to prevent PE while lysis is being performed. Acute venous thrombectomy is now rarely performed.

Mechanical devices for thrombus removal have been described but none are currently approved. Some of them have a jet, suction or a brush tip to allow disruption and aspiration of the clot. However all of these need IVC filters at the time of use to prevent PE.

Post-thrombotic syndrome (PTS)

This is a condition that appears up to several years after DVT, manifesting as chronic swelling, pain, varicose veins, venous eczema, pigmentation and venous ulcers. It probably occurs because of damage to deep venous valves, resulting in chronic venous hypertension. It affects up to 40% of patients after DVT and is more common after extensive iliofemoral DVT. There is evidence that long-term use of graduated compression stockings after DVT can reduce the incidence of PTS.

Summary

It is essential to define the preoperative risk of DVT and use best practice advice to reduce the risk in inpatients undergoing surgery. Treatment and care should take into account patients' needs and preferences. UFH, LMWH, fondaparinux and newer agents such as rivaroxaban and dabigatran are the main pharmacological agents currently used in prophylaxis and treatment of DVT. In the past decade, tremendous advances have been made with respect to the diagnosis and treatment of DVT. The use of invasive techniques to diagnose DVT has been completely replaced with accurate, yet noninvasive, diagnostic modalities. The therapy of DVT is undergoing exciting changes with the development of targeted antithrombotics with greater therapeutic efficacy and safety, as well as considerably greater ease of use.

References

1. National Institute for Health and Clinical Excellence. Venous thromboembolism: Reducing the risk of venous thromboembolism (deep vein thrombosis and pulmonary embolism) in patients admitted to hospital. NICE Clinical Guideline 92. January 2010 http://www.nice.org.uk

2. Geerts WH, Bergqvist D, Pineo GF, Heit JA, Samama CM, Lassen MR, Colwell CW; American College of Chest Physicians. Prevention of venous thromboembolism: American College of Chest Physicians Evidence-Based Clinical Practice Guidelines, 8th edn. *Chest* 2008; 133(6 Suppl): 381S–453S.

3. Rosendaal FR. Venous thrombosis: a multicausal disease. *Lancet* 1999; 353: 1167–73.

4. Anand SS, Wells PS, Hunt D et al. Does this patient have deep vein thrombosis? *JAMA* 1998; 279: 1094–9.

5. Bates SM, Kearon C, Crowther M et al. A diagnostic strategy involving a quantitative latex D-dimer assay reliably excludes deep venous thrombosis. *Ann Intern Med* 2003; 138: 787–94.

6. Hirsh J, Warkentin TE, Shaughnessy SG et al. Heparin and low-molecular-weight heparin: mechanisms of action, pharmacokinetics, dosing, monitoring, efficacy, and safety. *Chest* 2001; 119: 64S–94S.

7. Young T, Tang H, Aukes J, Hughes R. Vena caval filters for the prevention of pulmonary embolism. *Cochrane Database of Systematic Reviews* 2007, Issue 4. Art. no. CD006212. DOI: 10.1002/14651858. CD006212.pub3.

8. Watson LI, Armon MP. Thrombolysis for acute deep vein thrombosis. *Cochrane Database of Systematic Reviews* 2004, Issue 3. Art. no. CD002783. DOI: 10.1002/14651858.CD002783.pub2.

9. Comerota AJ, Gravett MH. Iliofemoral vein thrombosis. *J Vasc Surg* 2007; 46: 1065–76.

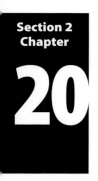

Final FRCS vascular topics

Infection in vascular surgery

Mike Clarke

Key points

- Infection of prosthetic vascular grafts is associated with a high mortality and morbidity
- Prosthetic grafts should be avoided if the risk of infection is high
- Early diagnosis requires a low index of suspicion
- The greatest chance of long-term success lies in complete removal of the infected prosthesis and revascularisation with autologous material
- A groin abscess in an intravenous drug abuser should be considered to be an infected false aneurysm of the femoral artery until positively excluded

Introduction

Managing the infective complications of arterial surgery represents one of the most complex challenges facing the vascular surgeon. Medical management alone seldom produces a satisfactory outcome but the removal of an infected prosthesis in a debilitated patient, possibly in the face of life-threatening haemorrhage, is rarely straightforward. The problem of then restoring distal perfusion may require innovative approaches whilst minimising the risk to the patient's life and reducing the likelihood of recurrent infection.

Epidemiology

Conventional surgical teaching is that 'clean' operative procedures should carry a post-operative wound infection rate of less than 1% (Table 20.1). Data from the Health Protection Agency (HPA) surveillance of surgical site infection rates however suggests that this is rarely achieved and approaches the sort of rates generally seen with clean-contaminated or contaminated procedures [1].

Causative organisms

Forty-six per cent of organisms seen in early postoperative infections following vascular procedures are staphylococcal, two-thirds of these being methicillin resistant *Staphylococcus aureus* (MRSA). Coagulase negative staphylococci are an unusual cause of early infection but may be more important in the development of late-presenting graft infections. *Enterococcus* and *Enterobacter* species are responsible for around 30% of early postoperative infections with the remainder consisting of *Streptococci*, *Pseudomonas*, anaerobes, fungi and other

Postgraduate Vascular Surgery: The Candidate's Guide to the FRCS, eds. Vish Bhattacharya and Gerard Stansby. Published by Cambridge University Press. © Cambridge University Press 2010.

Table 20.1 Incidence of infection following surgical procedures in England 1997–2005

Category	No. of operations	Infected (%)
Knee prosthesis	62 031	1.0
Total hip prosthesis	74 677	1.8
Coronary artery bypass graft	27 447	4.1
Vascular surgery	8 959	6.0
Large bowel surgery	14 296	9.2
Limb amputation	2 670	13.1

Table 20.2 Rates of Szilagyi grade III infection following arterial reconstruction by nature of graft and anatomical location

Graft type	Rate of grade III infection
Synthetic graft	1.9
Autogenous vein	0.4
Endarterectomies	0.2
Arterial allografts	0.4
Site of surgery	
Aorto-iliac	0.7
Aorto-femoral	1.6
Femoro-popliteal	3.0
Femoro-femoral	0.9
Other (intrathoracic, carotid, visceral)	1.0

bacterial species. Although MRSA is the commonest infecting organism, most studies suggest that outcomes are no worse with MRSA infection compared with other staphylococcal infections.

The HPA data refer specifically to infection rates during the original hospital stay and of these the vast majority relate to superficial wound infections. Nevertheless the data is in keeping with some historical series that have suggested the rate of vascular prosthesis implant infection may be as high as 7%.

Infection in following arterial reconstruction varies from simple superficial wound infection to deep infection involving the arterial conduit itself. The classification system proposed by Szilagyi in the 1970s remains relevant to vascular surgical practice today [2].

Grade I – dermis only.

Grade II – involvement of subcutaneous tissues.

Grade III – vascular graft involvement.

Although it is grade III infections that are of the greatest concern, it is recognised that early grade I and II infections are associated with the later development of grade III infections and so should always be taken seriously. Table 20.2 shows how rates of grade III infection vary by the nature of the conduit and the site of arterial surgery. As can be seen, prosthetic grafts are more at risk than autologous forms of reconstruction and risk is also increased by surgery involving the groin.

Prevention

Although not always possible, there is currently a keen focus on reducing infection rates in surgical patients. Some factors cannot be easily altered. Patient age and preoperative health status (including the presence of diabetes) have both been shown to be associated with higher instances of postoperative infection. Other risk factors include prolonged preoperative hospital stay, the presence of non-healing ulcers or other tissue loss, admission from a long-term care facility and excessive antibiotic usage.

Conduct of the operation

Surgical technique can go a long way to preventing infection following surgery. Simple measures include preoperative washing of patients; reducing theatre traffic to a minimum; careful attention to the handing of tissues; avoidance of excessive retraction with self-retaining retractors; preoperative marking of the long saphenous vein to avoid undermining skin flaps, careful skin closure without undue tension and with suture techniques that avoid devascularising the skin edges. Other factors that may help reduce perioperative surgical site infection include maintenance of normothermia during surgery and careful glycaemic control in patients with diabetes. Approximately 5% of patients undergoing arterial surgery will be colonised with MRSA prior to surgery. Preoperative screening for MRSA allows attempts at eradication therapy prior to admission and patients known to be colonised with MRSA should not be nursed alongside patients who are free from MRSA.

Antibiotic prophylaxis

It is important to develop a local antibiotic prophylaxis policy in conjunction with your microbiologists. Consideration should be given to observed patterns of infection in vascular patients as well as sensitivity and resistance patterns amongst organisms encountered. As well as routine prophylaxis, it is well worth the policy including an alternative regime for patients with known sensitivities or renal/liver impairment that precludes them from receiving the standard regime as well as an option for second-line prophylaxis for those patients requiring early re-exploration.

Diagnosis

Clinical presentation

Graft infections may present in a multitude of ways and it is important to maintain a high index of suspicion. For superficial grafts, the diagnosis may be relatively straightforward with, for example, an obviously infected false aneurysm within the groin or a discharging sinus overlying a graft. Any signs of bleeding should raise the possibility of anastomotic disruption and all too often a small herald bleed will be followed soon afterwards by major haemorrhage. The diagnosis of infection related to intracavity grafts can be somewhat more complicated. Patients presenting with upper gastro-intestinal haemorrhage following previous aortic surgery should be considered to have an aorto-enteric fistula until proven otherwise. In many cases however, the presentation is more subtle and may include pyrexia of unknown origin, general malaise and weight loss, vertebral osteomyelitis and hydronephrosis.

Laboratory investigations

Routine laboratory investigations can provide evidence in support of the diagnosis of graft infection but most are non-specific. They should, in the first instance, include: full blood count; erythrocyte sedimentation rate; C-reactive protein; urea and electrolytes; serum albumin; microscopy; culture and sensitivity of any wound or sinus discharge; and peripheral blood cultures.

Imaging

Imaging plays an essential role in the evaluation of patients with suspected arterial graft infection. In particular it can potentially confirm the presence of infection or the development of local complications, e.g. false aneurysm formation, hydronephrosis. In addition information can be obtained regarding proximal and distal vessels for planning reconstruction.

Ultrasound

Often useful in situations where a graft is placed superficially, ultrasound can quickly and easily detect the presence of peri-graft collections and the presence or absence of false aneurysms. In the carotid territory, a distinct rippling of the surface of an infected patch has been reported as being visible on ultrasound. Ultrasound guided aspiration of a peri-graft collection may provide the opportunity for microbiological confirmation of infection. In the absence of overt clinical signs of local infection one has to consider the possibility of introducing infection into an otherwise sterile field or precipitating other local complications and such aspiration should only take place under the guidance of a vascular surgeon.

Computed tomography (CT)

For intracavity grafts, CT remains the most useful method of imaging currently in use. The presence of a gas-filled fluid collection adjacent to the graft more than 3 months after implantation can be considered pathognomonic of infection. Such collections may be present in the first few weeks following implantation and at these times interpretation needs to be carefully considered alongside the clinical features. In these circumstances and if time allows, serial scans may be helpful in distinguishing normal postoperative change, which should progressively resolve versus progressive postoperative infection. Other features that may suggest infection include simple fluid collections, 'streaking' of surrounding fat planes or the presence of adjacent complications such as an anastomotic aneurysm.

In addition to confirming the diagnosis, CT angiography also offers the opportunity to outline the inflow and run-off vessels, thus avoiding the need for supplementary vascular imaging (Figure 20.1).

Angiography

Digital subtraction angiography provides little information on the presence or extent of infection. It can be helpful in providing detailed images of the run-off vasculature but rarely adds significantly more than CT.

Magnetic resonance (MR) scanning

Magnetic resonance offers many of the advantages seen with CT scanning including the diagnosis of intracavity graft infection and imaging of adjacent vasculature. T2 weighted

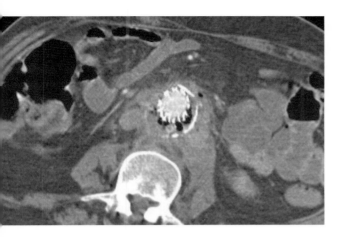

Figure 20.1 Computed tomography showing an infected aortic stent graft 2 years after insertion. Note the presence of gas within the aortic sac.

mages may be more sensitive in identifying peri-graft oedema prior to the development of a frank collection. There is, however, little firm data to support its use in place of CT, which s currently the more commonly utilised modality in UK practice.

Labelled white cell scans

Radionuclide-labelled white cell scintigraphy with technitium-99 and indium-111 have both been used in the diagnosis of vascular graft infection. They may be a useful adjunct to CT, particularly in confirming early graft infection although the results need to be interpreted with caution as although sensitive, the technique suffers from relatively low specificity.

Treatment strategies

In many instances, the ideal treatment strategy is excision of the infected prosthesis (if one is present), debridement of adjacent involved arterial wall and *in situ* reconstruction with autogenous vein. In the case of the infected lower limb prosthetic graft, the autologous saphenous vein is the most obvious choice, although in many cases, the reason for implanting a prosthetic graft in the first place has been the unsuitability of the saphenous vein. Consideration should be given to the contralateral long saphenous vein (LSV), if present, as well as short saphenous veins and upper limb veins.

In situ vein graft

Where the long saphenous vein is going to be of insufficient calibre, the superficial femoral veins can be successfully utilised. This is particularly so in replacing aortic grafts. The superficial femoral veins (SFVs) are frequently 10–12 mm in diameter and there are now a number of series that have demonstrated success in replacing infected aortic prostheses. As well as aortic replacement, the SFV is also a useful conduit when replacing infected femoro-femoral cross over grafts. The SFVs can be harvested down to popliteal level and may even be harvested when the LSV has already gone. At the proximal end, particular care should be taken to ensure that the profunda vein remains intact. Some leg swelling may occur after harvest of the SFV but this is rarely severe.

Excision and extra-anatomic bypass

In many instances, excision and extra-anatomic bypass would be considered the conventional approach to managing prosthetic graft infection. It has the advantage of removing the infected prosthesis whilst providing revascularisation without placing the new graft in the infected bed. In most instances it is necessary to use a second prosthesis for the extra anatomic bypass and there remains a relatively high rate of subsequent infection of the new prosthetic conduit.

Infected aortic grafts

Infection of a prosthetic aortic graft is invariably a catastrophic complication following aortic aneurysm repair. Presentation often occurs relatively late after the original surgery and may represent haematogenous seeding of the prosthetic graft or low-grade contamination from the time of implantation. Presentation varies. In some cases, patients present with features of chronic sepsis including general malaise, pyrexia of unknown origin and weight loss. Back pain and abdominal pain may be present but are not invariable and the diagnosis is frequently delayed. More acutely, patients may present with signs of gastrointestinal (GI) bleeding either from an aorto-duodenal fistula (with or without false aneurysm formation) or more commonly an erosion of the duodenum by the body of the graft. In this instance, the arterial anasatamosis is not involved but bleeding is from the eroded edges of the duodenum. In all patients with upper GI bleeding and a history of previous aortic surgery, the diagnosis of aorto-duodenal fistula should be considered until proven otherwise.

In patients presenting less acutely, time should be spent not only in investigation, but also in attempting to optimise the patient's status for surgery. Any surgery for an infected aortic graft is going to be a major undertaking and any time spent improving the patient's general condition will ultimately pay dividends. Positive blood cultures may allow administration of appropriate antibiotics and attention should be given to the patient's nutritional status, which may well be depleted by the effects of chronic sepsis.

The surgical strategy will to a large extent be determined by the general condition of the patient and the urgency for operative intervention (principally the presence of life-threatening haemorrhage). The key elements of the surgical approach are the safe excision of the infected graft and the provision of distal revascularisation.

Any revisional aortic surgery is demanding but particularly so in the presence of infection or when dealing with a proximal anastomotice false aneurysm. The ease by which proximal control can be established is largely determined by the length of aorta between the prosthetic graft and the origin of the renal arteries. In order to safely secure proximal control, some surgeons prefer to expose the aorta at the level of the diaphragm prior to dissecting out the infrarenal aorta. The lesser sac is entered by dividing the lesser omentum and the left lobe of the liver is retracted upwards to expose the crus of the diaphragm. In the emergency situation this can be split bluntly with scissors but in the elective setting can be progressively divided with diathermy. This exposes the most distal thoracic aorta above the coeliac axis where a clamp can be placed without closing it. Attention can then be turned to the infrarenal aorta, safe in the knowledge that if major haemorrhage is encountered, proximal control can be easily be achieved. An alternative means of securing rapid proximal control is to expose a more distal portion of the aortic graft and introduce an aortic occlusion balloon through a small arteriotomy in the graft.

Having achieved proximal control, distal control is generally more straightforward. If it is not possible to dissect out the iliac vessels, the graft can be divided and the iliac arteries controlled with Pruitt occlusion catheters or Fogarty-type catheters fitted with three-way taps.

Having excised the graft, the decision needs to be made about subsequent reconstruction. In the emergency setting, where the patient has been operated on for life-threatening haemorrhage, the decision will be dictated by the condition of the patient at this stage. If the patient is in extremis, the aortic stump should be over sewn and the patient returned to the intensive care unit in an attempt to stabilise them. If they recover sufficiently in the next few hours they may be returned to the operating theatre for lower limb revascularisation although it has to be accepted that if they survive many will face bilateral lower limb amputation.

In dealing with the infrarenal aortic stump, sufficient tissue should be debrided to allow safe ligation of the aorta and minimise the risk of the aorta subsequently giving way and leading to stump blow-out. The aortic stump is most securely closed in two layers with a non absorbable monofilament – a layer of interrupted mattress sutures and a second layer of continuous suture.

Where revascularisation is deemed appropriate, two options are available – extra-anatomic bypass or *in situ* replacement. The conventional approach is extra-anatomic bypass. Controversy exists as to whether this is by axillo-bifemoral or bi-axillo-femoral bypass. Furthermore, some authors advocate performance of the extra-anatomic bypass prior to graft excision to avoid the otherwise potentially prolonged period of lower limb ischaemia that occurs and the subsequent reperfusion effects. Others argue that pre-emptive insertion of the extra-anatomic grafts risks bacteraemic seeding at the time of excision of the infected aortic grafts and contributes to the 25% infection rate amongst extra-anatomic grafts inserted in the treatment of aortic graft infection. The other major concern with this approach is the risk of aortic stump blow-out. Historic series have reported blow rates of up to 40% although more recent practice would indicate a rate closer to 10%.

In situ graft replacement avoids the issue of an aortic stump and is thus particularly applicable when there is only a short infrarenal aortic segment although it does necessitate placing a graft in an infected bed. A number of series have reported good outcomes utilising prosthetic grafts treated to resist infection. The commonest way of doing this is to soak a polyester graft for 20 min in a rifampicin solution (60 mg ml^{-1}). The relative rarity of aortic graft infection means that most evidence comes from single-centre retrospective case series. One of the largest series of *in situ* prosthetic replacement grafts in 52 patients included a mix of rifampicin-bonded grafts and grafts covered with omental patches. In this series the perioperative mortality was 9% with 11% of patients developing recurrent infection of the aortic graft [3].

More recently, attention has turned to using autologous material for *in situ* replacement. Obviously, the LSV is of too narrow a calibre to be practicable but a number of series have now reported good outcomes using SFV [4]. The vein can readily be harvested from the subsartorial canal. Proximally it is divided immediately distal to its confluence with the profunda vein where the common femoral vein is formed. Distally, it is easiest to divide it just above the adductor hiatus – below this level there is an increasing number of geniculate branches to deal with, although if it is essential to obtain the maximum length then it is quite safe to harvest the entire above-knee popliteal vein in continuity. Postoperative leg swelling is reported to be minimal, even in cases where the LSV has been previously removed. In an adult, the femoral vein is generally 10–12 mm in diameter and can readily be fashioned to

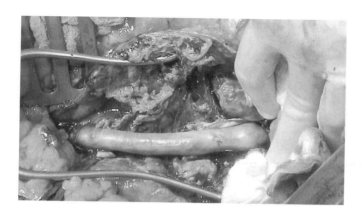

Figure 20.2 *In situ* reconstruction of a mycotic aortic aneurysm with superficial femoral vein.

allow anastomosis with the aorta. If necessary, both femoral veins can be harvested to allow construction of a Y-graft and it can also prove useful in the replacement of an infected aortic graft (Figure 20.2).

Another alternative to the autologous vein is fresh cryo-preserved human tissue. This is available from a number of sites around the UK including Oxford, Liverpool and Birmingham. The largest experience is with ascending aorta and aortic arch, which has been extensively used in paediatric cardiac surgery but material is now available from more distal aorta and superficial femoral artery. There is, as yet, little experience in the UK of using such grafts for the replacement of infected peripheral vascular grafts but reports from elsewhere suggest results comparable with autologous material [5].

Infected aortic endovascular grafts

Aortic stent grafts are not immune to infective complications [6]. A number of series have reported incidences of around 1%, similar to that seen following open aortic surgery. The mechanisms of presentation are also similar to those seen in infected open aortic grafts and include aorto-enteric fistula. Furthermore, the same principles of treatment apply – removal of the infected prosthesis, debridement of infected tissue and, where possible, distal revascularisation. In most cases removal of the infected stent graft is relatively straightforward as they do not become incorporated in the same manner as an open graft. Care must be exercised however when removing grafts with suprarenal fixation. It is easy to damage the suprarenal aorta whilst attempting to remove these devices and in some cases it is more judicious to detach and leave *in situ* the uncovered bare metal portion of the graft, which extends above the renal arteries.

Infected carotid patches

As with peripheral infection, infection related to a prosthetic carotid patch is generally a straightforward diagnosis. Presentation may be in the form of clear signs of acute infection with pain, swelling and erythema overlying the patch. In some cases the presentation is less acute and manifests as a discharging sinus or the presence of a false aneurysm. Rupture of a prosthetic patch is fortunately rare, as are recurrent neurological symptoms.

In most cases, first-line imaging is with Duplex scanning, to look for local features of infection and to confirm whether the internal carotid artery remains patent – an occluded nternal carotid is obviously considerably easier to manage. Magnetic resonance or CT angi-ography will give details about the distal carotid circulation. It can be very helpful to have an indication of the likely consequences of occlusion of the internal carotid artery as this is a very real risk following revisional surgery for infection. Information gathered at the time of the original operation can be helpful, e.g. if performed under local anaesthetic, did the patient tolerate the procedure without the need for a shunt? If this information is not available, then angiography with a trial balloon occlusion of the internal carotid artery can provide useful information.

As with infection of an arterial prosthesis elsewhere, the treatment strategy has to be considered in light of the patient's status, but successful eradication of infection generally requires removal of the infected patch. The operation should only be undertaken by sur-geons with considerable experience of carotid surgery. The patient should be warned of the relatively high risk of cranial nerve injury. The most difficult part of the procedure is usually obtaining adequate distal exposure to safely allow reconstruction. In patients with a low bifurcation and a short patch this is not too difficult but if difficulty is anticipated, naso-tra-cheal intubation allows the mandible to fully close and provides more room to manoeuvre than conventional intubation. When further access is required, some surgeons advocate approaching the distal internal carotid via an infratemporal fossa approach, usually in con-junction with an ear, nose and throat (ENT) surgeon.

Having established control proximally and distally, and following heparinisation of the patient, the patch can be opened and a suitable shunt inserted. In most cases we plan to attempt reconstruction with autologous vein and this can be reversed and 'pre-loaded' onto the distal limb of the shunt prior to insertion. In some circumstances and even with good distal exposure, the accessible part of the internal carotid artery (ICA) proves too friable to safely reconstruct. It is then necessary to ligate the artery and it is when faced with this situ-ation that knowledge of the patients likely tolerance of internal carotid ligation can aid the decision-making process as up to 50% of patients will suffer a stroke following acute ligation of the ICA.

In those patients where reconstruction is feasible, the choice between utilising the vein as a patch or interposition graft is largely determined by the amount of ICA wall left follow-ing adequate debridement of the edges of the original anastomosis. In a large proportion of cases, a patch is feasible and this is the simpler option. The vein that was loaded onto the shunt can be opened longitudinally and following excision of any valve leaflets can be used as a patch in the conventional manner.

If only a thin strip of back wall of the ICA remains, it is better to use the vein as an interposition graft. The distal ICA is transacted and the distal anastomosis fashioned first. Following completion of this anastomosis, the distal limb of the shunt is withdrawn into the vein graft and the anastomosis tested for adequate haemostasis. It is important to ensure this is satisfactory prior to undertaking the proximal anastomosis as access to the deep aspect of the graft is subsequently very difficult. The proximal anastomosis can then be completed, ideally incorporating the origin of the external carotid artery, although this is not always practicable, in which case the orifice of the external carotid can be over sewn.

Infected peripheral grafts

The diagnosis of peripheral graft infection is generally more straightforward than is the case with intracavity grafts. Patients generally have signs of localised sepsis including pain, swelling and erythema over the graft/anastomosis. There may be a purulent discharge from a wound sinus and any blood staining of the sinus should alert the surgeon to the possibility of incipient major haemorrhage. Anastomotic false aneurysm development is not always related to infection but even in the absence of other signs of sepsis, the possibility should always be borne in mind.

In most cases of peripheral graft infection, the underlying graft is prosthetic and successful treatment ultimately requires removal of the infected prosthesis. The anastomosis may be quite friable or there may have been false aneurysm development. It is therefore generally wise to ensure adequate proximal control prior to exposure of the anastomosis. With infrainguinal grafts in the groin, it is often possible to expose the inguinal ligament, the lower margin of which can then be carefully dissected upwards to provide exposure of the distal external iliac artery. If there is any doubt about the ability to safely gain control by this route (e.g. with extensive scarring, in very obese patients or with haemorrhage requiring rapid control) then an extraperitoneal approach to the external iliac artery should be followed.

Having achieved proximal and distal control the graft can then usually be detached from its anastomoses and removed. In some cases, the graft infection has resulted in the graft failing to become incorporated and removal from its track is relatively straightforward. It is often the case, however, that the graft has remained incorporated along a large proportion of its length. One useful technique is to utilise a Codman-style varicose vein stripper to remove the graft, however one has to weigh up the risk of ongoing infection in a graft remnant against that of damaging adjacent structures, e.g. the femoral vein in attempting to remove a well incorporated graft.

Revascularisation

In any case of arterial graft infection, amongst the most feared complications is that of recurrent infection with the possibility of life-threatening haemorrhage. Careful consideration therefore needs to be given as to whether the risks inherent in further attempts at arterial reconstruction are justified. In a proportion of cases, the limb in question will survive without further revascularisation. Experience of patients with infected false femoral aneurysms as a complication of drug misuse has shown that limb salvage can be maintained even following acute ligation of the common femoral artery. Factors that may indicate the possibility of achieving limb salvage without distal grafting include an already occluded graft, patients whose grafts were originally inserted for claudication and the ability to preserve flow down the profunda artery. Having taken down an infected common femoral anastomosis, it is necessary to excise a reasonable portion of the adjacent arterial wall. The atherosclerotic artery can harbour organisms and failure to adequately debride the artery wall can result in late haemorrhage, even when closed primarily. If necessary, the artery can be closed with a patch although this should ideally be autologous material. In many cases it is possible to find a short segment of vein to do this or alternatively, if the superficial femoral artery is occluded (which frequently it is) a segment can be excised, opened longitudinally and fashioned into a patch by removal of the occluded intima. Failing this, bovine pericardium may be used if no autologous material is available. Repair with further prosthetic material is a very high risk strategy (even if soaked in antibiotics or silver nitrate) and should be avoided.

It can be difficult to achieve sound wound closure of the groin, particularly when there has been extensive scarring. Detachment of Sartorius from the anterior superior iliac spine and mobilisation of its lateral border (to avoid devascularising it) allows the muscle to be 'rolled over' and tacked down to cover the common femoral artery.

Should distal revascularisation be deemed necessary then a number of options are available. Our own practice has changed over the years such that in nearly all cases prosthetic grafts are only utilised where no autologous material is available. There are, however, still some patients with an infected prosthetic infra-inguinal graft in whom the long saphenous vein is still present and suitable to use as a conduit. This includes a number of patients in whom the original operation record makes note of an 'unsuitable' vein! It is always worth re-examining the vein with Duplex to assess its suitability. Obviously, the search for a suitable vein should not stop at the ipsilateral long saphenous. The contralateral leg, short saphenous and upper limb veins should all be considered if necessary.

Interventional radiology techniques have advanced considerably over the years. Subintimal angioplasty, atherectomy catheters and remote endarterectomy have all increased the scope of disease that can be treated but by wholly or partial endovascular means and these can all be considered in cases where re-do bypass grafting with autologous vein is not feasible.

In cases where sepsis is confined to the groin and with no other options available, consideration may be given to extra-anatomic bypass. Iliopopliteal bypass via the obturator canal and axillo-popliteal bypass have both been utilised in these circumstances and it is worth remembering that both the above- and below-knee popliteal arteries can be approached by a lateral approach.

Many of the same principles apply to other peripheral grafts as apply to infra-inguinal grafts. Extra-anatomic grafts in particular have a relatively high incidence of graft infection. Although it is generally considered most appropriate to remove an infected graft, there have been some reports of successfully managing grafts *in situ*. This should ideally only be entertained when the infecting organism is of low virulence and the infection is confined to the mid portion of the graft, not involving the anastomoses. Surgical management includes adequate debridement of infected tissues, local application of antibacterial agents and adequate coverage of the graft, which may necessitate a vascularised myocutaneous flap.

Infected femoral pseudoaneurysms

Infected primary false aneurysms of the common femoral artery are perhaps worth a special mention. Invariably a consequence of intravenous drug abuse, they typically present as an apparent acute abscess in the groin. This can be a real trap for the unwary and in all such cases an underlying false aneurysm should be positively excluded prior to incision and drainage. There is often a mixed growth of organisms although staphylococci and Gram negative species are most common.

Direct exposure of the artery is potentially hazardous and made all the more difficult by the indurated and thickened tissues. The judicious approach is to establish proximal control via an extraperitoneal approach to the external iliac artery. On exposure there is often found to be a large defect in the anterior wall of the common femoral artery, which precludes primary repair. The very real risk of ongoing sepsis and recurrent haemorrhage means that in most cases the only prudent course of action is to ligate the common femoral artery without reconstruction. Contrary to expectations, the majority of patients will tolerate this with the affected limb surviving on a collateral circulation. In the unusual event of limb-threatening

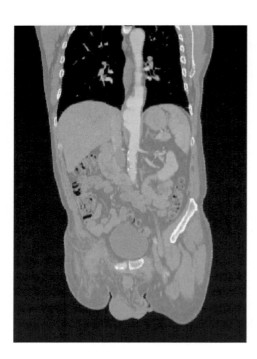

Figure 20.3 Computed tomography showing a saccular aneurysm of the distal thoracic aorta, strongly suggestive of a mycotic aetiology. The aneurysm was excised and repaired with an *in situ* cryo-preserved aortic arch homograft.

critical ischaemia developing, consideration may be given to an extra-anatomic ilio-popliteal bypass via the obturator canal although the safe option is a primary amputation.

Mycotic aneurysms

The term mycotic aneurysm is generally applied to any aneurysm with an infective aetiology. Historically, the commonest cause was septic embolisation in patients with infective endocarditis. Now a relatively rare cause, other aetiological mechanisms have come to the fore. There are a number of pathogenetic mechanisms including septic embolisation (into a small branch vessel or into the large vasa vasorum in the aorta), seeding of an established atherosclerotic plaque, secondary infection in an established aneurysm and rarely contiguous spread from local septic focus. Ultimately the infective process results in progressive destruction of the arterial wall with eventual aneurysm formation. Once established, the natural history of mycotic aneurysms is to progressively enlarge and eventually rupture.

As with graft infection, an appropriate index of suspicion is essential in making the diagnosis. In many patients, the 'vascular' presentation may occur some time after the initial septic episode or indeed a particular septic episode may not be apparent. In these cases the clue to the diagnosis often lies in the morphology of the aneurysm, which is frequently (but not invariably) saccular rather than fusiform (Figure 20.3).

The commonest causative organism seen in modern vascular practice is salmonella species although staphylococci, streptococci, haemophilus and pseudomonas are not infrequently cultured. Management is along similar lines to those for an infected prosthetic graft in the same anatomical location. One possible exception is the use of endovascular stents to treat mycotic aneurysms. This is a potentially attractive option in what is often a debilitated atient; published results demonstrate acceptable early outcome results [7]. There is, however, obvious concern about the development of late graft infection and as yet there is little ong-term follow-up data.

References

. Health Protection Agency. *Surveillance of Surgical Site Infection in England: October 1997 – September 2005.* London: Health Protection Agency, 2006.

. Szilagyi DE, Smith RF, Elliot JP et al. Infection in arterial reconstruction with synthetic grafts. *Ann Surg* 1972; **176**: 321–32.

. Oderich GS, Bower TC, Cherry KJ et al. Evolution from axillofemoral to in situ prosthetic reconstruction for the treatment of aortic graft infections at a single center. *J Vasc Surg* 2006; **43**: 1166–74.

. Gibbons CP, Ferguson CJ, Figelstone LJ et al. Experience with femoro-popliteal vein as a conduit for vascular reconstruction in infected fields. *Eur J Vasc Endovasc Surg* 2003; **25**: 424–31.

5. Brown KE, Heyer K, Rodriguez H et al. Arterial reconstruction with cryopreserved human allografts in the setting of infection: a single-center experience with midterm follow-up. *J Vasc Surg* 2009; **49**: 660–6.

6. Sharif MA, Lee B, Lau LL et al. Prosthetic stent graft infection after endovascular abdominal aortic aneurysm repair. *J Vasc Surg* 2007; **46**: 442–8.

7. Clough RE, Black SA, Lyons OT et al. Is endovascular repair of mycotic aortic aneurysms a durable treatment option? *Eur J Vasc Endovasc Surg* 2009; **37**: 407–12.

Vascular malformations

George Hamilton and Andrew Platts

Key points

- In the neonate differentiate between haemangioma and vascular malformation
- Clinical assessment is of prime importance
  - Is intervention or simple reassurance required?
  - Realistically manage patient and parent expectations
- Investigate by ultrasound, Duplex and magnetic resonance imaging (short T1 inversion recovery [STIR], T1 and T2 with selective use of magnetic resonance angiography and magnetic resonance venography)
- Invasive angiography rarely indicated except for complex arteriovenous (AV) malformations and planned embolisation
- Classify the malformation – extratruncular or truncular?
- The majority of congenital vascular malformations are venous – investigate for disseminated intravascular coagulation (DIC) in diffuse extensive capillary/venous malformations in the young child
- Malignant vascular malformations are rare
- Tailor treatment to the severity of the lesion – cosmesis, pain, function, asymmetry, tissue damage etc.
- Foam sclerotherapy will be suitable and repeatable for the majority of venous malformations
- Klippel–Trenaunay and Parkes-Weber syndromes will need multidisciplinary input – vascular and orthopaedic surgeons, paediatrician and dermatologist
- Look for and ablate ectatic and aneurysmal lateral marginal veins because of risk of thromboembolic disease
- Ethanol sclerotherapy and surgery for the minority usually extratruncular AV malformations
- The best care for patients of all age groups with congenital vascular malformations is provided by multidisciplinary groups (including plastic surgery) with a special interest

Introduction

Vascular malformations, currently most commonly termed congenital vascular malformations (CVMs), have a wide spectrum of clinical presentation and behaviour, ranging from

Postgraduate Vascular Surgery: The Candidate's Guide to the FRCS, eds. Vish Bhattacharya and Gerard Stansby. Published by Cambridge University Press. © Cambridge University Press 2010.

imple birthmarks to massive disfiguring lesions, which in a minority of patients can be ife threatening. Understanding the pathophysiology and anatomy of CVMs has been poor, esulting in clinical confusion with regard to treatment strategies and resulting poor outcomes. Since the 1990s, there has been a significant advance in understanding of the variety of CVMs, the introduction of a clinically relevant and useful classification system and significant improvement in their management.

Definition/classification of congenital vascular malformations

Neonatal/infantile haemangioma

Infantile and neonatal haemangioma usually appears after birth and rather than being a malformation is a vascular tumour arising from endothelial cells. Infantile haemangioma is characterised by early proliferation and growth can be rapid followed by spontaneous involution between 5 and 10 years. Haemangioma is relatively common with an incidence of 2–3% in newborn infants. The incidence of congenital vascular malformation is about 1% and because of its presentation also during the neonatal period, it is important to distinguish clinically between CVM and haemangioma. Congenital vascular malformation is characterised by malformed blood vessels while haemangioma is a localised vascular tumour behaving as described above.

Congenital vascular malformations

Congenital vascular malformations can be classified according to their make up as either arterial, venous, arteriovenous, lymphatic, capillary, and combined or mixed vascular malformation. Venous malformations are the most common form of CVM with 15–20% being mixed lesions, examples of which include the Klippel–Trenaunay syndrome and Parkes-Weber syndrome [1].

Eponymous syndromes

Early in the last century, before angiography was available, several clinical syndromes were described and named according to the clinician. Two eponymous syndromes, namely Klippel–Trenaunay and Parkes-Weber, continue to be used in modern times. This is largely because the syndromes describe the primary vascular malformation together with the secondary non-vascular pathologies.

Klippel–Trenaunay syndrome has venous, lymphatic and capillary components associated with soft tissue swelling, long bone growth, leg discrepancy and gigantism [2]. Parkes-Weber syndrome has capillary, venous and lymphatic malformation but is also characterised by arteriovenous shunting malformation (Table 21.1) [3].

The development of imaging modalities has led to a better understanding and classification of congenital vascular malformations.

Hamburg classification

This classification was based on a consensus established at the International Workshop in Hamburg in 1998 with subsequent modifications. The classification system is based on the insights achieved in determining the underlying pathophysiology, anatomical distribution both macroscopic and microscopic, the resulting underlying haemodynamic effects and

Table 21.1 Eponymous malformations

Klippel–Trenaunay syndrome
• Predominantly haemolymphatic (HLM)
• Venous, lymphatic and capillary malformation
• Vascular bone syndrome
Parkes-Weber syndrome
• Capillary, venous and lymphatic
• Arteriovenous shunting malformation (AVM)

Table 21.2 The Hamburg classification of congenital vascular malformations

A: Anatomical types
• Predominantly arterial defects
• Predominantly venous defects
• Predominantly arteriovenous (AV) shunting defects
• Predominantly lymphatic defects
• Combined vascular defects (Klippel–Trenaunay and Parkes-Weber syndromes)
B: Embryological types
• Extratruncular forms
Infiltrating, diffuse
Limited, localized
• Truncular forms
Aplasia or obstruction
Hypoplasia, aplasia, hyperplasia
Stenosis, membrane, congenital spur
• Dilation
Localized (aneurysm)
Diffuse (ectasia)

further differentiation relating to their time of development in the embryo. The classification is summarized in Table 21.2 with the first component (A) being classification into one of five types based on the vascular pathophysiology, namely arterial, venous, lymphatic, arterio-venous and combined vascular malformations.

The second very important component of the classification (B) is based on the embryological stage at which the malformation develops and divides malformations into either extra-truncular or truncular.

This part of the classification is particularly important in terms of management and prognosis in that the clinical behaviour of the two forms is predicated at the embryological stage at which the malformation develops and at which development arrest occurs.

Extra-truncular congenital vascular malformations

Extra-truncular cardiovascular malformations arise during the earlier phase of embryological development. At this stage, vascular cells are primarily angioblasts derived from mesenchymal cells. These are similar to stem cells, which at any stage of life can be stimulated to proliferate. These stimuli can be hormonal, such as menarche, adolescence and pregnancy, or as a response to trauma or surgical intervention. Extra-truncular malformations most commonly are diffuse and infiltrating in nature, less commonly more localised but typically having compressive effects on adjacent tissues and organs. A further clinically important feature is their high propensity for recurrence if treatment is sub-optimal. In general extra-truncular malformations have greater morbidity, worse prognosis and present a greater therapeutic challenge.

Truncular congenital vascular malformations

These malformations develop later in the embryological vascular development. They are therefore constituted of cells that have lost their primitive stem cell-like properties, in particular the potential to proliferate. These malformations may present as persistent foetal remnants, such as the sciatic vein, or a defectively developed structure, often occlusive, with a combination of stenotic, aneurysmal or web-like disease. The classification therefore further subdivides truncular lesions in to obstructive or dilated. Truncular lesions are much less likely to recur when treated.

Mulliken classification of cardiovascular malformations

This is a different system that characterises malformations as either slow flow or fast flow. This further haemodynamic classification is clinically useful but the Hamburg classification remains predominant, particularly with its ability to predict the clinical outcome for treatment according to the malformation being either extra-truncular or truncular.

Differential diagnosis

Most commonly presentation takes place in the peri-natal period. A congenital vascular malformation having developed in the later stages of the foetus is an abnormal vascular lesion present at birth. A haemangioma is most commonly not present at birth but develops suddenly within the first 4 weeks of the neonatal period with rapid early growth, stimulation and then regression between the ages of 5 and 10 years. The first step in the differential diagnosis is therefore to exclude the diagnosis of haemangioma (Table 21.3).

Classification of a congenital vascular malformation is the next step in the process of differential diagnosis and as described above is made by applying the Hamburg classification. The presence of an AV component predicts a more virulent and unpredictable clinical course with higher morbidity. It is therefore also extremely important to investigate every vascular malformation for the possibility of an arteriovenous component. Initially this may not be clinically obvious but declares itself during follow up.

Investigation

After the initial steps of clinical assessment by history taking and examination, the first step in the diagnostic process is by non-invasive assessment, primarily in the vascular laboratory. Duplex ultrasonography based on colour Doppler imaging and spectral waveform analysis primarily provides anatomical and haemodynamic information. This methodology can reliably demonstrate arterial and venous components and define the anatomy and extent of the lesion, in particular the presence of feeding arteries and draining veins. When there is deeper involvement of anatomical structures, such as in the chest, abdomen or pelvis, or involvement of long bones, Duplex sonography may be limited in its diagnostic potential (Table 21.4).

Table 21.3 Differential diagnosis

- Haemangioma occurs in 2–3% of neonates, rising to 10% at the end of the first year
  - Vascular tumour
- Congenital vascular malformation occurs in 1%
  - Congenital stable malformation that grows commensurately
- Venous malformations are the most common congenital vascular malformations (CVMs)
  - 15–20% are mixed lesions (Klippel–Trenaunay and Parkes-Weber syndromes)

Table 21.4 Investigation

- Ultrasound
  - Excellent screening tool, central to correct diagnosis
    - Flow characteristics of the lesion can be defined
    - Arterial, venous or combined
  - High flow or low flow
  - Confirms complications, such as thromboses
- Computed tomography (CT)
  - Excellent anatomical detail with contrast for arteriovenous (AV) malformations
- Magnetic resonance imaging (MRI)
  - Excellent anatomical detail of surrounding tissues
  - Confirms venous nature of the lesion
  - Excellent for picking up complications or occult features

Magnetic resonance imaging (MRI) is the second component of the initial diagnostic process for all malformations. STIR, T1 and T2 weighted studies will provide excellent anatomical detail of the extent of the cardiovascular malformation, differentiate between high and low flow lesions and is particularly valuable in the diagnosis of venous malformations. In addition, MR angiography and venography can be added to the above MRI investigation for further anatomical detail. Computed tomography contrast scans are also valuable for assessment, in particular of malformations involving bone, the thorax, abdomen and pelvis. Three-dimensional reconstruction of CT angiograms is particularly useful in the diagnosis of arteriovenous malformations (Figure 21.1).

Lympho-scintigraphy is the investigation of choice for assessment of lymphatic or haemo-lymphatic malformations and MR lymph-angiography may also be used to provide further anatomical detail of the extent of the lymphatic malformation.

Simple bone X-ray is indicated where there is limb asymmetry in the presence of vascular-bone syndrome, and MRI can confirm the presence of bony or articular involvement.

In cases of deep seated haemangioma or congenital vascular malformations, MR and CT imaging are important. This will be needed to differentiate between various hamartomatous pathologies and most importantly to exclude the possibility of sarcoma. Where there is still doubt, CT-guided needle biopsy is of value in these cases.

Angiography and venography are important, more invasive investigations currently used in planning interventional or surgical treatment of symptomatic vascular malformations.

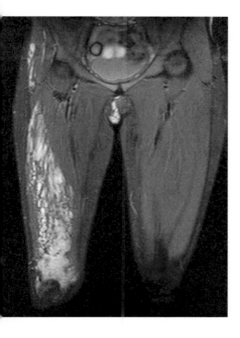

Figure 21.1 Magnetic resonance imaging (MRI) revealing the extent of a venous malformation with diffuse involvement of the thigh muscles and the right labium majorum.

Basic haematological investigations are of course important but should include coagulation studies to detect the possible presence of a consumptive coagulopathy, which could complicate extensive extra-truncular lesions or large marginal veins. Large marginal veins and venous aneurysms have a high risk of venous thrombosis. Coagulopathy is found in children with extensive haemangiomas and in these children anticoagulation might be required.

Diagnosis summary

Diagnosis in the vast majority of malformations is based on careful clinical assessment and examination, Duplex sonography with STIR, T1 and T2 weighted MRI. In very young children more complex investigations, which require sedation or general anaesthesia, can be delayed where the malformation is clinically assessed as unlikely to be aggressive [4]. Earlier management principles focused on aggressive surgical excision of these lesions. The poor outcomes in the absence of the clinical insight given by the Hamburg classification resulted in a move to more conservative treatment. Currently, treatment outcomes are much improved and are focused on a multidisciplinary approach. This will involve disciplines such as paediatric dermatology, vascular surgery, plastic and reconstructive surgery, orthopaedic surgery, head and neck surgery, ENT surgery. The outcome of multidisciplinary assessment will be focused on dealing with the primary malformation and subsequently on dealing with the secondary affects, particularly on the vascular and musculoskeletal systems.

Indications for treatment

Many malformations presenting in children will not need initial treatment but rather careful monitoring of their development and or regression. This will require careful documentation of clinical history, photographic and non-invasive assessment.

Table 21.5 Indications for intervention

Prevention of harm
– Heart failure
– Consumptive coagulopathy
– Ischaemia of limb, skin, etc.
– Compression of airway, etc.
– Bleeding
Treatment of symptoms
– Pain
– Unpleasant pulsation – tinnitus or bruit
Treatment of signs
– Unsightly vessels or swelling
– Limb or facial asymmetry
– Cosmesis

Absolute indications for intervention are in most cases clear and include bleeding from arteriovenous or venous malformations, progression of high output heart failure in arteriovenous malformations, persistent lymphatic leakage with infection or sepsis from lymphatic or haemo-lymphatic malformations, and chronic venous insufficiency secondary to venous or haemo-lymphatic malformations. Vascular malformations situated in potentially life-threatening regions such as next to the airway or significantly compromising limbs, or vital functions such as seeing, hearing, eating, are also indications for intervention. Relative indications for treatment include severe unremitting pain, non-healing ulceration, lesions causing deep vein thrombosis, such as in the marginal vein with its associated risk of thromboembolic disease, haemathrosis where the lesions involve the knee joint, and cosmetically unacceptable lesions.

In venous malformations, the most common presentation, early aggressive treatment is only indicated in situations as highlighted above but also where the vascular bone syndrome results in limb gigantism. The treatment plan for diffuse extra-truncular lesions has to be very carefully formulated because of its progressive nature and high potential for recurrence (Table 21.5).

In treatment of all malformations the management of expectation of the patient and parents is key. It must be made clear that multiple interventions may be required to control and deal with the effects of the malformation and it is also important to stress that control rather than cure is the likeliest outcome in the majority of patients [5].

Surgical treatment

The old principle of surgical ligation of a feeding or draining vessel rarely applies and indeed ligation of a feeding artery is absolutely contraindicated since this will deny the possibility of endovascular treatment to future recurrences. Surgical treatment is frequently combined with embolization in AV malformations, or may be required after sclerotherapy in predominately venous malformations. The policy of preoperative and postoperative

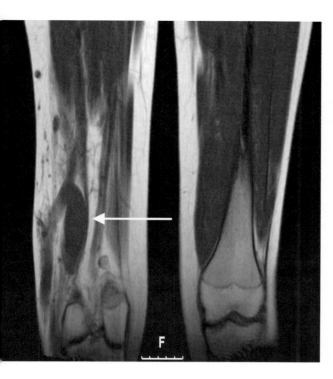

Figure 21.2 The aneurysmal marginal vein in the lateral aspect of the right leg of this young woman was removed with preoperative marking and intraoperative Duplex localisation of the deep draining veins for ligation. These venous ectasias have significant potential for thromboembolic complications [6].

mbolo-sclerotherapy allows treatment of complex and infiltrating congenital vascular malformations that previously were beyond surgical therapy (Figure 21.2).

In general, the truncular forms will be best treated by surgery, particularly venous malformations such as the marginal vein in the Klippel–Trenaunay syndrome and in venous aneurysms [7]. Surgery to vascular malformations can be either haemodynamic or ablative. Haemodynamic surgery is designed as the first step in dealing with the vascular malformation where restoration of arterial blood flow around an infiltrating lesion, e.g. a femoro-popliteal bypass graft, or a venous bypass to restore venous drainage, is required. After haemodynamic surgery has been successfully achieved excisional or ablative surgery can be performed. Complete ablative resection of CVMs has greater success when the malformation is superficial to the deep fascia of any muscle and not invading into major muscles, bone or into the thorax, abdomen or pelvis [8]. Secondary surgery to limb length discrepancy (epiphysiodesis) can then take place, usually between the ages of 3–7 years, by the orthopaedic service.

The more extensive excisional surgery will in many cases involve the reconstructive plastic surgeons. Where there is gross deformity and marked compromise of function in a limb, then primary amputation may be the best option, resulting in early optimisation of function (Figure 21.3).

Endovascular therapy

Embolisation using coils or liquid embolic agents such as glues and Onyx™ are useful in dealing with the arterial component of AV malformations. In extensive venous malformations coils and glues are not indicated because of the diffuse nature of the lesion and the

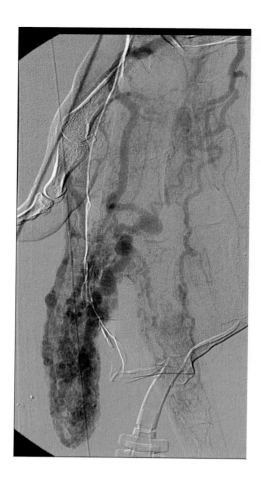

Figure 21.3 This extensive and progressive extratruncular malformation flared up after trauma; primary amputation of the index finger resulted in an excellent symptomatic and functional outcome.

high propensity for these structures to be flushed out of the malformation. Although glue is effective, it leaves a hard cast within the obliterated malformation that may be uncomfortable or unsightly. Coil and glue embolization will rarely be effective in the more diffuse extra-truncular lesions. Sclerotherapy by injection of various agents is of value in many malformations, both arteriovenous, venous, truncular and extra-truncular. These sclerosants act by their toxic effects resulting in endothelial destruction, thrombosis and fibrosis. The important factors to be considered are the strength of the sclerosant, the length of time that the sclerosant is in contact with the vein wall and the area of contact between sclerosant and endothelium. A mainstay of treatment with sclerosants is post-injection compression. There are several sclerosants in use [9].

Ethanol

Absolute ethanol has been used for many decades. It is a very potent sclerosant so much so that it can cause vessel necrosis and have local toxic effects. These include severe pain, swelling with compartment syndrome, damage to surrounding structures, in particular nerves and in more superficial lesions overlying skin necrosis. In addition ethanol has potent systemic side effects including cardiac arrhythmias and pulmonary hypertension secondary to pulmonary vasospasm. The reported incidence of complications including cardiovascular collapse and death has been reported to be as high as 28%.

Ethanol is therefore a very powerful sclerosant but with potentially devastating side effects and should only be used in more aggressive generally extra-truncular malformations and after multidisciplinary assessment of the therapeutic options. Ethanol injection is particularly useful in dealing with diffuse extra-truncular lesions causing significant complications. The core or nidus of the lesion must be identified and targeted with the ethanol injection to achieve a good result.

The ethanol is injected either directly under careful fluoroscopic control or by a catheter. General anaesthesia is required and careful attention to postoperative monitoring and analgesia is essential. The maximum dose of ethanol should not exceed 1 ml kg^{-1} of body weight.

Other sclerosing agents

Polidocanol, tetradecyl sulphate, sodium morrhuate and ethanolamine have been used in the treatment of cardiovascular malformations. They are particularly valuable in dealing with venous malformations and treatments can be repeated many times, in many cases without general anaesthesia.

Technique

In arteriovenous malformations catheter delivery is most commonly used. In venous malformations direct-injection sclerotherapy is used. Duplex ultrasonography is very useful in imaging the malformation and very frequently multiple needles are used. Under fluoroscopy, contrast is injected to define the extent of the malformation and also to assess its volume. The volume identified of sclerosant is injected – it is important to be able to monitor the spread of the sclerosant into the malformation. This is not a problem with the foam sclerosant but when a 'neat' sclerosant solution is being used, this should be mixed with contrast. The aim is to compress the draining vein and then to inject additional sclerosant to fill as much of the malformation as possible. With the use of multiple needles injections continue until the sclerosant begins to drain from the other needles (Figure 21.4). Compression

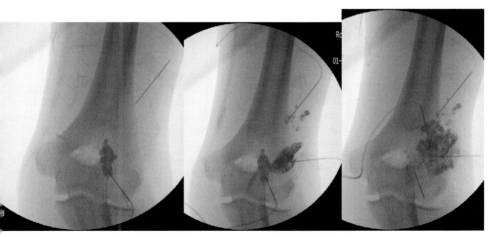

Figure 21.4 Using three separate needles the components of this venous malformation of the elbow were sequentially filled with foam sclerosant to treat the entire malformation; immediate compression was applied.

is then applied. Using foam, intravenous sedation and pain relief may be all that is required. With the injection of 'neat' sclerosants and certainly ethanol, general anaesthesia will be required. More recently, with major venous malformations, a transvenous placement of an occlusion balloon catheter into a large draining vein has been used, alternatively in more superficial lesions tourniquets are useful for occluding draining veins. These manoeuvres aid in maximal filling of the malformation with the sclerosant.

The results of injection sclerotherapy have been good with the modern focus being on the use of foam sclerosant (this is prepared by mixing 'neat' sclerosant with either air or carbon dioxide at a ratio of 1 : 10). There are several outcome reports with success particularly in reduction of the pain associated with venous malformations. The complication rate is low mainly with transient skin pigmentation and a very low incidence of skin necrosis. Multiple episodes of injection sclerotherapy are required in the majority of patients with venous malformations [10].

Summary

Over the last decade there have been significant advances and improvements in the management of the difficult condition of congenital venous malformations. Central to this success is the clinical classification of these disorders, in particular into truncular and extra-truncular lesions. The multidisciplinary approach is of absolute importance with the vascular/endovascular surgeon and interventional radiologist central to the team. Embolo-sclerotherapy has proved to be a major advance in the management of these conditions, particularly venous malformations. It has also revolutionised the approach to high flow and extensive malformations, facilitating surgical excision of life-threatening lesions or those associated with severe complications. Advances in devices and agents such as coils, glues and sclerosant foam have also reduced the morbidity of treatment and widened the indications. Ethanol remains the most effective sclerosant but is toxic and has significant side effects. The current drive is towards finding alternatives to ethanol.

Most patients referred to a multidiscipline unit will not require treatment but benefit from the reassurance that their disease is unlikely to progress, that it is not a tumour and that if symptoms do develop they have established contact with a unit that is able to deliver all aspects of the care that they may need.

References

1. Lee BB, Laredo J, Lee TS, Huh S, Neville R. Terminology and classification of congenital vascular malformations. *Phlebology* 2007; **22**: 249–52.
2. Gloviczki P, Driscoll DJ. Klippel–Trenaunay syndrome: current management. *Phlebology* 2007; **22**: 291–8.
3. Comi AM. Update on Sturge-Weber syndrome: diagnosis, treatment, quantitative measures, and controversies. *Lymphat Res Biol* 2007; **5**: 257–64.
4. Lee BB, Laredo J, Lee SJ, Huh SH, Joe JH, Neville R. Congenital vascular malformations: general diagnostic principles. *Phlebology* 2007; **22**: 253–7.
5. Lee BB, Laredo J, Kim YW, Neville R. Congenital vascular malformations: general treatment principles. *Phlebology* 2007; **22**: 258–63.
6. Mattassi R, Vaghi M. Management of the marginal vein: current issues. *Phlebology* 2007; **22**: 283–6.
7. Loose DA. Surgical management of venous malformations. *Phlebology* 2007; **22**: 276–82.

8. Maftei N, Howard A, Brown LC, Gunning MP, Standfield NJ. The surgical management of 73 vascular malformations and preoperative predictive factors of major haemorrhage – a single centre experience. *Eur J Vasc Endovasc Surg* 2009; **38**: 488–97.

9. Rosenblatt M. Endovascular management of venous malformations. *Phlebology* 2007; **22**: 264–75.

10. Bergan J, Cheng V. Foam sclerotherapy of venous malformations. *Phlebology* 2007; **22**: 299–302.

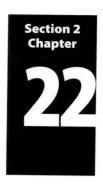

Final FRCS vascular topics

Vasospastic disorders and vasculitis

Mohammed Sharif, Jonathan Smout and Gerard Stansby

Key points

- Understanding of the nomenclature used for the classification of vasospastic disorders into primary and secondary Raynaud's phenomena is essential
- The management of these disorders requires a multidisciplinary team approach involving physicians, rheumatologists and vascular specialists
- Treatment of Raynaud's includes general supportive measures, pharmacotherapy and correction of underlying disorders
- Vasculitis is associated with a range of medical conditions and can present as digital ischaemia
- A diagnosis of vasculitis is suggested by constitutional symptoms and confirmed by raised inflammatory markers, autoantibodies and biopsy of the skin lesions
- Immunosuppressive therapy is the mainstay of treatment in vasculitic disorders

Introduction

Raynaud's phenomenon refers to a clinical state characterised by episodic vasospasm, usually involving the distal small arteries of the upper limb although sometimes toes and feet are also affected. In addition, there are other vascular disorders characterized by inflammatory changes in the arterial wall, known as 'vasculitidies', which can present with digital ischaemia.

Vasospasm (Raynaud's phenomenon)

Maurice Raynaud first described this clinical picture in 1862. The classical presentation of Raynaud's phenomenon is characterised by a sequence of colour changes in the following order:

- pallor, reflecting initial vasospasm;
- cyanosis as a result of deoxygenation of stagnant blood during maximum vasospasm;
- rubor, representing inflow of oxygenated blood and reactive hyperaemia as the vasospasm subsides.

Episodes usually last for 30–60 min. However, some patients present with only cold hands and do not exhibit the classical triple colour response although they demonstrate a similar blood flow pattern to classical vasospasm. The factors triggering these changes and the parts of the body affected are listed in Table 22.1.

Postgraduate Vascular Surgery: The Candidate's Guide to the FRCS, eds. Vish Bhattacharya and Gerard Stansby. Published by Cambridge University Press. © Cambridge University Press 2010.

Table 22.1 Triggering factors and the parts of the body affected by Raynaud's phenomena

Factors provoking a vasospastic episode
• Cold exposure
• Emotional stress
• Vibration – hand arm vibration syndrome (HAVS)
• Industrial chemicals
• Tobacco smoke
• Trauma
• Drugs
Parts of the body affected by vasospasm
• Fingers (commonest)
• Toes
• Nose
• Ear lobes
• Tongue
• Nipples

Epidemiology

The overall incidence of Raynaud's phenomena is 11.8% with women affected nine times more often than men. In certain geographical areas that are prone to a cold and damp climate, 20–30% of the population is affected. A familial predisposition has also been reported, which is more likely if the age at onset is less than 30 years.

Raynaud's phenomenon has particularly been described as a complication of occupations involving vibrating tools such as pneumatic drills and vibrating saw chains, in which context it is also referred to as 'vibration white finger'. Over 50% of people using these tools may ultimately show symptoms of the disease. The underlying mechanism appears to be a high-frequency vibration, which exposes the small digital arteries in the fingers to severe stress. This leads to inflammatory changes and fibrosis in the arterial wall. Since 1985, hand arm vibration syndrome (HAVS) has been listed as an industrial disease in the UK and these patients might be eligible for compensation provided they fulfil disease specific criteria.

Chronic exposure to cold temperature at the industrial level has also been associated with vasospastic disorder and up to 50% of workers dealing with alternate cold and hot water exposure manifest some symptoms of vasospasm.

Nomenclature used in vasospastic disorders

- Raynaud's phenomena (RP) – a blanket term used to describe all vasospastic disorders.
- Primary Raynaud's disease (RD) – vasospastic symptoms manifested on their own without any underlying systemic disease process.
- Secondary Raynaud's syndrome (RS) – vasospasm associated with another known disease entity.

Most people with mild symptoms would usually present to their general practitioner and usually have primary RD. Those with more severe forms are more likely to have secondary RS. It should be noted that sometimes the symptoms of vasospasm are present for many years in advance of diagnosis of the associated secondary RS cause. The differentiation between primary RD and secondary RS is helpful in planning the initial treatment but is sometimes difficult, requiring a sound clinical knowledge of the diseases associated with secondary RS as listed in Table 22.2.

Pathophysiology

Although the exact mechanism of RP is not completely understood, a number of key factors are implicated in its aetiology and pathogenesis. These include:

1. neurogenic alterations;
2. haemodynamic changes;
3. inflammatory and immune regulation;
4. mechanical;
5. genetic predisposition.

For simplicity, we have described these different mechanisms separately. However, in actual practice, there is likely to be a complex interaction between them [1].

Neurogenic alterations

Patients with RP have an increased sensitivity to cold and show increased vasospastic tone in response to cold exposure and other triggering factors. This vascular neurogenic response can occur in the absence of an obstructive arterial lesion. The vasospastic response is explained on the basis of enhanced sensitivity of both alpha and beta adrenergic receptors in the peripheral sympathetic nervous system controlling the arterial tone.

Haemodynamic changes

Normal vascular tone depends on interactions between the flowing stream of blood (cellular and plasma components) and the endothelial lining of the vessel wall. Patients with RP show changes in these microvascular components, which trigger an obstructive and vasospastic response. These include the following:

- Changes in blood and blood components:
  - Platelet activation and aggregation leads to formation of platelet plugs, causing obstruction to the blood flow and release of thromboxane A2 resulting in vasospasm.
  - Activated leukocytes release free radicals causing further vasoconstriction.
  - Red cells become stiff and obstruct the vessel lumen resulting in further obstruction to microcirculation.
  - Plasma viscosity is increased as a result of an increase in plasma proteins.
- Changes in endothelial function:
  - Patients with RP show signs of endothelial dysfunction, such as activation of von Willebrand factor (VWF), which promotes clotting and activates platelets.
  - Tissue plasminogen activator (tPA) activity is reduced, resulting in less effective fibrinolysis and a prothrombotic state in patients with RP.

Table 22.2 Disorders associated with secondary Raynaud's syndrome

Connective tissue diseases (CTD)	Drugs
• Systemic sclerosis	• β-blockers
• Systemic lupus erythematosis	• Cytotoxic drugs
• Henoch–Schönlein purpura	• Anti-migraine drugs including ergotamine
• Scleroderma (CREST* syndrome)	Industrial
• Sjögren's syndrome	• Hand arm vibration syndrome
• Rheumatoid arthritis	• Vinyl chloride
• Mixed connective tissue disease	• Frozen food workers
Obstructive	Circulating globulins
• Atherosclerosis	• Malignancy
• Buerger's disease (thromboangitis obliterans)	• Multiple myeloma
• Microemboli	• Cryoglobulinaemia
• Thoracic outlet syndrome (cervical rib/band)	Miscellaneous
Myeloproliferative disorders	• Chronic renal failure
• Leukaemia	• Reflex sympathetic dystrophy
• Myeloid metaplasia	• Hypothyroidism
• Polycythemia rubra vera	

CREST = Calcinosis, Raynaud's syndrome, Esophageal dysfunction, Sclerodactyly, Telangiectasia.

Inflammatory and immune regulation

Patients with an underlying connective tissue disorder manifest the most severe symptoms of RS. It is a reflection of an intense systemic inflammatory and immune response involving the connective tissues in general including the connective tissue in the arterial wall. The vessel wall in these cases shows a mixture of inflammatory cells including neutrophils, lymphocytes and plasma cells.

Mechanical

Vibration white finger disease seen in patients exposed to high-frequency vibration tools is associated with mechanical damage to vessel wall and secondary inflammatory changes.

Genetic predisposition

RP is reported in patients with Scleroderma and CREST (Calcinosis, Raynaud's syndrome, Esophageal dysfunction, Sclerodactyly, Telangiectasia) syndrome showing a familial association with class II MHC antigens. In addition, primary RD has been seen in monozygotic twins.

Clinical presentation

Key points in the clinical assessment and diagnosis are:
- The clinical picture is episodic with each episode lasting from a few minutes to an hour.
- The RP is usually triggered by exposure to cold or emotional upset.

- Usually fingers and sometimes toes are affected. The distribution of involved digits could be asymmetrical with one or more digits affected at one time although all digits can be affected in one particular patient.
- Involvement of one limb only suggests a possible local cause such as a cervical rib.
- Patients either show a biphasic or triphasic response of colour changes or associated symptoms.
- The first phase is observed after initial exposure to the triggering factor and is associated with vasospasm characterized by clinical feature of pallor. Some patients would experience cold hands and numbness at this stage as a result of reduced blood flow to the digital arteries.
- The initial phase is followed by cyanosis and/or rubor because of reperfusion and is sometimes associated with pain and paraesthesias.
- Other parts of the body can be affected as described earlier, including ear lobes, nose and nipples.
- A cyanotic episode without preceding pallor is not usually because of RP.

Laboratory investigations

A number of laboratory tests, including blood flow measurement, blood tests and radiological investigations, can be helpful during investigation of patients with RP.

- The diagnosis of RP is mainly clinical, based on a history of biphasic/triphasic colour changes in response to cold exposure or emotional upset along with physical examination if the presentation is during an acute episode.
- Laboratory investigations are mainly aimed at differentiating primary RD from secondary RS by identifying any underlying systemic disease.
- Digital blood flow measurement is usually not required to make a diagnosis of RP unless the clinical assessment is inconclusive. The methods used for assessing digital blood flow include strain gauge plethysmography and computerized thermography, as outlined in Table 22.3.
- Nail fold capilloroscopy has been established as a corner stone in the diagnosis of connective tissue disease (CTD) in patients with RP.
- The relevant blood tests include the following:
  - Full blood count, urea and electrolytes, C-reactive protein (CRP), erythrocyte sedimentation rate (ESR) and urinalysis to detect renal dysfunction and anaemia of chronic illness.
  - An autoantibody screen, which should include rheumatoid factor and antinuclear antibodies.
  - Cryoglobulins and cold agglutinins are required only if there is a clinical suspicion of a prothrombotic state.
  - Thyroid function test if suspecting hypothyroidism as an underlying cause of RP.
- Abnormal nail fold capilloroscopy combined with an abnormal autoantibody test predicts CTD in 90%.
- A baseline upper extremity arterial Duplex scan should be carried out to exclude an underlying occlusive arterial disease.
- A plain chest radiograph can demonstrate basal pulmonary fibrosis seen in CTD and cervical rib if present.

Table 22.3 Investigative techniques used for the assessment of blood flow in patients with RP

Investigation	Technique	Interpretation
Digital systolic blood pressure measurement (measurements taken before and after cooling hands at 15°C)	Two techniques used for measuring blood pressure, strain gauge plethysmography and photoplethysmography	>30 mmHg drop in systolic pressure on cooling is considered significant Avoid testing for 2–3 hours after an acute episode, as the fingers would still be in a state of reactive hyperaemia
Nail-fold capilloroscopy	Microscopic examination of the nail bed for abnormal blood vessels.	Abnormal enlarged, dilated and tortuous blood vessels indicate possibility of CTD Beware that similar changes can occur in diabetes and nail fold trauma
Computerized thermography	Skin temperature is assessed as a marker of blood flow during different phases of RP.	Caution is required in interpreting the results as both the arterial as well as venous flow can affect the skin temperature

CTD, connective tissue disease.

Management

Patients with primary RD usually have mild or moderate symptoms and do not require specific drug treatment. However, they should be given general advice, reassurance and written information such as that provided by the Raynaud's and Scleroderma Association, UK. Any causative drug, such as β-blockers, should be replaced with alternatives and any underlying disease such as hypothyroidism should be treated. Good symptomatic control is possible with these measures, despite the non-availability of a definite cure. Figure 22.1 outlines the management algorithm in patients with RP.

General supportive measures

These are suitable for patients with RD showing mild to moderate symptoms without an underlying disease process. The key points are:

- Reassurance, explanation and information leaflets.
- Stop smoking.
- Electric gloves and stockings.
- Special shoes with broad and padded fitting (Abel shoes). These are available from the hospital appliance departments.
- Meticulous attention to areas of skin breakdown, ulcers and infection.

Pharmacological therapy

This should be reserved for more severe symptoms, which affect quality of life or work, as outlined in Figure 22.1.

Calcium channel blockers

Nifedipine is the most effective and commonly used vasodilator, either by oral or sublingual route for a quick action. Other drugs include diltiazem and amlodipine but they are less effective and have fewer side effects than nifedipine because of less vasodilatory properties.

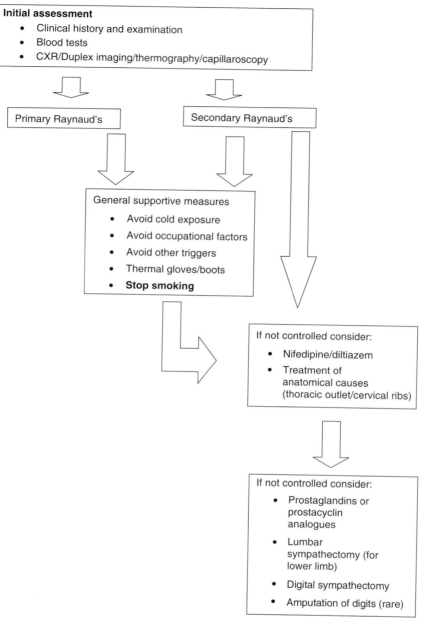

Figure 22.1 Algorithm for the management of Raynaud's phenomenon.

Peripheral vasodilators

These include naftidrofuryl, inositol nicotinate, pentoxifylline and moxisylyte. Patients with primary RD benefit more from these agents than those with secondary RS. A combination of low dose nifedipine and one of the peripheral vasodilators may avoid the adverse effects of both while achieving maximum symptomatic relief [2].

Prostaglandins (PGI2 and PGE1)

These are powerful vasodilatory agents with additional antiplatelet activity and cytoprotective effects. Iloprost is a synthetic analogue with a longer half-life and is commonly used as an intravenous infusion over a period of 6 hours for 5 days during the course of one treatment. The dose is titrated against the individual response and the maximum dose is adjusted at a rate lower than the dose, causing headache, hypotension and flushing (maximum permissible daily dose is 2 ng kg^{-1} min^{-1}). A single course of treatment may provide relief for several months.

Sympathectomy

Cervical and lumbar sympathectomy using phenol injection can sometimes relieve symptoms of upper and lower extremity RP, respectively. However, it should be reserved only as a last option for those with severe symptoms who do not respond to other methods of treatment. The results of sympathectomy are not always predictable. Thoracoscopic cervical sympathectomy, in particular, is less effective and is associated with a higher rate of relapsing symptoms with only one-third achieving a long-term benefit [3]. In addition, there are frequent side effects and for this reason it is not recommended as routine. Digital sympathectomy can be helpful in alleviating the symptoms associated with chronic digital ischaemia in patients with severe RP [4].

Vasculitidies

Vasculitis is characterised by inflammatory changes in the vessel wall, which can affect either the arteries or veins and results in destruction of the normal architecture of the vessel wall. The three commonest vasculitic disorders that vascular surgeons may be involved with are Takayasu's arteritis, Giant cell arteritis and Buerger's disease. In this section we will consider these common vasculitidies.

Takayasu's arteritis

Takayasu's arteritis (TA) produces segmental and patchy granulomatous inflammation of the arterial wall. The condition was first described by Mikito Takayasu in 1908, and is of unknown aetiology. The inflammatory process produces medial thickening and intimal kinking. These changes result in stenoses, occlusion and aneurysmal dilatation. Takayasu's arteritis predominantly affects the aorta and its major branches.

Clinical presentation

Takyasu's arteritis classically affects young women (90% women, and most aged between 15 and 30 years at onset). The condition usually presents with systemic symptoms and loss of normal supra-aortic pulses; hence the term 'Pulseless disease'. In simple terms the condition evolves from an acute pre-pulseless phase to a chronic pulseless phase; although not all patients progress on to the chronic phase. The pre-pulseless phase can be divided into the early prodrome followed by the occlusive phase. The subclavian vessels are most commonly affected followed by the aorta and carotid vessels. Raynaud's phenomenon is commonly associated with TA.

Diagnostic criteria

Various criteria have been designed to aid the early diagnosis of TA. These include the American College of Rheumatology (ACR) criteria, the Ishikawa classification and more

Table 22.4 Modified Ishikawa classification for the diagnosis of Takayasu's arteritis (TA) [5]. The presence of two major or one major and two to four minor criteria suggests a high probability of TA.

Three major criteria:

1. Left mid-subclavian artery lesion

2. Right mid-subclavian artery lesion

3. Characteristic symptoms and signs of at least 1 month duration

Ten minor criteria:

1. High ESR (>20 mm h^{-1})

2. Carotid artery tenderness

3. Hypertension

4. Aortic regurgitation or annuloaortic ectasia

5. Pulmonary artery lesion

6. Left mid common carotid lesion

7. Distal brachiocephalic trunk lesion

8. Descending thoracic aorta lesion

9. Abdominal aorta lesion

10. Coronary artery lesion

ESR, erythrocyte sedimentation rate.

recently a modification of the Ishikawa classification (Table 22.4). The modified classification had a sensitivity of 92.5% with a specificity of 95% for the diagnosis of TA in 106 patients who had TA, as shown on angiograms compared to 20 control subjects [5].

Investigations

Clinical diagnosis of TA can pose diagnostic difficulty in view of its varied presentation. Various non-invasive imaging studies can help not only in making an early diagnosis but are also helpful in monitoring the progress of the disease and response to treatment. Conventional angiography, on the other hand, can only provide luminal details. Ultrasound can identify the early morphological changes in the vessel wall characterized by circumferential thickening. Oedema or enhancement of vessel wall on computed tomography (CT) or magnetic resonance imaging (MRI) is considered a sign of active inflammation. However, this may not lead to the characteristic morphological changes of TA and, on the other hand, vessels showing no inflammatory changes can later develop TA.

Sometimes it is difficult to differentiate between oedema of chronic inflammation and chronic fibrosis in the vessel wall based on CT or MRI alone. Positron emission tomography (PET) with labelled ^{18}Fluorodeoxyglucose may provide better diagnostic imaging for evaluation of active inflammation in the vessel wall [6].

Treatment

Takayasu's arteritis is initially managed with high-dose steroids, with or without immune modifying drugs such as azathioprine and methotrexate. A quarter of the patients do not enter into remission. Where surgical intervention is being contemplated the patient should ideally be in remission, although if this cannot be achieved surgery may be necessary to prevent end organ damage. Bypass surgery should be performed to and from disease free areas of the artery, with biopsies taken from anastomotic sites. Aneurysm formation tends to occur at a later stage, and the indications for intervention will depend on conventional factors such as aneurysm size, rate of growth and the presence of distal embolisation.

Restenosis after intervention has been observed in upto one third of the patients with TA. This can be minimised by delaying the intervention until the patient is in remission and starting immunosuppressive treatment after the intervention [7].

Giant cell arteritis (temporal arteritis)

A surgeon's most frequent encounter with giant cell arteritis (GCA) is during the request for temporal artery biopsy. Giant cell arteritis is a systemic inflammatory vasculitis predominantly affecting extracranial medium- and large-sized arteries. The inflammatory infiltrate consists predominantly of mononuclear cells with giant cell formation. Although a variety of causative factors have been implicated (genetic, immune, infective) the exact aetiology for GCA remains unknown. The inflammation can be segmental in distribution and for this reason the biopsy results should be interpreted with caution. The vertebral, superficial temporal and ophthalmic arteries are the vessels most commonly involved. Less commonly the disease affects larger vessels such as the aorta, subclavian arteries and branches of the abdominal aorta [8].

Clinical presentation

The condition rarely presents before the fifth decade and affects women twice as often as men. Involvement of the ophthalmic artery can result in ischaemic optic neuropathy, which can result in sudden blindness and hence the condition is treated as a medical emergency. Presenting symptoms often include following:

- fever;
- new onset headache often seen as the hallmark symptom (usually temporal or occipital in location);
- scalp tenderness;
- jaw or tongue claudication;
- visual disturbances;
- tinnitus;
- peripheral neuropathy;
- aneurysm formation, if a large vessel is affected.

Investigations

The majority of patients with GCA have an elevated ESR. Traditionally temporal artery biopsy has been performed to confirm the diagnosis, although a negative biopsy does not exclude the disease. Ultrasound imaging of the temporal arteries is becoming more widely available as a diagnostic tool as an alternative to biopsy. It shows a dark halo (oedema) surrounding the diseased vessel – 'halo sign'. Although not universally accepted, the combination of ultrasound evidence of inflammatory process plus a good clinical history is taken by some clinicians to be diagnostic.

Management

Giant cell arteritis is managed with high-dose corticosteroid therapy to induce remission and to reduce the inflammatory changes in the vessel wall. The presence of visual symptoms warrants immediate treatment with corticosteroids, as prompt treatment reduces the rsik of permanant visual impairment. Constitutional symptoms, vascular symptoms, and inflammatory markers (ESR) can guide immunosuppressant therapy. Therapeutic surgical intervention is confined to managing consequences of the disease such as aneurysm formation.

Buerger's disease

Buerger's disease (thromboangiitis obliterans) is an inflammatory disease that predominantly affects medium- and small-sized arteries. Leo Buerger first described the condition in 11 amputated limbs of patients of Jewish descent in 1908, and he termed the disease thromboangiitis obliterans. The special features of the disease [9] include following:

- The pathological changes are distinct from atherosclerosis with minimal atheroma formation and more cellular infiltrate along with a striking perivascular inflammatory reaction resulting in occlusion of the vessel lumen.
- These inflammatory changes can be observed in both the arterial as well as the venous system.
- Both the upper and lower extremities can be affected, although lower limb disease occurs more frequently.
- Tobacco exposure is strongly associated with the initiation and progression of Buerger's disease, although the exact pathological mechanism is not known.
- Smoking cessation is the only way to stop the disease progression and nearly one-half of those who continue to smoke end up with a major amputation.

Clinical presentation

The disease usually affects men at the age of <45 years. Unlike patients with atherosclerotic disease, patients with Buerger's usually present with rest pain and tissue loss, rather than claudication. This reflects the involvement of more distal vessels. The prevalence of Buerger's disease is higher in patients of Middle or Far Eastern descent. The disease is historically rare in women, although this pattern is changing as is reflected by the increasing proportion of female smokers.

The tissue loss typically involves painful ulceration or necrosis of the digits of the hands and feet. As the disease progresses it may involve more proximal vessels, although it would be very unusual to lose proximal pulses from Buerger's disease alone. Involvement of the small vessels results in vasospastic symptoms. Patients may also present with sepsis or extensive foot infections where local infections of necrotic tissue are neglected. The venous inflammatory changes can cause a superficial thrombophlebitis.

Several diagnostic criteria have been suggested to aid correct diagnosis. These include the following:

- Exclusion of other causes of limb ischaemia (hypercoagulability, emboli, diabetes, etc.).
- Tobacco use (previous or current).
- The presence of distal extremity arterial disease.
- Young age of onset (<45).

The presence of additional features such as upper limb disease, phlebitis migrans, Raynaud's phenomena, and radiological signs strengthen the diagnosis.

nvestigations

The radiological appearance of Buerger's disease comprises of relatively normal arteries to the knee level, abrupt occlusions of the tibial vessels and 'corkscrew' collaterals feeding the distal vessels at the ankle. It is often helpful to look at the images of the unaffected limb, as these hallmark radiological features may already be present in the asymptomatic limb. It should be remembered that the similar angiographic features could also be seen in diabetes and other connective tissue disease.

There are no specific laboratory tests for Burger's disease. The primary role of laboratory tests is to exclude other causes of occlusive arterial disease. Likewise echocardiography is useful to exclude a proximal embolic source.

Management

Medical

The absolute goal in managing Buerger's disease is to stop smoking completely and permanently. Aspirin should be prescribed for its antiplatelet effects, and analgesics for pain control. Prostaglandin infusions (iloprost) may help to control the symptoms. However, it is uncertain if it could alter the progression of tissue loss. Patients should be educated about foot care, prevention of injury and avoidance of cold exposure.

Surgical

Given the pattern of small- and medium-vessel occlusive disease, the options for surgical revascularisation in Buerger's are extremely limited. Any significant co-existing proximal atherosclerotic arterial disease should be treated to improve the inflow. Attempting to intervene with revascularisation is probably futile while the patient continues to smoke. Local amputation is often required to treat necrosis, non-healing ulcers or intractable pain. Distal ischaemic lesions will often auto-amputate, and it is usually helpful to await demarcation even if surgery is planned. Antibiotics may be needed intermittently for any infective episodes.

Behçets's disease

Behçet's disease (BD) is a multisystem inflammatory condition that can affect both arteries and veins. The disorder was first publicised by the Turkish dermatologist Hulusi Behçet in 1937, who described a syndrome of aphthous ulceration, genital ulceration, and uveitis. Behçet's disease has historically been noted to occur more frequently along the old silk trading routes of the Middle East and in Central Asia; hence, the name 'Silk Road' disease. No specific causative factor has been noted, although it is seen more commonly in individuals with HLA-B51 gene.

Veins are affected more often than arteries. When large arteries are involved, inflammatory changes affect the vasa vasorum, resulting in medial destruction and fibrosis. Subsequent damage to the arterial wall can lead to aneurysm formation.

Clinical presentation

BD is a chronic inflammatory condition characterised by episodes of recurrence and remission. International diagnostic guidelines emphasise the importance of the following features for the diagnosis:

- oral (aphthous) ulcers;
- genital ulcers;

- skin lesions;
- uveitis.

Venous involvement is manifested by thrombophlebitis of the superficial and deep veins. These changes are not wholly confined to the peripheral vasculature and can also involve the visceral and central veins. Arterial involvement is manifested by aneurysmal disease, which necessitates intervention due to the risk of rupture. Occlusive disease can occur in BD and tends to affect medium- and small-sized arteries.

Investigations

There is no specific diagnostic test for BD. The disease occurs more commonly in HLA-B51 individuals, and this gene is more prevalent in the Middle East. The 'pathergy' test can be helpful in the diagnosis of BD but is not 100% specific. The test involves a needle prick to the forearm. The presence of a papule (>2 mm in diameter) 1 to 2 days after the test constitutes a positive result. Investigation for aneurysmal or venous disease would follow standard investigative pathways.

Management

Steroid therapy is utilised to ease the symptoms and reduce the inflammatory changes of the disease. Anti-tumour necrosis factor (TNF) therapy is beneficial in the management of uveitis, skin and mucosal symptoms. Aneurysm formation in BD necessitates surgical intervention due to the risk of rupture. False aneurysms at the anastomotic sites are more common in BD as compared to atherosclerotic disease. Similarly, inflammatory changes can occur at the site of previous arterial surgery.

Connective tissue disorders

In this section, we will discuss some common connective tissue disorders affecting the vascular system, including Marfan's syndrome and Ehler–Danlos syndrome.

Marfan's syndrome

Marfan's syndrome is an autosomal dominant connective tissue disorder. One-quarter of the affected population has a new genetic mutation. The underlying genetic defect arises from mutations of the fibrillin-1 (FBN1) gene based on chromosome 15. Fibrillin is a complex structural protein that serves as substrates for elastin in the aorta and other connective tissues. Abnormalities of these microfibrils results in weakening of the aortic wall and cardiac valves. In addition the normal fibrillin-1 protein has a role in vascular smooth muscle development by binding to transforming growth factor beta (TGF-β). The role of angiotensin II receptor blockers has been investigated in modifying the vascular changes induced by TGF-β.

Clinical presentation

The major manifestations of Marfan's syndrome include the following:

- mitral valve prolapse;
- aortic root dilatation;
- aortic aneurysm formation;
- aortic dissection;

- dural abnormalities;
- lens dislocation (ectopia lentis).

External features include tall stature, arachnodactyly, dolichostenomelia (limbs disproportionately long compared with trunk), joint hypermobility, scoliosis, pectus excavatum, high arched palate and dental crowding.

Investigations

Genetic investigations have a limited role in the diagnosis of Marfan's syndrome as not all FBN1 mutations are associated with Marfan's syndrome. In addition, genetic testing is not available in all centres. The diagnosis is currently made on the basis of family history and clinical features, with or without molecular testing if available. The 'Ghent' diagnostic criteria consist of major and minor features based on the systems involved. To be diagnosed with Marfan's syndrome using the Ghent criteria requires two major criteria and one minor criterion affecting different systems or if there is a family history one major criterion and one minor criterion.

Major criteria include:

- Aneurysmal aorta.
- Dissection of aorta.
- Dislocation of the lens.
- Family history of the syndrome.
- At least four skeletal problems, such as:
  - pectus carinatum or pectus excavatu;
  - arm span greater than height;
  - reduced upper to lower segment ratio – this is when the length of the torso (from shoulders to legs) is shorter than the length of the legs;
  - positive wrist sign – this is when the thumb and little finger overlap when you grasp the other wrist;
  - positive thumb sign – this is when you put your thumb on your hand and it extends beyond the palm;
  - curvature of the spine (scoliosis) with a curve greater than 20°;
  - spondylolisthesis;
  - flat feet (pes planus);
  - protrusion acetabulae on hip X-ray;
- Dural ectasia of spinal cord – shown on CT or MRI.

Minor criteria include:

- myopia;
- unexplained stretch marks;
- loose joints;
- long, thin face;
- high, arched palate.

Patients with Marfan's syndrome should be regularly screened for cardiac complications and aortic dilatation to allow prophylactic intervention against potentially fatal complications.

Management

Open surgical repair of descending thoracic and abdominal aortic dilatation is considered a reliable treatment option in patients with Marfan's syndrome and has resulted in improved survival based on studies carried out over the last decade. It still remains the first choice of treatment. Thoracic endovascular stenting for aneurysmal disease and dissection in patients with Marfan's syndrome has been increasingly used in recent years but the published studies in this area are limited to small numbers. Further larger studies are required with long-term follow up to show a conclusive benefit of thoracic endovascular stenting in Marfan's syndrome [10]. In particular there is a worry about the durability of endografting since the majority of these patients are young. It is also essential that the follow up in these patients should include monitoring for new aneurysmal disease or anastomotic aneurysms.

Loeys–Dietz syndrome

Loeys–Dietz (LD) syndrome is a recently discovered autosomal dominant disorder with many of the clinical features of Marfan's syndrome. The disorder originates from a defect in the gene responsible for coding the transformation of growth factor β-receptors (TGF-β 1 or 2). The two genetic defects result in a similar syndrome and the condition was previously considered to be a subtype of Marfan's syndrome.

Clinical presentation

The main clinical features of LD syndrome include:

- arterial aneurysms;
- arterial tortuosity (often in the carotid vessels);
- hypertelorism (widely-spaced eyes);
- bifid or broad uvula.

This combination of major features is usually seen together in other connective tissue disorders. As with Marfan's syndrome, aneurysms occur at young age and frequently involve the aortic root. LD syndrome has been classified into two subtypes, depending on the craniofacial involvement. Many of the other features seen in LD are also seen in Marfan's syndrome as previously described.

Ehlers–Danlos

Ehlers–Danlos (ED) syndrome is a connective tissue disorder that results in impaired strength, elasticity, and healing of the tissues. The condition is thought to have an incidence of 1 : 10 000, and is usually inherited as an autosomal dominant disease. ED syndrome is caused by abnormalities of collagen synthesis. The clinical picture depends on the type of collagen defect and the distribution of that type of collagen in the individual tissues. There are at least six phenotypes with considerable overlap between them. This often makes the exact categorisation difficult in up to half of the patients. Type IV ('vascular' type) ED syndrome is of most relevance to the vascular surgeon as it involves the abnormalities of type III collagen [11].

Clinical presentation

ED syndrome ('vascular' type) often presents with arterial or visceral rupture and the diagnosis is only made at post mortem. An arterial rupture is either spontaneous or follows minor trauma, with or without the presence of an underlying aneurysm. Aneurysms often involve multiple sites and arterial dissection is common. There is a high risk of bleeding complications and aneurysm formation following surgical intervention in these patients in view of the tissue friability.

Clinical findings include:

- thin translucent skin;
- easy bruising;
- hyperextensible skin;
- hypermobile joints;
- high and narrow palate;
- dental crowding;
- abnormal wound healing and scars;
- aneurysm formation;
- varicose veins;
- arteriovenous fistulae.

Investigations

The combination of the clinical features listed above in addition to a family history of the disease or history of a family member unexpectedly dying at a young age should alert the clinician to the possibility of ED syndrome. To confirm the diagnosis, collagen typing can be performed on cultured skin fibroblasts. Investigations for vascular involvement should be non-invasive as conventional diagnostic angiography carries an unacceptably high risk of haemorrhagic complications.

Management

Treatment for ED is currently confined to the identification and treatment of complications. Patients should also receive lifestyle advice to avoid trauma. As previously noted surgical or endovascular intervention should be avoided unless absolutely necessary due to the friability of the tissues and bleeding complications.

Investigations

The characteristic facial features and clinical findings will usually suggest the diagnosis. Genetic tests provide more definitive confirmation of the disease. Patients with LD syndrome should be placed under long-term CT or MR follow up to detect aneurysm formation at an early stage.

Management

Murine laboratory research has suggested that angiotensin II receptor blockade can reduce the formation of aortic aneurysms in Marfan's syndrome. This observation is particularly relevant in LD where the abnormality in TGF-β activity is the fundamental defect. Therapy with angiotensin II receptor blockers such as losartan reduces the potential complications caused by increased TGF-β.

Pseudoxanthoma elasticum

Pseudoxanthoma elasticum (PXE) is a rare genetic condition with an incidence of 1 : 50 000. The condition involves progressive calcification and fragmentation of elastic fibres contained within the dermis of the skin, retina and cardiovascular system. More recent studies have suggested that this may be a systemic metabolic condition. The cardiovascular and gastrointestinal complications are the major causes of morbidity and mortality. Vascular calcification involves the intimal and medial layers of the vessel wall containing the elastic fibres. The cardiovascular complications of PXE often occur later than the cutaneous and haemorrhagic complications. The gastrointestinal bleeding complications result from the fragility of the calcified submucosal vessels.

Clinical presentation

The condition is usually first manifested with cutaneous lesions on the lateral part of the neck (often symmetrical). These lesions have the appearance of small yellow papules and occur in a linear or reticular pattern. The lesions can coalesce and form plaques and take on the appearance of 'plucked chicken' skin. The skin lesions also commonly occur in the folds of major joints such as the axillae. As the skin disease progresses it often becomes lax, wrinkled and hangs in the form of thick folds. Other clinical features of PXE include:

- gastrointestinal haemorrhage;
- intermittent claudication;
- ischaemic heart disease;
- retinal haemorrhages;
- haematuria.

Investigations

Blood tests are carried out for anaemia, renal impairment and baseline lipid levels. Urine should be tested for haematuria. Whenever possible, vascular imaging should follow a non-invasive course because of the risk of haemorrhagic complications after conventional angiography. The cardiac function should be assessed before vascular intervention in view of the high risk of cardiac complications.

Management

Patents should be counselled regarding changes in lifestyle to reduce the risk of complications. There is no specific treatment at present to halt or reverse the disease progression. Best medical therapy should be instituted to reduce the cardiovascular risk, although caution should be exercised with antiplatelet therapy due to the haemorrhagic risk.

References

1. Bakst R, Merola JF, Franks AG Jr, Sanchez M . Raynaud's phenomenon: pathogenesis and management. *J Am Acad Dermatol* 2008; **59**: 633–53.
2. Vinjar B, Stewart M. Oral vasodilators for primary Raynaud's phenomenon. *Cochrane Database Syst Rev* 2008; **16**: CD006687.
3. Thune TH, Ladegaard L, Licht PB. Thoracoscopic sympathectomy for Raynaud's phenomenon – a long term follow-up study. *Eur J Vasc Endovasc Surg* 2006; **32**: 198–202.
4. Kotsis SV, Chung KC. A systemic review of the outcomes of digital sympathectomy for treatment of chronic digital ischaemia. *J Rheumatol* 2003; **30**: 1788–92.
5. Sharma BK, Jain S, Suri S, Numano F. Diagnostic criteria for Takayasu's arteritis. *Int J of Cardiol* 1996, **54**(Suppl): S141–7.
6. Pipitone N, Versari A, Salvarani C. Role of imaging studies in the diagnosis and follow-up of large-vessel vasculitis: an update. *Rheumatology* 2008; **47**: 403–8.
7. Park MC, Lee SW, Park YB, Lee SK, Choi D, Shim WH. Post-interventional

immunosuppressive treatment and vascular restenosis in Takayasu's arteritis. *Rheumatolgy* 2006; **45**: 600–5.

8. Salvarani C, Cantini F, Hunder GG. Polymyalgia rheumatica and giant-cell arteritis. *Lancet* 2008; **372**: 234–45.

9. Małecki R, Zdrojowy K, Adamiec R. Thromboangiitis obliterans in the 21st century – a new face of disease. *Atherosclerosis* 2009; **206**: 328–34.

10. Cooper DG, Walsh SR, Sadat U, Hayes PD, Boyle JR. Treating the thoracic aorta in Marfan syndrome: surgery or TEVAR? *J Endovasc Ther* 2009; **16**: 60–70.

11. Germain DP. Clinical and genetic features of vascular Ehlers–Danlos syndrome. *Ann Vasc Surg* 2002; **16**: 391–7.

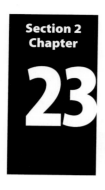

Final FRCS vascular topics

23 Critical care considerations and preoperative assessment for general and vascular surgery

Ian D. Nesbitt and David M. Cressey

Key points

- Perioperative cardiac complications are the most serious risk to delineate and pre-emptively manage
- Discussions between anaesthetist, surgeon and cardiologist are frequently required on a case-by-case basis
- Critical care is an essential and rapidly developing support to many surgical procedures

Introduction

'Good surgeons know how to operate, better surgeons know when to operate, and the best surgeons know when not to operate.' This aphorism reflects the intertwined nature of surgery, anaesthesia and critical care. Poor patient selection or preparation for a particular surgical procedure cannot be entirely compensated for by good anaesthesia or critical care. The purposes of preoperative assessment include the identification and management of individual patient risks as well as appropriate resource allocation.

Sixty per cent of patients undergoing major vascular surgery have significant coronary artery disease (CAD). Similarly, CAD is common among patients having non-vascular procedures, so an understanding of the important principles of investigation and management is important for all surgeons and anaesthetists. This section will therefore concentrate particularly on cardiovascular assessment, although other disease states are also considered.

Preoperative assessment

General preoperative assessment

When considering an individual patient, the degree of CAD is often difficult to adequately assess by history and examination alone (e.g. because of limitations in exercise capacity due to claudication, general fatigue or the time limited nature of an emergency presentation). However, a good history and examination can allow specific directed investigations to be carried out. Examples include: echocardiography for patients with suspected aortic stenosis and cardiopulmonary exercise testing for patients with poor functional reserve. Individual history taking can be combined with population based information such as the Heart Outcomes Preventation Evaluation (HOPE) study and Reduction of Atherothrombosis for

Postgraduate Vascular Surgery: The Candidate's Guide to the FRCS, eds. Vish Bhattacharya and Gerard Stansby. Published by Cambridge University Press. © Cambridge University Press 2010.

Table 23.1 Some risk scoring systems

Risk score	Comments
Association of Anesthesiologists (ASA)	General scoring system with significant variation in scoring between different clinicians
Goldman Index	Developed >30 years ago: superseded by later systems
Detsky Score	Principally concerned with perioperative cardiac event prediction
Lee Revised Cardiac Risk Index	See Table 23.2 for additional details
V-POSSUM	Specific vascular surgical score developed in the UK
Parsonnet Score	Scoring system for cardiac surgery

Continued Health (REACH) registry (which show that a history of peripheral vascular disease strongly predicts adverse cardiovascular outcomes) to help direct other investigations or management.

Risk assessment and scoring systems for surgery

Aside from a general preoperative assessment, more sophisticated investigations may have additional benefits. It is important to assess the risk of a particular procedure, not only from a patient's viewpoint (adequate information is required for informed consent) but also from a medical and organisational perspective. This includes appropriate targeting of resource and therapy, e.g. preoperative investigation and physiological optimisation; efficient use of critical care beds; consideration of conservative management rather than operative intervention, and also comparisons of observed versus expected outcomes, which may be used for wider comparative purposes (Table 23.1).

In all these scores, cardiac failure and recent myocardial infarction are the strongest indicators of postoperative cardiac complications. Aortic stenosis is a strong independent predictor of perioperative complications: a gradient of 25–50 mmHg increases operative risk fivefold, and a gradient greater than 50 mmHg increases risk sevenfold.

The Revised Cardiac Risk Index (RCRI) performs best as a predictor in real life practice, and is detailed in Table 23.2.

Ideally a scoring system allows accurate and individualised prediction of the outcome from a particular operation for each patient, with low false positive and negative rates. No scoring system yet allows this. Others use population based historical outcomes to prospectively stratify patients. These can be useful to discuss general risks with patients, but are too imprecise to be used to attempt individual predictions.

Attempts to improve the prognostic ability of preoperative investigations have yielded mixed results. It is increasingly recognised that static testing, such as resting echocardiography, may provide information on valvular anatomy or pulmonary artery pressures, but has little *prognostic* value in vascular surgery. Dynamic testing such as dobutamine stress echocardiography (DSE) adds value to preoperative investigations, but even this has limited prognostic ability, and there is much current interest in cardiopulmonary exercise testing (CPX).

Cardiopulmonary exercise testing involves a combination of exercise electrocardiography (ECG), usually on a bicycle, with concurrent measurement of exhaled CO_2 and oxygen consumption (Figure 23.1). These allow calculations of anaerobic threshold (AT)

Table 23.2 Revised Cardiac Risk Index (RCRI)

Criteria	Details
Ischaemic heart disease	Angina, myocardial infarction, previous PCI or CABG
Heart failure	History of or examination compatible with left ventricular failure. Paroxysmal nocturnal dyspnoea
Cerebrovascular disease	Previous TIA or CVA
Insulin dependent diabetes	
Chronic renal impairment	Creatinine > 177 mmol l^{-1} (2 mg dl^{-1})
High risk surgical case	Thoracic, abdominal or pelvic vascular operation

No RCRI criteria = low risk (0.4–1% risk of cardiac complications).
1–2 RCRI criteria = intermediate risk (2–7% risk).
3+ RCRI criteria = high risk (>9% risk).
PCI, percutaneous coronary intervention; CABG, coronary artery bypass grafting; TIA, transient ischaemic attack; CVA, ceresro vascular accident.

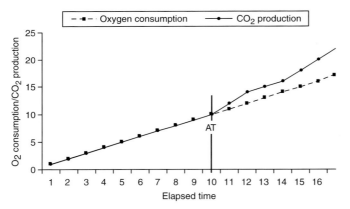

Figure 23.1 Cardiopulmonary exercise (CPX) testing. During gentle (aerobic) exercise, O_2 consumption and CO_2 production are similar, so the graphs have a similar slope. During strenuous (anaerobic) exercise, CO_2 production is greater than O_2 consumption, so the CO_2 graph has a steeper slope. The transition between aerobic and anaerobic metabolism is the anaerobic threshold (AT), and reflects the integrated ability of the cardiorespiratory and cellular mechanisms to manage an increased workload. Aside from training and general conditioning, a variety of cardiac and respiratory disease states produce diagnostic patterns in CPX data.

and development of any myocardial ischaemia during exercise. An AT below 11ml min^{-1} kg^{-1} is considered an indicator of high-risk cases, although more complex evaluations are increasingly being developed, based on nature of surgery, early versus late ischaemic changes and absolute AT [1]. It is likely that prognostic cut-off values will vary between population groups and surgical centres (e.g. the average AT for major surgery at the authors' institution is 9.5ml min^{-1} kg^{-1}, with a mortality/morbidity rate below the UK average).

These investigations can be used to aid decision making regarding intraoperative and postoperative care. For example, a patient with a high AT having aortic reconstruction may be suitable for a level 2 (HDU type) bed postoperatively, while a patient with a poor AT having similar surgery may be much more likely to require a level 3 (ITU type) bed, with consequent implications for hospital resource management.

Preoperative decision making requires more than simply assessing risk. If possible, the perioperative risks should be reduced or eliminated. This may involve optimising the patients' condition. Typically, this includes achieving control of co-morbidities including blood pressure, diabetes, dyslipidaemia and consideration of β-blockade (see below).

The actual investigative and management pathways will vary between institutions, but ultimately, success depends on good communications and relationships between radiology, anaesthesia, critical care and surgery. There is an increasing role for pre-assessment clinics (PACs) as co-ordinators of investigations and optimisation, but to be successful, PACs require strong leadership and clear strategies. Agreed inter-departmental policies are an important part of this e.g. anticoagulation, major bleeding, cross matching, based partly on national recommendations such as National Institute of Health and Clinical Excellence (NICE) guidelines for preoperative investigation.

Co-ordination of complex cases, e.g. decisions about staging of carotid and coronary surgery, proximal thoraco-abdominal aortic aneurysms requiring partial or complete cardiopulmonary bypass, staged visceral re-vascularisation should be carried out in specialist centres with an adequate volume of work to achieve good results. Increasingly unfit patients are presenting for carotid, thoracic and abdominal endovascular procedures, and again require expert multidisciplinary team assessment, if possible.

Specific management of other co-morbidities

Pulmonary disease

Obstructive pulmonary diseases (asthma, emphysema and bronchitis) should have long-term drug therapy optimised. Typically, this is based on multi-modal anti-inflammatory drugs and bronchodilators. Particular attention to pre-existing pulmonary disease is required if surgery involves deflating a lung for surgical access.

Restrictive lung disease may be intrinsic, e.g. fibrosis, or more commonly extrinsic, e.g. due to kyphosis or obesity. Treatment options for the specific restrictive lung disease may be limited, but may influence the choice of regional versus local or general anaesthesia for a particular surgical procedure.

As with cardiovascular diseases, close liaison with the anaesthetist and intensive care team is required to optimally manage patients with significant lung disease. Pulmonary hypertension (PHT) and cor pulmonale are important risk factors for postoperative death, and patients with severe lung disease should have PHT actively excluded by echocardiography.

Epidural anaesthesia may reduce postoperative respiratory morbidity and reduce length of ICU stay, but has implications for some drug therapies in the perioperative period (see below).

Obesity

Obesity is a multi-system disease with implications for both anaesthetic and surgical approaches. Patients with obstructive sleep apnoea may require postoperative respiratory support in critical care rather than immediate transfer to a ward environment, since respiratory complications are more common in the obese. Local services will dictate where these patients are managed.

Diabetes

In addition to predisposing to macro- and microvascular disease, diabetes is a significant risk factor for many postoperative complications, including renal failure, myocardial infarction and death. The long-term benefits of good diabetic control are well established, but the optimal details of short-term perioperative diabetic control are less clear. Tight (4.4–6.6 mmol l⁻¹) glycaemic control may improve outcomes in selected (predominantly cardiac surgical) patients, but less rigid control (perhaps below 10 mmol l⁻¹) is more practical and possibly safer among a general patient population. Traditionally, type 2 diabetics undergoing minor surgery are placed early on an operating list, and simply omit any morning hypoglycaemic agents. Type 1 diabetics may either take their normal insulin or have a glucose-potassium-insulin (GKI) infusion started, depending on the timing and nature of surgery and the local policies in use.

All diabetics having major surgery should have a GKI started preoperatively and continued until enteral feeding is established again.

Hypertension

Systemic hypertension is a risk factor in the long term for cardiovascular and cerebrovascular complications, but the evidence that perioperative outcomes are worse unless hypertension is severe (perhaps >180/100 mmHg) is weak. Local agreements about how an individual patient with hypertension is managed will depend on multiple other factors.

Permanent pacemakers (PPMs) and implantable cardiac defibrillators (ICDs)

An increasing number of patients present for surgery with pacemakers or ICDs. Aside from the traditional indications such as sick sinus syndrome and complete heart block, PPMs/ICDs may now be indicated as treatment of choice for diseases as diverse as refractory atrial fibrillation, vasovagal syncope, and post myocardial infarction ventricular dysfunction, as well as in survivors of first presentation life-threatening arrhythmias.

It is important to know what type of device is in use prior to surgery. This allows planning both for deliberate actions and emergency management, should device interference occur. Patients may be a source of useful information in this respect, and a 12 lead ECG is mandatory, but recent device interrogation by a pacemaker clinic is most helpful.

Some PPMs and ICDs may require re-programming or deactivation prior to anaesthesia. Unipolar diathermy should be avoided if possible, as should prolonged periods of continuous diathermy during surgery. This reduces the electromagnetic interference, which may reset the PPM to a backup mode, or trigger inappropriate defibrillation by an ICD. Postoperatively, the device may need re-programming, and should be rechecked before the patient is discharged.

Percutaneous coronary interventions (PCIs), coronary stents and cardiac surgery

More than 90% of PCIs involve insertion of at least one stent, the majority of which are drug eluting stents (DESs). Although DESs may have a short-term advantage over bare metal stents (BMSs) regarding early stent thrombosis, they carry the disadvantage of requiring prolonged (at least 9–12 months post procedure) dual antiplatelet therapy to prevent late stent thrombsosis, which has a high mortality rate.

Percutaneous coronary intervention usually involves large doses of anticoagulant and antiplatelet agents. Intravenous heparin has a relatively short (dose dependent) half-life but glycoprotein IIb/IIIa inhibitors such as abciximab or tirofiban may have activity up to 48 hours (and can inhibit the activity of any transfused platelets). This and the condition precipitating PCI have obvious implications for the conduct of surgery and anaesthesia.

In the emergency situation, vascular emergencies may present around the time of a PCI e.g. retroperitoneal haemorrhage due to vessel injury during angiography. Additionally some patients requiring vascular interventions will have had a relatively recent PCI for intercurrent active CAD.

Although no specific rules apply to management, since the risk–benefit will depend on the nature and urgency of surgery, major elective surgery in patients with a DES in place may be best deferred for at least 12 months. Patients having PCI with BMS or PCI alone should have at least 6 weeks delay. Patients who have undergone coronary artery bypass grafting should have non-cardiac surgery delayed for at least 30 days, if possible.

For emergency cases, or those where regional anaesthesia is considered essential, a platelet transfusion may reduce major bleeding without substantially increasing the risk of stent thrombosis. Recommended platelet target levels are between 50 and 80 000 μl^{-1}

This is a rapidly evolving area of practice, and recommendations change frequently, so focused discussion is essential when faced with such situations.

Specific management of drug therapy

The scientific understanding of atherosclerosis has changed over recent years, from a simple mechanical obstructive model to one of a variable and ongoing inflammatory pathological process with central involvement of platelet activation and aggregation. This and the observed hypercoagulable state following surgery have implications for both drug management and surgical interventions.

Antiplatelet agents

Aspirin

This inhibits thromboxane A2 to reduce platelet aggregation, although up to 40% of patients may be aspirin resistant. In general, the risk of excess perioperative haemorrhage is sufficiently low to recommend that, for most surgery, aspirin should be continued if possible. Prostate and intra-cranial operations may have a higher bleeding rate, so the use of aspirin should be discussed with the anaesthetist involved.

Clopidogrel

This pro-drug, when activated, inhibits fibrinogen binding to platelet glycoprotein IIb/IIIa receptors and reduces platelet aggregation. A small proportion of patients are clopidogrel resistant, but generally, a loading dose takes several days to exert its full effect, and the antiplatelet effect lasts for up to 7 days. During this time, any transfused platelets are also affected, although often to only a small degree. Frequently, clopidogrel is used as either combination therapy with aspirin, or as monotherapy for patients intolerant or resistant to aspirin. A significant indication for antiplatelet therapy is to prevent coronary stent thrombosis – untreated, around 20% of stents thrombose, with a 20% mortality. Premature cessation of antiplatelet therapy is a major concern, although it is difficult to precisely quantify the risk for most individual patients.

Generally, in cases where the risks of bleeding are small, and the risk of thrombosis high, dual antiplatelet therapy should be continued. For patients with a high risk of bleeding, discussion between anaesthetist, cardiologist and surgeon is essential. Although no firm evidence exists, the emphasis is on continuing antiplatelet therapy whenever possible. This poses a potential problem for many procedures where epidural or central neuraxial blockade (CNB) is used.

Oral anticoagulants

Many vascular patients take warfarin. New oral anticoagulants, such as the direct thrombin inhibitor dabigatran and the direct factor Xa inhibitor rivaroxaban, are now available, and are likely to replace warfarin. These drugs may be easier and safer to manage from a patients perspective (predictable fixed dosing without intensive monitoring), but emergency reversal may be more problematic.

Patients with mechanical heart valves should have an individual assessment of risk from surgical haemorrhage against risk of cardiac thrombotic complications. This will depend on the nature and location of the heart valve and the planned surgery. Traditional perioperative management involves stopping warfarin 3 or 4 days before surgery, and using heparin infusion until a few hours preoperatively, then re-starting the heparin postoperatively until adequate oral intake allows rewarfarinisation.

Statins

There is some evidence from retrospective and case control studies (e.g. The Statins for Risk Reduction in Surgery [StaRRS] study) that statins reduce mortality following major surgery possibly due in part to stabilisation of inflammatory atherosclerotic plaque. No prospective trials have confirmed this observation, and any proposed mechanism of action is currently putative. Nonetheless, patients with dyslipidaemias should have lipid-lowering therapy started, irrespective of their need for surgery.

β-Blockers

The role of β-blockade in the perioperative period remains uncertain. Initial small trials showed an all-cause reduction in mortality, but the more recent POISE study showed that myocardial protection was more than balanced by all-cause mortality and stroke [2, 3]. Patients already taking β-blockers should probably continue these in the perioperative period, but starting β-blockers in the immediate preoperative phase for patients with uncomplicated coronary artery disease should not be considered routine practice at present.

Angiotensin converting enzyme inhibitors (ACEIs) and angiotensin II antagonists

Angiotensin converting enzyme inhibitors are first-line therapy for heart failure. Angiotensin II receptor (AT II) antagonists may be used as an alternative or additional treatment. There is uncertainty regarding the optimal management of these drugs in the perioperative period. Patients continuing these drugs may be more susceptible to hypotension during anaesthesia, and to renal impairment and possibly even postoperative death. This is perhaps most marked in hypovolaemic patients. However, patients stopping ACEI or ATII antagonists may be at risk from non fatal cardiac complications. If ACEIs are withheld preoperatively, this should be for at least 12 hours. Angiotensin II receptor antagonists should be withheld for at least 24 hours due to their longer half life.

Management of emergency or acute cases

Increasingly, carotid surgery should be carried out in an acute setting, and many vascular patients present as emergencies. Time to investigate, treat or stabilise may be limited, and patient outcome then depends on the expertise and functioning of the whole team. Outcomes are better when experienced teams, who have practiced and worked together over prolonged periods, carry out these complex tasks, rather than random on-call teams of varying abilities. This has implications for centralisation of services and specialisation of staff, which are beyond the remit of this chapter.

Radiologic embolisation for control of bleeding is possible under local anaesthesia in selected emergency cases to avoid the risks of general anaesthesia and open surgery. Again, this has wider implications for service provision beyond the scope of this chapter.

Critical care considerations

Critical care issues cover a wide range of topics both in examinations and clinical practice relevant to many surgical specialties. Some topics (e.g. brain death, organ donation) are covered elsewhere in this book. Others should be taken from source documents due to their regular revision. Examples include cardiac arrest management, treatment of common arrhythmias and anaphylaxis. These topics are clearly and concisely set out on the Resuscitation Council UK website (http://www.resus.org.uk, see the guidelines page for a link to the algorithms for a concise revision aid). A precise knowledge of current algorithms is vital not just for examination purposes but for everyday clinical practice. It is reasonable to expect a senior surgical trainee to have a clear understanding of these areas of emergency management.

Practical procedures often associated with critical care are central venous line insertion, chest drain insertion and vascular access for haemodialysis. Indications for the procedure, common complications and the details of surface anatomy and actual insertion technique have all been asked in the exit examination and candidates should have a clear understanding of these. These areas are covered in the Care of the Critically Ill Surgical Patient (CCrISP) course and the handbook for that course sets them out well.

Definitions of levels of critical care

Critical care can be considered as a spectrum from enhanced ward care, including support from Critical Care Outreach services, up to the advanced multiple organ support provided in an intensive care unit. In 2000, the Department of Health produced a document 'Comprehensive Critical Care' defining critical care into levels 0 to 3 (see Table 23.3).

In some hospitals each level of care is provided for in distinct clinical areas. This is the traditional model of acute surgical ward (level 1), high dependency unit (HDU, level 2), which may be directly supervised by the surgical directorates or managed as a step-down unit from intensive care by the intensivists, and intensive care or intensive therapy units (ICU or ITU level 3). Many hospitals are now moving to a system of integrated critical care units (ICCUs) with all the enhanced level beds [4, 5] in one location.

Definitions of organ failure

Most critical care therapy supports failing organ systems to allow time for other treatments and the patients own defence mechanisms to generate recovery. Multiple organ dysfunction syndrome (MODS) describes what is often a secondary injury to tissues caused by a host inflammatory response to a primary insult. It is characterised by a progressive loss of function in several different organ systems and its treatment is the core of ICU care. Deterioration of any organ ranges from reduced to complete loss of function and there are many definitions of exactly what constitutes organ failure. One set of definitions used in several large trials of sepsis treatment is summarised in Table 23.4 along with definitions of

Table 23.3 Levels of critical care

Level 0	Patients whose needs can be met through normal ward care in an acute hospital
Level 1	Patients at risk of their condition deteriorating, or those recently relocated from higher levels of care, whose needs can be met on an acute ward with additional advice and support from the critical care team
Level 2	Patients requiring more detailed observation or intervention including support for a single failing organ system or postoperative care and those 'stepping down' from higher levels of care
Level 3	Patients requiring advanced respiratory support alone or basic respiratory support together with support of at least two organ systems. This level includes all complex patients requiring support for multi-organ failure

acute lung injury (ALI) and acute respiratory distress syndrome (ARDS). The Sepsis-related Organ Failure Assessment (SOFA) score is another widely used measure of organ failure [5]. Calculated daily it can be used as a measure of severity of illness and response to treatment.

Monitoring and therapeutic measures for specific organ failure

All critical care measures must be built on a foundation of sound basic care. Treatment of any organ failure needs to start with an assessment of airway, breathing and circulation (A, B, C) as per CCrISP or Advances Trauma and Life Support (ATLS) guidelines and these should always be followed with immediate treatment of any deficit detected. A full physical examination including measurement of pulse, blood pressure, respiratory rate, pulse-oximetry and temperature is also mandatory. Critical care therapeutic options for specific organ system failure are set out below.

Respiratory failure

Immediate measures to treat respiratory failure begin with optimal positioning of the patient (e.g. sitting up in bed or in a chair to improve chest expansion). Oxygen should be used in all acutely breathless patients. If there is a strong suspicion of chronic lung disease likely to include carbon dioxide retention then arterial blood gas analysis (ABG) to monitor this will be required soon after commencing oxygen. If sputum retention is suspected then urgent physiotherapy may be required. When clinical signs suggest an active chest infection then appropriate antibiotics should be started immediately, ideally after obtaining a sputum specimen. Other treatable causes for breathlessness should be sought and rectified, such as excessive pain or anxiety, pneumothorax, pleural effusion and cardiac arrhythmias.

For a patient who remains breathless or tachypnoeic, or whose peripheral oxygen saturations remain depressed in spite of supplemental oxygen, ABG analysis is appropriate. Arterial blood gas analysis results will provide information on pH, oxygen and carbon dioxide levels, base deficit, bicarbonate and often lactate. Respiratory failure can be differentiated into types 1 and 2 on the basis of pO_2 and pCO_2 (Table 23.4).

Standard mixed concentration (MC) oxygen face masks can deliver up to a maximum of around 60% oxygen regardless of how high a flow rate of oxygen is used due to entrainment of air around the sides of the mask during rapid inspiration. The addition of a non-rebreathe bag to the mask allows more oxygen to be drawn from the bag during inspiration and may increase inspired oxygen concentration to approximately 80%. For CO_2-retaining patients

Table 23.4 Indicators of organ dysfunction

Type I respiratory failure	pO_2 less than 8 kPa with normal or reduced pCO_2
Type II respiratory failure	pO_2 less than 8 kPa with elevated $pCO_2 > 6.7$ kPa; assistance with ventilatory effort required
Acute lung injury (ALI)	Acute onset
	$PaO_2/FiO_2 < 300$ mmHG (despite normal pCO_2 and regardless of PEEP)
	Bilateral diffuse infiltrates on CXR
	No apparent cardiogenic cause (pulmonary capillary wedge pressure < or = 18 mmHg or 2.4 kPa if measured, or no clinical evidence of left atrial hypertension
	Known triggering event or risk factor
Acute respiratory distress syndrome (ARDS)	Same as ALI except oxygenation $PaO_2/FiO_2 < 200$ mmHg (despite normal $PaCO_2$ and regardless of PEEP)
CVS	Systolic arterial pressure < 90 mmHg despite adequate fluid resuscitation and/or vasopressor requirement
	pH < 7.3 or base deficit >5 in association with lactate >1.5 × upper limit of normal
Renal	Urine output < 0.5 ml kg^{-1} for more than 1 hour despite adequate fluid resuscitation
Haematological	Platelet count < 80 000 mm^{-3} (or 50% fall in 3 days)

PEEP, positive end expiratory pressure; CXR, chest X-ray.

needing tightly controlled oxygen venturi masks will ensure a maximum inspired oxygen concentration is delivered independent of oxygen flow rate and inspiratory effort.

If levels of oxygen greater than 80% are required then a tight-fitting mask is needed to prevent entrainment. The use of continuous positive airway pressure (CPAP) may further enhance oxygen delivery. CPAP (delivered via a nasal or face mask or hood device) increases functional residual capacity (FRC) by preventing airway pressure falling to zero during expiration. A rise in FRC reduces ventilation-perfusion mismatch thereby improving gas exchange. Continuous positive airway pressure requires a cooperative patient with a patent airway and intact airway reflexes. Above CPAP pressures of 20 cmH$_2$O insufflation of the stomach may occur with a risk of vomiting and aspiration. Oxygenation may be improved by CPAP but CO$_2$ removal may not be improved with its use. In some cases a reduced work of breathing may permit improved respiration and affect pCO$_2$ but this is not a predictable response.

For patients with rising pCO$_2$, or need for high oxygen concentrations in the presence of impaired airway protection or impending exhaustion intubation and positive pressure, ventilation may be indicated. A cuffed tube placed in the trachea will allow a degree of protection of the airway from aspiration and the application of airway pressure in excess of 20 cmH$_2$O without risk of gastric insufflation. Intermittent positive pressure ventilation (IPPV) can be delivered as a pressure controlled volume limited ventilation (i.e. bilevel positive airway pressure [BIPAP]) or as a volume controlled pressure limited ventilation (conventional intermittent mandatory ventilation [IMV], which may be synchronised with patients own respiratory efforts [SIMV]). Currently accepted methods include the use of high positive end expiratory pressure (PEEP) to enhance FRC and thus oxygenation in conjunction with low tidal volumes (maximum 6 ml kg^{-1} body weight tidal volume) as per the ARDSNET study to reduce volutrauma damage to the lungs in ALI [6].

Limiting tidal volumes may lead to rising pCO$_2$ but in the absence of marked acidaemia this is considered an acceptable side effect of this ventilatory strategy, described as permissive hypercapnia.

Prolonged oral or nasal intubation may lead to long-term injury to vocal cords and to ischaemic mucosal damage of the trachea leading to stenosis. Tracheostomy has long been an established alternative. With the advent of percutaneous dilational techniques there has been an increase in the use of tracheostomy and also a tendency to perform it earlier in a patient's ITU stay. Additional advantages include a reduced need for sedation, which in turn may reduce vasopressor requirements and direct access to the trachea for suctioning in a patient who is awake and able to cough, communicate and cooperate with physiotherapy. This may speed the process of weaning from ventilation.

Cardiac failure

Standard assessment of the cardiovascular system begins with clinical examination and non-invasive assessments including ECG and echocardiography, supplemented by invasive methods including arterial and central venous access, and cardiac output estimation by one of several methods. Therapy builds from optimisation of cardiac filling and correction of rhythm abnormalities to inotropic and vasopressor regimes and perhaps cardiac-assist devices such as intra-aortic balloon pumps. These therapies aim to ensure optimum oxygen delivery to end organs. Global oxygen delivery is a product of the haemoglobin concentration in the blood, the oxygen saturation of that haemoglobin and the cardiac output. Dissolved haemoglobin makes up a very small percentage of oxygen content of the blood. Therapeutic measures need to ensure each of these aspects is optimised. Less predictable or amenable to treatment is tissue-level oxygen flux. Microcirculatory abnormalities and impaired enzyme function may reduce oxygen delivery at cellular level. This is particularly seen in severe sepsis.

The effectiveness of treatment of circulatory impairment at end-organ level can be assessed by simple means including Glasgew Coma Scale (GCS) for adequacy of cerebral perfusion or urine output and creatinine levels for renal perfusion. Assessment of adequacy of global oxygen delivery can be estimated from lactate levels although local ischaemia or liver failure may complicate this. Oxygen saturations of less than 70% on a central line venous sample may indicate inadequate oxygen delivery.

To maximise cardiac function, left ventricular filling, myocardial contractility, and afterload (systemic vascular resistance [SVR]) should be optimised. Starling's curve relates increased stretch on myofibrils to contractility of those fibres. It can be extrapolated to predict the effect of increasing left ventricular filling on myocardial contractility. With increased filling, myocardial contractility increases up to a certain point. Thereafter further increases in volume lead to a decrease in contractility and a failing heart. In a normal heart central venous pressure, which estimates right atrial pressure will be a reasonable measure of left atrial pressure and therefore left ventricular filling. Where valves are damaged or pulmonary resistance is increased this may not be true. Pulse contour analysis of arterial pressure traces using complex algorithms are a surrogate measure of left ventricular filling, in particular showing what effect fluid boluses have on stroke volume (SV). If a bolus causes less than a 10% rise in SV then further filling may not benefit contractility and may even have adverse effects.

A variety of methods are available to estimate cardiac output itself. The gold standard remains pulmonary artery flotation catheter methods using dilutional calculations but risks associated with these, including death, mean their use is declining. Less invasive methods include oesophageal Doppler (ODM), lithium dilution (LiDCO) and pulse contour cardiac output analysis (PiCCO). Each method has its own problems and none necessarily gives an exact measure of cardiac output. Most clinicians accept that the measure is an estimate and are more interested in the dynamic effects of interventions on the reading to demonstrate improvements or otherwise.

Once cardiac filling is optimised, contractility can be further assisted by ensuring a suitable electrolyte and pH balance in the myocardial tissues. Calcium, potassium, phosphate and magnesium are all essential factors for muscle contraction and should be closely monitored and optimised. Severe acidosis can have a detrimental effect on contractility and pH should be normalised whenever possible (see renal failure below). Effective contraction is also enhanced by sinus rhythm and any new onset arrhythmia should be corrected.

Thereafter contractility can be augmented by the use of positive inotropic agents. The most commonly used are epinephrine (adrenaline) and dobutamine with strong agonist actions on β1-adrenoreceptors. Although cardiac output influences global oxygen delivery, the systolic blood pressure determines localised perfusion of tissues such that a very low systolic pressure is likely to be harmful. Drugs such as dopamine and dopexamine are known to be positive inotropes but are often used in lower doses by clinicians who believe they can improve specific regional blood flow (in particular renal and splanchnic) but the evidence for this is not strong. Their other adverse side effects (tachyarrhythmia, dopaminergic receptor stimulation) make these two drugs less attractive as pure inotropes.

Profound vasodilation in severe sepsis may reduce systolic pressure to harmful levels even in the presence of a high cardiac output. Drugs acting as α-adrenoreceptor agonists can produce vasoconstriction to improve overall tissue perfusion pressure and tissue oxygen delivery. Norepinephrine (noradrenaline) and phenylephrine are first-line vasopressor agents. Vasopressin and terlipressin are second-line agents, which may supplement the actions of norepinephrine. In patients with severe sepsis and vasopressor resistant hypotension low-dose steroids (50 mg hydrocortisone IV qds) may reduce vasopressor requirements but effects on outcome are unclear.

Renal failure

Classically causes of renal failure can be divided into pre-renal, renal and post-renal. Pre-renal causes arise when an insufficient oxygen supply is available to the kidneys. Optimisation of the cardiovascular system, as described above, is key to preventing or limiting pre-renal injury. Clearly, ensuring patency of renal vessels is of primary importance. Thereafter optimal filling, maintenance of cardiac output and adequate mean arterial pressure (with vasopressors if needed) are the only proven therapies that reduce the degree and duration of renal failure from this cause.

Treatable causes of renal failure usually involve removal or avoidance of nephrotoxic agents. Non steroidal anti-inflammatory drugs (NSAIDs), aminoglycocides and iodinated contrast media are commonly encountered in critical care but should be avoided when feasible.

In the specific case of renal failure following rhabdomyolysis, hydration and a forced alkaline diuresis may limit injury (myoglobin is precipitated in the collecting tubules at acid pH). Sodium bicarbonate infusion may be needed to achieve this. Furosemide should be used with caution, if at all.

As a general rule, diuretics increase urine volumes and are useful in patients with volume overload but do not reduce the occurrence of or duration of renal failure. Their use in patients with developing acute renal failure may worsen outcome by causing hypovolaemia.

Mannitol has been used, particularly in the context of aortic surgery as a 'reno-protective' measure. It is an osmotic diuretic and may produce an increase in urine volume, but there is minimal evidence to support any effect on onset or severity of renal impairment.

Dopamine and dopexamine have both been used at 'renal' doses to try to enhance the perfusion of the reno-splanchnic vascular systems. Again, the evidence for efficacy is limited.

Contrast induced nephropathy (CIN)

This usually occurs within 72 hours of exposure to iodinated contrast media. It is usually transient, resolving in 7–10 days, but is occasionally permanent and is associated with an increased morbidity and mortality. Contrast induced nephropathy is dose dependent and use of high osmolar contrast media carries an increased risk. Using the lowest possible dose of contrast media and adequate pre-procedure hydration will reduce the incidence of nephrotoxicity. N-acetyl-cysteine or sodium bicarbonate infusions are used in some centres to reduce contrast injury but the evidence for this is weak.

Post-renal causes of renal failure consist of obstruction to outflow of urine, this may be an occluded ureter post-surgery, prostatic hypertrophy or tumour or other forms of bladder outflow obstruction. In most patients with impending renal failure an ultrasound of the renal tract is a mandatory part of investigation. Bladder catheterisation, both as a monitoring and also a therapeutic measure, is usual in patients with renal impairment.

Established acute renal failure

Acute renal failure leads to raised levels of urea and creatinine, the potential for fluid overload and worsening acidosis and hyperkalaemia. This combination, if left untreated, will result in arrhythmias and eventually death.

For treatment of severe hyperkalaemia calcium gluconate or calcium chloride 10 mmol IV, should be given immediately. These act as membrane stabilisers to reducing the risk of life-threatening ventricular fibrillation. Urgent reduction of serum potassium can be achieved by pushing the potassium ions into the intracellular space using dextrose and insulin (15 IU actrapid in 50 ml 50% dextrose over 15 min) and by correcting the acidosis. Salbutamol either IV or nebulised can also effectively reduce serum potassium in the emergency situation. Intravenous sodium bicarbonate infusion will increase serum pH as long as the patient maintains an ability to increase ventilation to remove the extra carbon dioxide this generates. Potassium is driven into the intracellular space by alkalosis. Chelating agents such as calcium resonium (for adults 30 g given as a PR enema) will further help to remove potassium from the serum.

Definitive treatment is still likely to be required. Intermittent haemodialysis (IHD) or continuous veno-venous haemofiltration (CVVH) can provide this.

In a haemodynamically stable patient IHD over 3–4 hours via a twin lumen venous access line (vascath) will clear acidosis, hyperkalaemia and uraemia rapidly. The rapid fluid shifts involved with this make it difficult to achieve in the more unstable patient. Many units prefer to use CVVH in this group.

In a CVVH circuit venous blood is pumped into a filter with a pore size suitable to allow water and small molecules to pass through whilst preventing the passage of most proteins, cells and platelets. In this ultrafiltrate, waste such as urea and creatinine along with a mixture of electrolytes and water are separated out and diverted to a waste bag. The volume removed is carefully measured and then replaced with a balanced solution of water and electrolytes. Potassium is added separately as required. The replacement fluid is either lactate buffered (which remains stable for long periods) or 'lactate-free' bicarbonate buffered (which requires mixing immediately prior to use). Units treating patients with liver impairment tend to use lactate free fluid as the liver is the main site of lactate metabolism. If a greater degree of clearance is required there is an option to apply a counter-current flow of the balanced solution through the filter with the aim of increasing the concentration gradient for solutes to exit into the waste flow (haemodiafiltration).

Continuous veno-venous haemofiltration, as its name implies, is run as a 24 hours-a-day process. By adjusting the amount of fluid replaced into the patient relative to the volume of ultrafiltrate removed it is possible to remove water to achieve the desired daily fluid balance. In unstable patients the fluid shifts and haemodynamic effects of CVVH are better tolerated. There may also be less injury to the kidney during the filtration process due to the greater haemodynamic stability than with IHD.

Nutrition

Postoperative patients and those with sepsis and systemic inflammatory response syndrome (SIRS) usually mount a highly catabolic response. Significant loss of muscle mass and strength may prolong ICU and hospital stay, inadequate nutrition may also affect wound healing. As such, nutrition is a vital part of their critical care therapy. The average catabolic patient in ITU will need a daily calorie intake of around 1600 kcal day^{-1}. Where possible, the route of delivery should be via enteral feeding. Early enteral feeding even at low levels (10 ml hour^{-1}) has been shown to increase splanchnic blood flow and there is better maintenance of gut mucosal anatomy.

In the unconscious patient this might be nasogastric (NG) or percutaneous endoscopic gastrostomy (PEG) tube delivered. Many ICU patients develop gastroparesis for a variety of reasons and post-pyloric feeding should be considered early in a patient with high gastric aspirates not responding to prokinetics. With foresight, nasojejunal tubes can be sited during a laparotomy using direct manipulation. Later insertion of post-pyloric tubes using blind techniques or with endoscopy causes delay in feeding and is not without risk.

A range of feeds is available, each with its own benefits, and the choice should be tailored to the individual. Osmolite is a standard feed with 1 kcal ml^{-1}. Nepro is a low volume feed with 2 kcal ml^{-1} with low potassium, sodium and phosphate loads suitable for those with renal failure. Pulmocare and oxepa have a high fat : carbohydrate ratio so generate less CO_2 on metabolism, which may be useful for those with severe respiratory failure. Impact has relatively high protein content with added arginine, fish oils and omega 3. It may be beneficial in immunocompromised patients with sepsis. Other feeds exist and the choice should be made in consultation with a dietician.

Where it is not possible to feed via the gut then total parenteral nutrition (TPN) is used. A dedicated central venous access port and exemplary aseptic technique is needed when using

Table 23.5 Definitions in critical illness

SIRS (systemic inflammatory response syndrome)	Requires two of: • Pyrexia > 38oC or hypothermia < 36oC • Tachycardia > 90 bpm (in absence of β-blocker) • Tachypnoea > 20 breaths per min or PaCO$_2$ < 4.3 kPa (32 mmHg) or a requirement for mechanical ventilation • White cell count > 12 000 cells mm-3 or < 4000 cells mm-3
Sepsis	SIRS + documented source of infection
Severe sepsis	Sepsis plus altered organ perfusion or evidence of dysfunction in one or more organs
Septic shock	Refractory hypotension in addition to the above in the presence of systemic infection
MODS (multiple organ dysfunction syndrome)	Presence of altered organ function in acutely ill patients such that homeostasis cannot be maintained without intervention. Usually involves two or more organ systems

TPN. Line-related sepsis leading to septicaemia is a particular problem associated with TPN as the solution provides ideal growth media for bacteria. The solution used for TPN should be tailored to the individuals' biochemical and nutritional needs although 'off-the-shelf' preparations are available. Due to the high lipid content of TPN fluids, fatty infiltration of the liver is relatively common and liver function tests should be measured regularly.

Severe sepsis

Definitions of SIRS, sepsis, severe sepsis and MODS are often a topic of discussion in the examination situation and definitions are presented in Table 23.5. For a summary of the management of sepsis the European surviving sepsis campaign editorial sets out an extensive discussion of treatment options. A succinct summary can be derived from Tables 23.3–23.5 of this paper [7]. Treatment revolves around source control to eradicate the infection site with supportive therapy to maintain organ function during recovery. It is vital to liaise closely with the microbiology department and send regular culture specimens to screen for infection, identify pathogens and establish antibiotic sensitivities. Discussion of detailed antibiotic use is beyond the scope of this chapter.

Specific therapy for severe sepsis may include activated protein C (aPC). The exact role of this drug is unclear at present, since the initial encouraging results from a large international trial have not been upheld in daily practice. A new trial is underway to clarify the issue.

Tight glycaemic control (blood glucose 4.5–6.0 mmol l^{-1}) in patients with severe sepsis was thought to be beneficial initially [8]. However a recently published Australian study suggested very tight control may be deleterious, in part due to hypoglycaemia [9]. Current thinking supports blood glucose control between 6–10 mmol l^{-1} in septic patients.

Despite all the currently available treatment options for severe sepsis with MODS the mortality rate remains high (approximately 25% ITU mortality, 40% hospital mortality).

Finally it must always be remembered that the goal of any treatment is to allow the patient to return home with an acceptable quality and quantity of life. If the chances of achieving this become minimal then consideration of the appropriateness of continuing that therapy is vital. This is certainly the case in ICU where many life-prolonging treatments are available in the face of severe illness. National mortality figures for those admitted to ICU show that for all-cause admissions 18% die in the ICU with overall hospital mortality being 27%. For elective and emergency surgery these figures are 2.8 versus 7% and 14.4 versus 24.4%, respectively (Intensive Care National Audit & Research Centre Case Mix Programme ICNARC CMP) data 2008). Where prognosis is poor a change to palliation should be seen as an active decision in the course of ICU care. Appropriate use of palliative care schemes such as the Liverpool Care Pathway may give dignity and ensure relief from unnecessary suffering for patients at the end of their lives.

References

1. Cardiopulmonary Exercise Testing Website. www.cpxtesting.com (accessed 2 April 2009).
2. Deveraux PJ, Beattie WS, Choi, PT-L, et al. How strong is the evidence for th use of perioperative ß-blockers in non-cardiac surgery. *BMJ* 2005; **331**(7512): 313–21.
3. POISE Study Group, Deveraux PJ, Yang H, et al. Effects of extending release metoprolol succinate in patients undergoing non-cardiac surgery (POISE Trial): a radomized controlled trial. *Lancet* 2008; **371**(9627): 1839–47.
4. Auerbach A, Goldman L. Assessing and reducing the cardiac risk of non cardiac surgery. *Circulation* 2006; **113**: 1361–76.
5. Vincent JL et al. The SOFA (Sepsis-related Organ Failure Assessment) score to describe organ dysfunction/failure. *Intensive Care Med* 1996; **22**: 707–10.
6. The Acute Respiratory Distress Syndrome Network. Ventilation with lower tidal volumes as compared with traditional tidal volumes for acute lung injury. *N Engl J Med* 2000; **342**: 1301–8.
7. Dellinger RP et al. Surviving Sepsis Campaign International Guidelines for Management of Severe Sepsis and Septic Shock 2008. *Intensive Care Med* 2008; **34**: 17–60.
8. Van den Berghe G, Wouters P, Verwaest C, et al. Intensive insulin therapy in critically ill patients. *N Engl J Med* 2001; **345**: 1359–67.
9. The NICE SUGAR Study Investigators. Intensive versus conventional glucose control in critically ill patients. *N Engl J Med* 2009; **360**: 1283–97.

24 Access surgery

David C. Mitchell and William D. Neary

Key points

- Planning for vascular access in renal failure needs to begin at least 6 months prior to the predicted onset of dialysis
- Surgery should be aimed at the most distal veins first to preserve the more proximal ones
- Autologous arteriovenous (AV) fistula are the most durable form of access
- Most access procedures can be performed under local anaesthesia as day case surgery
- A good access programme should have an individual to coordinate investigations and surgery
- Surveillance improves access graft function and longevity

Introduction

Vascular access is required in those patients where frequent repeated access to the circulation is required. The vast majority need this for haemodialysis to treat renal failure. Other examples are for plasmapharesis, injection of antibiotics (e.g. cystic fibrosis) or drugs (e.g. in chemotherapy for neoplasia).

The focus of this chapter will be on the provision and maintenance of vascular access for haemodialysis, but the principles of access placement and surveillance hold good for patients with alternative requirements.

Diagnosis of need for access placement

At first sight this appears straightforward. Those patients with end-stage chronic kidney disease will need dialysis and should have access placed. As AV fistula have the lowest morbidity and failure rate, once established, this is regarded as the 'ideal' form of access. Many fistula and all grafts will require surveillance and some may need interventions to keep them functioning adequately. It serves little purpose to place a fistula some years in advance and then spend a lot of resources maintaining it, never to see it used. Conversely patients who present needing dialysis without established access have worse survival. For this reason the National Service Framework in the UK identified that access needs to be placed some months in advance of its anticipated need [1].

Studies show that using serum creatinine as a measure of severity of renal failure is not very accurate. This is because renal function can vary significantly for the same creatinine

Postgraduate Vascular Surgery: The Candidate's Guide to the FRCS, eds. Vish Bhattacharya and Gerard Stansby. Published by Cambridge University Press. © Cambridge University Press 2010.

depending on age, race and body mass. A better measure is the glomerular filtration rate (GFR), but measurement of this is time consuming. Most centres use estimated GFR (eGFR), which is calculated using one of several formulae from the combination of plasma creatinine, age, sex and race. This method is sufficiently reproducible in adults to give reliable trends of renal function over time.

There are opinions as to how best to decide the timing of access placement. Some recommend the use of a single eGFR measurement as a trigger, with figures between 15 and 25 being those most commonly used. Studies in some centres, including our own, have shown that eGFR is a good predictor of cardiac death, but a poor predictor of time to onset of dialysis. The best predictor of the need for renal replacement therapy (RRT) (i.e. dialysis or transplantation) is a combination of rate of creatinine fall and clinical decision by a nephrologist. There are inaccuracies associated with each approach. As a result, some access will be placed and never used. The key to an efficient service is to maximise those starting with established access, whilst minimising unnecessary operations. Those units wanting to start a high proportion of their patients using an established fistula will have a significant redundancy rate built into their surgical programme to achieve this.

Organising an access service

Most Western medical services recognise that access surgery should ideally take place some months prior to the anticipated date of first use. This allows for delays in providing operating time and also for revisional surgery should the first procedure prove inadequate.

Superficially organisation of an access service appears straightforward. The patient is seen, a diagnosis of impending need for dialysis is made and a referral made for surgery. Unfortunately many patients will not have suitable visible veins for fistula placement and will need preoperative assessment with a Duplex scan. Those with identified veins and patent arteries will need to be assessed to determine the likelihood of success.

Successful access surgery is dependent on both arterial (i.e. flexibility and size) and vein quality (size, continuity, distensibility). Where the patient has had previous central lines, the central veins will need checking for stenosis that may jeopardise the success of the procedure by obstructing blood flow in the access.

Once all the information is available, an operating list space will need to be identified and surgery will be performed. Following surgery, some assessment of the success of the procedure is needed and the patient will need to be reviewed to ensure that the fistula is suitable for dialysis. In those where the fistula is not able to be used within a few weeks, further surgical or radiological procedures will be required to make the fistula suitable for use.

The solution to meeting these challenges and delivering a timely service is best addressed by having a defined pathway of care [2] and a multidisciplinary team able to respond to the varying needs of the patient. A central figure in the service is the 'access co-ordinator' who provides a link between patient, dialysis unit and the hospital team.

Timing of access placement

Patients need to come to dialysis with functioning access. This requires timely placement, ideally about 6 months ahead of the anticipated date of first dialysis. The access co-ordinator should be informed by the medical team of the proposed date for starting RRT. This will trigger placement on the waiting list. If suitable veins are visible, adjacent to a palpable arterial pulse, then no further preoperative planning is required. At this stage the patient can be listed for surgery. Routine surgical clinical review serves to impose delays without improving care and is best focused on difficult clinical problems. If no suitable veins and arterial pulse can be identified in the clinic, then ultrasound scanning should be undertaken to facilitate planning of surgery.

If a fistula is planned, placement should occur as soon as the patient is within 6 months of the anticipated RRT date. If no suitable veins are identified, and placement of central venous catheter or access graft is planned, then these can be inserted much closer to the time of RRT commencement, as the time required before they can be used is much shorter.

From this, it is clear that planning needs to begin at least 6 months prior to the anticipated RRT date. This will ensure that the patient comes to RRT with appropriate access for their needs.

Types of vascular access

There are three routes used for establishing vascular access. These are the arteriovenous fistula (AVF), a prosthetic access graft or a central venous catheter (CVC). Each has their own advantages and disadvantages (see Table 24.1).

Choosing which type of access to place requires experience and a good understanding of the needs of the patient. There are some principles that govern the choice of access.

1. Fitness of the patient

    Both AVF and grafts require a good blood flow both to maintain patency and to be useable for dialysis. Patients with failing hearts, or those unable to increase their cardiac output to maintain access flow, will not be suitable for these types of access. In this situation, a decision has to be made to use a CVC or not to embark upon haemodialysis.

2. Adequacy of vessels

    The state of both arteries and veins needs to be considered when planning vascular access. The most commonly encountered difficulty is an absence of suitable veins due to previous cannulation. Duplex scanning is a valuable resource for identifying suitable veins. Most surgeons are reluctant to use veins below 2–2.5 mm in diameter in adults, although smaller veins have been used successfully [3].

    The population coming forward for access surgery is steadily ageing. Many will have diabetes. Both diabetes and chronic kidney disease lead to vascular calcification. While small amounts of vessel wall calcification may not prejudice the success of surgery, heavily calcified (i.e. rigid) arteries are unable to increase flow to allow fistula maturation or to maintain graft patency. Arteries need to be an adequate size and again 2–2.5 mm diameter would be regarded as the lower limit for successful access placement.

3. Handedness

    A 4-hour dialysis session is unpleasant enough without rendering patients unable to use their dominant hand. For this reason it is customary to place access in the non-dominant limb wherever possible. If no suitable vessels are identified, then it is acceptable to use the dominant limb after discussion with the patient.

4. Central vein stenosis or occlusion

    Patients with previous CVC placement, pacemakers or port-a-caths may have stenosis of their central veins. In these patients, imaging of the central veins is advised. Ultrasound may show normal respiratory phasicity suggesting adequate patency. If there are doubts about the veins in the root of the neck, then arm venograms are a good method of imaging the central veins.

Table 24.1 Advantages and disadvantages of vascular access procedures

	AVF	Graft	CVC
Ease of placement	Variable depending on state of veins Easy LA procedure for primary wrist and elbow AVF, more complex for transposition procedures	Variable, often needs GA or loco-regional block	Usually straightforward unless CV stenosis
Advantages	Usually LA day case procedure (75%) Robust once established Resistant to thrombosis and infection Revision rate about 15% pa	Can bridge long distance between artery and vein Usually easy to establish provided vessels adequate	Insertion under LA, tunnelled if required for more than 3 weeks Not dependent on good cardiac output Can be used immediately for dialysis
Disadvantages	May take months to mature for use Difficult to establish, only about 55% will be useable 1 year after formation May need revising to promote maturation	Needs a couple of weeks to become incorporated prior to use (unless designed for immediate use) Prone to thrombosis, mostly due to venous intimal hyperplasia More susceptible to infection than AVF Revision rates about 85% pa	Vulnerable to sepsis Associated with higher mortality than AVF Venous stenosis around catheter may preclude future access placement in limb

AVF, arteriovenous fistula; CVC, central venous catheter; LA, local anaesthesia; GA, general anaesthesia.

5. Patient preference

Some patients may have a strong preference for certain types of access. Younger patients may be particularly sensitive about the cosmetic appearance of a fistula and may request brachio-cephalic AVF, thigh grafts or CVC. It is the role of the medical team to make patients aware of the advantages and disadvantages of their choices and then to support them in providing acceptable access.

Operative techniques

The choice of operation is based on the factors above. The ideal access is usually an AVF in the distal part of the non-dominant limb. An AVF has the advantage of being robust, thrombosis and infection resistant when compared to the alternatives. Arteriovenous fistula requires the least maintenance of any type of access. The principle issue with AVFs is the difficulty faced in establishing them. This may take more than one operation. In our unit 55% of AVFs are useable at one year after a single operation. This rises to 84% after two operations. Only a small number of patients require more than two operations. It is this need for a second procedure in a substantial minority that dictates that patients planned for AVF formation need to start on their surgical pathway some months prior to the onset of dialysis.

Patients may anticipate more than one operation to maintain access over the lifetime of their renal failure. It is in their interests to minimise the trauma associated with surgery and to plan the simplest procedure compatible with a good outcome. For this reason, local or regional anaesthesia is preferred wherever possible. Many procedures can be carried out in the day case facility, minimising hospital time. A survey of the workload in our unit (about 450 operations a year) identified that about 75% are done as day case procedures under local anaesthesia.

Arteriovenous fistula (AVF)

These should be fashioned as end of vein to side of artery anastomoses. At the wrist or in the anatomical snuffbox, some surgeons prefer end-to-end anastomoses. The results from the two approaches seem to be broadly similar. At the wrist a long anastomosis is preferred. This reduces narrowing from intimal hyperplasia and maximises flow in small vessels. Prolene sutures are commonly used. There is a suggestion in the literature that the use of external clips for the anastomosis may produce technically superior anastomoses [4]. The clips are considerably more expensive than sutures, which may influence surgeon's choice.

More proximal AVFs are fashioned using the end-to-side configuration, but more care needs to be taken to keep the anastomosis at about 8 mm length. Larger anastomoses are prone to develop very high flows, which may steal blood from the distal part of the limb. In some cases high flows (usually of $2 \, l \, min^{-1}$ or more) can precipitate high output cardiac failure.

When the easily accessible superficial veins (cephalic and forearm basilic) are exhausted then attention may have to focus on the deeper veins (arm basilic and great saphenous). These veins may form good quality AVFs but need transposing towards the skin to make them accessible to dialysis needles. Most surgeons will undertake to transpose and form the AVF at a single operation. Occasionally the vein may be a bit small and then it is acceptable to perform a simple end-to-side anastomosis and await vein enlargement before subjecting the patient to the bigger transposition operation. The results of either approach are broadly equivalent, with greater success rates (at about 75% primary patency) from basilic vein transposition.

Arteriovenous access grafts

The commonest material used is polytetrafluoroethane (PTFE), but many types of access graft material can be used. Some grafts are designed with self sealing coatings to allow immediate cannulation after placement. Grafts may be placed in any configuration between a suitable artery and vein. Where they are placed over muscle (upper limb and thigh) it is important to place them superficially to the deep fascia as peri-graft haematomas can cause compartment syndrome if the graft is placed too deeply.

A graft of 6 mm diameter is usually adequate for dialysis. Smaller grafts may prove difficult to puncture accurately with dialysis needles. The exception is the stepped graft where the arterial end is deliberately of lower calibre. This is to try and reduce turbulent flow, which is thought to contribute to venous intimal hyperplasia and graft failure. The larger upper part of the graft is the portion that is used for dialysis.

A number of variations have been employed to try to reduce the narrowing seen at the venous end. Grafts with pre-dilated venous ends are sold commercially, but there is no good vidence of superior outcome from their use. Vein cuffs may be used, as for lower limb arte-ial bypass, but their efficacy remains unproven.

Where grafts are placed, they may need subsequent removal for sepsis. This can be very difficult operation, particularly around the artery in an infected groin. Complete emoval of all graft material is required to eliminate infection. It is the authors' preference o place a vein interposition cuff between artery and graft to facilitate subsequent removal. he dissection of the infected graft goes down to the cuff:graft anastomosis. A clamp can e placed across the cuff, which is then oversewn avoiding the need to formally dissect he artery.

entral venous catheters (CVCs)

he main advantage of CVCs is that they can be placed and used immediately. They are the nainstay of providing dialysis in acute kidney injury and in those with chronic kidney dis-ase who present acutely before placement of permanent access.

The catheters should be placed in large central veins using a Seldinger technique under ltrasound guidance. It is preferable to use the jugular veins. This avoids damage to the ubclavian veins from the trauma of placement, or subsequently due to scarring of the vein round the catheter. Narrowing of the subclavian vein may jeopardise the placement of ccess distally within the limb.

Central venous catheters are prone to infection, so if it is anticipated that the catheter ill remain in place for more than a week or two, a tunnelled catheter should be placed. The atheter has a cuff, which is situated just within the tunnel and reduces migration of micro-rganisms along the catheter. Eradication of methicillin-resistant *Staphylococcus aureus* MRSA) carriage is an important part of reducing sepsis related to CVC use.

are of access after placement
on-maturation of AVF

significant minority of AVF fail to mature. There is evidence that early identification and orrection of abnormalities significantly improves maturation rates [5]. Flow rates increase ignificantly within minutes of AVF formation, and reach near maximal levels within 2–7 ays. A Duplex scan at 1–2 weeks will detect those with low flow that are very unlikely to nature to use. This allows early intervention. The commonest cause of non-maturation is tenosis in the 'swing' segment of the fistula, where the vein is mobilised to swing across the artery. Revision or angioplasty are equally effective at correcting the abnormality, lthough angioplasty may need to be repeated more often to obtain the same result [6].

Large tributaries may split the flow leaving no single vein large enough to use for dialysis. dentification and ligation of such tributaries can improve maturation rates significantly.

Finally an increasingly common problem is with an AVF that is too deep to needle due patient obesity. The solution here is to mobilise the AVF up under the skin (disconnecting nd reconnecting the anastomosis if need be) to allow improved access.

arly failure of grafts

his should be a rare occurrence if patients have been carefully assessed and selected for graft lacement. The commonest cause is a technical surgical failure and failure within 24 hours hould stimulate the surgeon to re-explore the graft. Occasionally it will become apparent that the artery or vein was insufficient for the procedure, but often a technical problem a one or another anastomosis can be corrected to improve access function. Sometimes i longer grafts and those with loop configurations, a kink in the tunnelling is responsible fo early failure.

Surveillance of access

Vascular access requires surveillance following placement to ensure that it functions cor rectly. This is of vital importance to patients as the access is their lifeline, without whicl they are unable to dialyse. Each type of access has its own particular needs, but the commor theme of surveillance is to detect abnormalities before access failure and to resolve then before the access becomes unuseable. There is debate about the value of surveillance witl some studies suggesting improved outcomes and others not [7, 8].

The problem of failure is most acute with grafts. This is usually due to stenosis at the venous anastomosis and this is the first place to focus on if surgical re-exploration i planned. Whether thrombectomy is performed with catheters or at open operation, it i vitally important to treat any stenosis or the graft will probably clot again. One exceptior to this is the overdialysis or patients, or volume depletion secondary to fluid loss (diarrhoe and/or vomiting). In this situation the thrombosis is consequent on low flow states and sim ple thrombectomy plus re-adjustment of dialysis dose will suffice.

AVFs are less likely to fail, although there is some evidence that surveillance and inter vention may prolong the life of established AVFs [8]. They degrade rapidly after thrombosis Arteriovenous fistulae need to be declotted rapidly, within 48–72 hours (unlike grafts) i they are to be salvaged after failure. Central venous catheters tend to clot but can often b resuscitated with endovascular techniques. There is no formal surveillance programme fo CVCs and this may in part reflect the fact that many of the CVCs are placed temporarily a a bridge to more permanent access.

Techniques for the surveillance of grafts and AVFs centre on clinical assessment, flov estimation and assessment of dialysis efficacy. It is not the purpose of this chapter to provid an in-depth critique of various techniques. The variety of methods speaks for the fact tha none is perfect. It is up to individual units to select a method that suits the needs of thei patients and then to understand both its advantages and shortcomings.

Clinical surveillance revolves around thrill detection in the access and recognition o significant abnormalities. Thrill detection can be performed by the patient, and patients ar told to report loss of thrill immediately. This is an indication for immediate review and con firmation of thrombosis/critical stenosis at the earliest opportunity. Other factors that ar detected clinically are infection (rigours, redness and pain over access), aneurysm formatior and vascular steal syndrome. Some stenoses may be detected by noting a change in the char acter of the thrill/turgidity of the AVF along its length.

While clinical surveillance may detect significant abnormalities, the most commor clinical problem encountered with access is thrombosis. Ideally the abnormality leading t thrombosis (usually a stenosis) should be detected before it is clinically problematic. Tw strands of investigation have emerged with this aim in mind. One centres on intra-dialyti measurements of flow or recirculation within the access. The other relies on external Duple: scanning to detect abnormalities at an early stage.

The advantage of intra-dialytic measurement is it avoids extra visits to hospital. Flow ca be measured in the fistula by ultrasound dilution techniques. These have been shown to b

oth reproducible and sensitive. Significant deterioration in flow rates triggers investiga-
ion by ultrasound and interventions as appropriate. Similarly, rising rates of re-circulation
within the access (i.e. dialysing the blood within the access, rather than the patient) should
trigger investigation by ultrasound and then either angioplasty or surgery as appropriate.

Duplex ultrasound surveillance works in the same way as aneurysm or lower limb bypass
raft surveillance. The patient is scanned at regular intervals, looking for evidence of stenosis
r change in volume flow. There are no clear cut-off figures at which intervention becomes
ssential. Most clinicians will be concerned with a fall in flow rate of 20% or more or an
bsolute flow of less than 600 ml min^{-1}. Duplex will often demonstrate the site of abnormal-
ty, allowing a directed choice of therapy. Once again such choices are best determined by
nultidisciplinary teams.

Managing failing access

Failing AVF

Reducing flow or dialysis efficacy may be related to stenosis formation, often at the anas-
omosis, sometimes at the site of fistula damage from needling. The treatment options lie
etween angioplasty and surgery to revise any stenotic segments. The evidence suggests that
utcomes are broadly similar, but that angioplasty may need to be repeated more frequently.
Overall, costs of treatment are similar. For early failure due to anastomotic stenosis in wrist
stula, surgical revision gives good results. However in brachio-cephalic fistula and mature
stula with scarring from dialysis, mobilisation of vein may be more difficult. In this situa-
ion, angioplasty is probably to be preferred.

Some fistulae exhibit rapid aneurysmal enlargement. If this is throughout the fistula,
hen ligation may be the preferred option. Often the aneurysm is associated with a down-
tream stenosis. Aneurysm growth may be arrested by dilating the stenosis.

Failing arteriovenous graft

Grafts usually work well initially unless there is some technical problem with their place-
nent. Subsequent reduction in flow is most commonly due to stenosis at the venous anasto-
nosis. Angioplasty is effective at prolonging graft survival and American studies have shown
hat with repeated interventions the longevity of grafts can approach that of AVF.

When angioplasty is unsuccessful, or if the graft has been clotted for a few days and
annot be lysed successfully, surgical revision can be effective. Once declotted, the graft
an be extended with a short extra segment, to an undamaged vein distal to the original
nastomosis.

Graft infection can be very difficult to eradicate. The simplest approach is graft removal,
ut this often needs to be followed by temporary CVC placement risking catheter infection.
ocalised infection at needling sites and small abscesses can be managed by antibiotics and
ocal graft excision with adjacent skip grafting. This is not always successful but may salvage
particularly valuable access.

Failing central venous catheter

he commonest cause of failure is clotting or obstruction to flow by the development of a
heath of fibrin around the catheter tip. Clotted catheters can be re-opened by a passage of

guidewires and small wire brushes. Fibrin sheaths can be difficult to remove. One technique is to pass a Dormier basket from the groin, close it around the catheter and strip the fibrin sheath away. An alternative is to change the CVC over a wire, which sometimes improves flow.

Central venous catheters are the most susceptible form of access to infection. The best management is to remove the CVC and treat the patients with antibiotics for a few days until better. A new catheter can then be placed, ideally in a new location or at the same site if there is no overt inflammation. Patients can develop severe complications from catheter sepsis including infective endocarditis, arthritis and discitis, so early aggressive antibiotic treatment of infection is important to minimise the risk of complications.

Vascular steal syndrome

This is a problem peculiar to fistulae and grafts. In the limb, a proportion of blood flow is directed through the access. It is not uncommon to see reversed flow in the artery beyond the anastomosis. This is not usually a problem at the wrist as the ulnar or interosseous arteries provide adequate flow to the hand. At the elbow, reversed flow in the brachial artery may be asymptomatic, providing collateral vessels at the elbow to maintain adequate flow to the hand.

If the collateral flow is inadequate, the patient may complain of coolness, numbness and tingling, or overt pain. If this occurs rapidly after access placement (i.e. on waking or the anaesthetic block wearing off) this is a clinical emergency. Once neurological deficit is present, it is difficult to reverse it, even with access ligation. This aggressive version of steal is called 'ischemic monomelic neuropathy" and usually leaves a permanent deficit.

True vascular steal usually presents within a few days, but can present later in AVFs if they enlarge or if there is progressive arterial narrowing. Symptoms are not always present at rest and may sometimes only be present after a period of dialysis.

Diagnosis can be clinical by arm elevation, demonstrating blanching with colour being restored by temporary access occlusion. Digital:brachial pressure (DBI) measurements can help and a DBI of less than 0.6 is strongly associated with steal syndrome.

The management of vascular steal is to restore flow to the distal part of the limb. This can be achieved by access ligation, but this leaves the patient without their lifeline. Attempts to place access in another limb risks re-creating the problem elsewhere. For this reason, other attempts are often made to improve blood flow to the hand. This can be achieved by banding the access and reducing flow, but banding is difficult to get exactly right and symptoms may persist or the access may clot. Extending the access distally or proximally may increase resistance and allow improved flow distally. The distal revascularisation and interval ligation (DRIL) procedure ligates the artery just distal to the access. The artery is then bypassed from at least 8 cm proximal to the access, creating two flow channels, one to the access and one to the distal limb. Occasionally simple distal ligation may suffice, by abolishing the reversed arterial flow beyond the access [9].

Conclusion

Access surgery requires not only good vascular specialist skills, but also requires good service organisation. A well organised service will correctly identify those in need of access, investigate them appropriately to plan the best procedure for the patients and will then undertake surgery in a timely manner.

Once surgery is completed, it is necessary to provide quality assurance by both assessing access adequacy and providing surveillance where needed. A well-organised team will need to review scans and flow measurements regularly and decide on appropriate management of those accesses at risk of failure. A service will need to be provided to deal with those accesses that fail in a timely manner to ensure continuing provision of dialysis for the patient.

References

. Renal NSF part 1. http://www.dh.gov.uk/ en/Publicationsandstatistics/Publications/ PublicationsPolicyAndGuidance/ DH_4070359 (accessed 19 September 2010).

. Winearls C, Fluck R, Mitchell D, Gibbons C et al. The organisation and delivery of the haemodialysis access service for maintenance haemodialysis patients. Joint Publication Vascular Society/ Renal Association British Society for Interventional Radiology, August 2006. http://www.vascularsociety.org.uk/Docs.

. Wong V, Ward R, Taylor J et al. Factors associated with early failure of arteriovenous fistulae for haemodialysis access. *Eur J Vasc Endovasc Surg* 1996; **12**: 207–13.

. Zeebregts CJ, Kirsch WM, van den Dungen JJ, Zhu YH, van Schilfgaarde R. Five years' world experience with nonpenetrating clips for vascular anastomoses. *Am J Surg* 2004; **187**: 751–60.

. Tordoir JH, Rooyens P, Dammers R et al. Prospective evaluation of failure modes in autogenous radiocephalic wrist access for haemodialysis. *Nephrol Dial Transplant* 2003; **18**: 378–83.

6. Tessitore N, Mansueto G, Lipari G et al. Endovascualr versus surgical preemptive repair of forearm arteriovenous fistula juxta-anastomotic stenosis: analysis of data collected prospectively from 1999 to 2004. *Clin J Am Soc Nephrol* 2006; **1**: 448–54.

7. Robbin ML, Oser RF, Lee JY et al. Randomized comparison of ultrasound surveillance and clinical monitoring on arteriovenous graft outcomes. *Kidney Int* 2006; **69**: 730–5.

8. Tessitore N, Lipari G, Poli A et al. Can blood flow surveillance and pre-emptive repair of subclinical stenosis prolong the useful life of arteriovenous fistulae? A randomized controlled study. *Nephrol Dial Transplant* 2004; **19**: 2325–33.

9. Bourquelot P, Guadric J, van Laere O. Surgical techniques for steal treatment. In: Tordoir J, ed. *Vascular Access*. Turin: Publ Edizioni Minerva Medica, 2009.

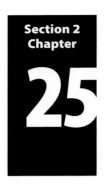

Final FRCS vascular topics

Basic outline of solid organ transplantation

Mathew Jacob, Jeremy French and Derek Manas

Key points

- Solid organ transplantation is now commonplace and is the standard of care for patients with end-stage organ failure
- Indications have changed over time and there are few absolute contraindications
- Equity of access to transplant waiting lists is paramount and selecting the correct recipient and donor pair will optimise the outcome
- The surgical techniques for all organ transplantation are now well established and standardized and as a result there has been a year-on-year improvement in 1-year survival. Most receipnts die because of co-morbidity or poor organ function
- Live donor transplantation for both kidney and liver recipients has become an extremely important source of donor organs
- Complications are general to surgical patients but indeed each organ has its own specific risks
- Immunosuppression has advanced hugely over the past 10 years and, as a result, the overall attrition rate due to acute rejection has reduced considerably
- The biggest problem facing transplantation today is the donor shortage. In 2008, the organ donor taskforce set up by the Minister of Health has set out a plan to increase donation by 50%
- Until this happens, transplantation will always have to deal with the ethical dilemmas of allocation, utilization and fairness

Introduction

Solid organ (liver, pancreas and kidney) transplantation is an important treatment modality for end-stage organ failure. Indeed if a vital organ such as the liver fails, transplantation is the only management option currently available.

Organ transplantation increases life expectancy and quality of life (for the recipient and their family), but is not without risk. Since the pioneering days of solid organ transplantion (kidney 1950, liver 1963) there have been many advances, both surgical and medical, resulting in considerable reduction in overall risk.

While these advances clearly are beneficial in terms of graft and patient survival, these successes have lowered the threshold for acceptance of patients onto transplant waiting lists worldwide, thus significantly contributing to the observed increased demand.

Postgraduate Vascular Surgery: The Candidate's Guide to the FRCS, eds. Vish Bhattacharya and Gerard Stansby. Published by Cambridge University Press. © Cambridge University Press 2010.

Table 25.1 Disease-specific indications for liver transplantation

Primary recipient disease	
Cirrhosis	Secondary sclerosing cholangitis
• Primary biliary cirrhosis	Alpha-1-antitrypsin deficiency
• Secondary biliary cirrhosis	Budd–Chiari syndrome
• Cryptogenic	Wilson's disease
• Alcoholic	Biliary atresia
Non-alcoholic fatty liver disease	Other congenital biliary abnormalities
Chronic active hepatitis (autoimmune)	Acute/subacute fulminant hepatic failure (FHF)
Chronic viral hepatitis B	Primary hepatocellular carcinoma in cirrhotic liver
Chronic viral hepatitis C	Primary hepatic malignancy
Congenital hepatic fibrosis	Inborn errors of metabolism not in chronic liver failure (CLF) group
Primary sclerosing cholangitis	

The fact that the demand for donor organs outstrips supply creates ethical and medical considerations specific to transplantation such as: selection and de-selection criteria; waiting list prioritisation; national organ sharing schemes; development of organ donation and retrieval methods; and the concept of transplant benefit.

This chapter will explore some of these issues as well as giving an overview of the medical and surgical technical aspects of transplantation.

Indications

Liver transplantation (LT)

Following the death of a young woman with liver failure, a colloquium was set up in the UK in 1999 to establish guidelines for the selection of patients for LT. It was agreed that livers donated for transplantation should be considered a national resource. Patients should be considered for transplantation if they had an anticipated length of life (in the absence of transplantation) of less than one year or an unacceptable quality of life. It was also agreed that patients should be accepted for transplantation only if they had an estimated probability of being alive 5 years after transplantation of at least 50% with a quality of life acceptable to the patient. The British Society of Gastroenterology has published clinical guidelines on the indications for referral and assessment in adult liver transplantation [1]. The common indications for liver transplantation are shown in Table 25.1.

Special considerations

Alcohol-induced liver disease may be associated with significant damage to cardiovascular and neurological systems, as well as the risk of patients reverting back to alcohol abuse, resulting in them not complying with medication or follow-up schedules and thus damaging the new liver. A multidisciplinary approach is required to select those patients who are likely to comply; all potential recipients, once accepted onto the waiting list, have to enter into a written contract with the transplanting centre not to return to alcohol consumption after transplantation.

Illegal drug use is not a contraindication to transplant if the patient will comply with the required schedules. However, continued intravenous drug use is considered a contraindication.

Age in itself is not a contraindication, although the survival rate after transplant of the over 65s is significantly worse than that of younger patients.

Self-inflicted conditions such as overdose of paracetamol would only be contraindicated if there were good reasons to believe that the patient would, despite appropriate support, return to their pre-morbid lifestyle that would lead to liver failure or result in a quality of life unacceptable to the patient.

Co-morbid medical or psychiatric conditions are relevant if they affect the patient's quality of life or prospect for survival post transplant. Patients in whom early graft damage from recurrent disease can be anticipated such as recurrent hepatitis C virus (HCV) and hepatitis B virus (HBV) infections should only be transplanted as part of an agreed protocol of treatment. There are well-developed protocols now for prevention of recurrence. With the advent of effective treatment, those co-infected with human immunodeficiency virus (HIV) may be suitable candidates for transplantation.

Re-grafts will need special consideration dependent on the circumstances that gave rise to the need for the re-graft. This is because the results after early re-graft are poor and of only limited benefit.

Where potential liver allograft recipients have suffered from previous extra-hepatic malignancy, the decision to proceed for liver transplantation depends on the probability of malignancy recurring following liver transplantation. Some immunosuppressive agents may encourage the growth of malignancy. In patients with primary hepatic malignancy (HCC), there are agreed criteria that predict a high probability of tumour persistence after transplantation: these include number and size of lesions. More than three liver tumours with a maximum diameter of 5 cm indicates that HCC is likely to persist following liver transplantation. However, these criteria are under regular review.

Currently in the UK, patients with cholangiocarcinoma are not appropriate candidates for transplantation.

It has also been agreed that if the condition of patients awaiting a liver transplantation deteriorates to the extent that the probability of a 5-year survival may fall below 50%, they will be removed from the waiting list but only after full discussion with them. Such patients – although in greatest need – are at greatest risk of not benefiting after transplantation.

Kidney transplantation

With the tremendous improvements in transplant management most patients with kidney failure can be considered for transplantation. Diseases that may be indications for renal transplantation are listed below:

Glomerulonephritis

1. Idiopathic and post-infectious crescentic
2. Membranous
3. Mesangiocapillary (Type I)
4. Mesangiocapillary (Type II) (dense-deposit disease)
5. IgA nephropathy
6. Antiglomerular basement membrane
7. Focal glomerulosclerosis
8. Henoch–Schönlein

Chronic pyelonephritis (reflux nephropathy)

Hereditary
1. Polycystic kidneys
2. Nephronophthisis (medullary cystic disease)
3. Nephritis (including Alport's syndrome)
4. Tuberous sclerosis

Metabolic
1. Diabetes mellitus
2. Hyperoxaluria
3. Cystinosis
4. Fabry's disease
5. Amyloid
6. Gout
7. Porphyria

Obstructive nephropathy
Toxic
1. Analgesic nephropathy
2. Opiate abuse

Multisystem diseases
1. Systemic lupus erythematosus
2. Vasculitis
3. Progressive systemic sclerosis

Haemolytic uraemic syndrome
Tumours
1. Wilms' tumour
2. Renal cell carcinoma
3. Incidental carcinoma
4. Myeloma

Congenital
1. Hypoplasia
2. Horseshoe kidney

Irreversible acute renal failure
1. Cortical necrosis
2. Acute tubular necrosis

Trauma

All patients between the ages of 2 and 70, who require dialysis or expect to require dialysis within the next 12 months, will be considered for transplantation. It is important to satisfactorily resolve other co-morbidities to increase the safety of the transplant. Patients must be evaluated early to allow them to consider their options for renal replacement therapy. This is particularly valuable since living donor kidney transplantation can be considered and timed appropriately to serve as renal replacement therapy, obviating the need for dialysis and access surgery. Live donation has increased significantly over the past 5 years with the advent of the laparoscopic donor operation. As a result, live donors now contribute up to 50% of the kidneys for transplantation in most large programmes in the UK.

Most patients are listed for a cadaver kidney when their creatinine clearance (Clcr), calculated by the Cockcroft–Gault formula, is less than 30 ml min^{-1}. The Cockcroft–Gault formula for calculation of the Clcr is now considered to be superior to actual measured creatinine clearance, as determined by 24-hour urine collection, due to inherent inaccuracies and collection difficulties. The creatine clearance formula is as follows:

Clcr (ml min^{-1}) = ((140 – age)(weight in kg))/(creatinine (mg dl^{-1}) ×72)

For women, the result is multiplied by 0.85.

Although all causes for kidney failure can be considered for transplantation, some causes of kidney failure, such as certain types of glomerulonephritis, may occasionally recur in the new transplant. In most cases, transplantation is worthwhile since recurrence is usually very slow to develop. These risks are discussed with patients on a case-by-case basis. Patients with primary oxalosis require combined kidney-liver transplantation since without metabolic correction of oxalosis with liver transplantation, recurrent kidney disease would be very rapid.

Diseases that may recur in renal transplants are:

- diabetes mellitus;
- systemic lupus erythematosis;
- IgA nephropathy;
- focal segmental glomerulosclerosis;
- membranous glomerulonephritis;
- membranoproliferative glomerulonephritis;
- amyloidosis;
- cystinosis.

Contraindications for kidney transplantation

There are certain absolute contraindications to renal transplantation:

1. disseminated or untreated cancer;
2. severe psychiatric disease;
3. unresolvable psychosocial problems;
4. persistent substance abuse;
5. severe mental retardation;
6. un-reconstructable coronary artery disease or refractory congestive heart failure.

Relative contraindications:

- Treated malignancy. The cancer-free interval required will vary from 2 to 5 years, depending on the stage and type of cancer.
- Substance abuse history. Patients must be involved in drug-free rehabilitation. This includes negative random toxicology screens.
- Chronic liver disease. Patients with chronic hepatitis B or C or persistently abnormal liver function testing must be seen by a hepatologist prior to consideration.
- Cardiac disease. All patients over the age of 55 or those with a history of diabetes, hypertension, or tobacco abuse must have dobutamine stress echocardiography, or exercise or pharmacologic stress cardiac scintigraphy. Any patient with a history of a positive stress test or history of congestive heart failure must have cardiology evaluation prior to consideration.

Structural genito-urinary abnormality or recurrent urinary tract infection. Urologic consultation is required prior to consideration.

Past psychosocial abnormality. Social work or psychiatry evaluation, as appropriate.

Aorto-iliac disease. Patients with abnormal femoral pulses or disabling claudication, rest pain or gangrene will require evaluation by a vascular surgeon prior to consideration. Patients with significant aorto-iliac occlusive disease may require angioplasty or aorto-iliac grafting prior to transplantation.

Special consideration needs to be given to:

morbid obesity;

antibody status;

re-transplantation;

HIV-positive recipients.

ndications for simultaneous pancreas-kidney (SPK) transplantation patients with insulin-dependent (type 1, juvenile diabetes) diabetes who have end-stage renal disease (ESRD) and require dialysis or expect to require dialysis in the next 12 months may be considered for SPK transplantation. Special care is taken to exclude recipients with type 2 diabetes. Candidates with a strong family history, or late age or gestational onset, have a C-peptide level determined after glucose loading. Only those individuals with C-peptide levels of 0.2 ng ml^{-1} are further considered for transplantation. In addition, evidence of at least one type of progressive secondary diabetic complication including: diabetic retinopathy, diabetic neuropathy, diabetic gastroparesis and accelerated atherosclerosis should be present.

ndications for pancreas transplantation (solitary pancreas transplant, pancreas transplant alone, pancreas after kidney)

Patients with insulin-dependent (type 1, juvenile diabetes) diabetes may be candidates for pancreas transplantation if they have secondary diabetic complications that are progressive despite the best medical management. This includes patients for whom the indication is brittle diabetes and hypoglycaemic unawareness with evidence of frequent hypoglycaemic events, despite an attempt at optimal medical management. Patients with brittle diabetes as the primary indication should have evidence of impairment of employability, hypoglycaemic-induced accidents involving themselves or small children in their care. Usually there is evidence of frequent emergency care for hypoglycaemia or diabetic ketoacidosis. In some cases these patients will have received a prior kidney transplant, usually from a living donor (living donor kidney transplant alone, LDKTA). Absolute and relative contraindications for pancreas transplantation are similar to those for kidney transplantation. Special consideration needs to be given to the cardiovascular system because of the high incidence of asymptomatic coronary artery disease in this population. All type 1 diabetic patients require dobutamine stress echocardiography.

Allocation and ethics of organs for transplantation

There is no doubt that there is a spectrum of ethical dilemmas within transplantation. These range from more straightforward issues, such as the allocation of scarce resources, to complex issues such as financial reward for organ donation and xenotransplantation.

The system of allocation of organs for transplantation in the UK varies with the individual organ. Factors common to different organs, which are important in allocation, are ABO blood group compatibility (all organs) and the comparative sizes of donors and recipient (liver, heart, heart/lung and lung). Other important considerations when allocating specific organs include: tissue matching (histocompatibility) in kidney transplantation; the MELD (Model for End-stage Liver Disease) score for liver transplantation; the quality of the donor organ and how appropriately it matches a particular recipient, especially as it relates to marginal donors and recipients; and the concept of transplant benefit, currently being applied to lung transplantation in the USA.

All patients who are waiting for transplants in the UK are registered on the National Transplant Database held by UK Transplant – now part of an organisation linked with the National Blood Service called National Blood and Transplant (NHSBT).

Currently UK Transplant run organ-specific national allocation schemes with an overarching principle of ensuring patients are treated equally. Donated organs are allocated in a fair and unbiased way, based on the patient's need and the importance of achieving the closest possible match between donor and recipient. Kidneys are allocated according to a national waiting list based on a weighted scoring system, which includes waiting time, time on dialysis, sensitization levels and tissue match. Liver grafts are allocated to the centre which prioritizes locally based on the MELD/UKELD score (bilirubin, INR, creatinine and serum sodium) equating to how 'sick' the potential recipient is. This has been validated in the USA to predict survival up to 3 months post transplant. Currently no potential recipient can be registered for a liver transplant unless they meet the minimum listing criteria, which is a UKELD score of 49 [2]. A national allocation system for liver transplantation operates for patients with acute liver failure deemed to have less than 72 hours to live. These patients are categorized as 'super-urgent'. Pancreas grafts are currently allocated to the retrieving centre unless there is a potential recipient nationally who was previously sensitized but has been shown to be suitable for a particular graft. These are patients usually those who have transplanted previously and are awaiting a 'window of opportunity'.

Some patients have a greater clinical need, resulting in others waiting longer. Donation rates are greater in some ethnic groups, while in other ethnic groups the need for transplantation is greater. Utilitarian principles therefore compete against duty-based ones.

Organ donation and transplantation are covered by the Human Tissue Act 2004 in England, Wales and Northern Ireland and by the Human Tissue (Scotland) Act 2006. Consent, or authorisation in Scotland, is the fundamental principle of both acts and is required before organs can be removed from the deceased, stored and used. Consent is also required from live patients offering organs, but is covered by common law.

The number of people needing organ transplants in the UK is far greater than the number of donor organs available (Figure 25.1). In the financial year 2007–8 there were 2385 organs transplanted from 809 deceased donors with a further 839 live donor transplants, but there were 7655 patients on the active waiting list. This list grows at 8% per year, with approximately 1000 potential recipients dying each year while waiting or becoming too ill for a transplant.

This means there has to be a system in place to ensure that patients are treated equally and that donated organs are allocated in a fair and unbiased way, based on the patient's need and the importance of achieving the closest possible match between donor and recipient. The underlying ethical principles are straightforward in that organs should be allocated irrespective of age, gender, race, religion or social standing. But the reality is more

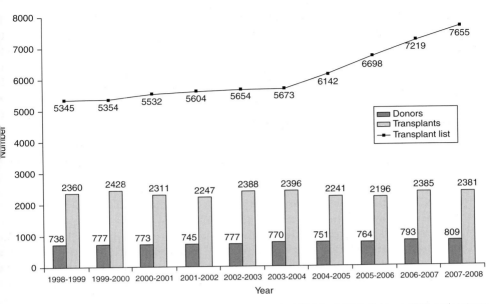

Figure 25.1 The number of deceased donors and transplants in the UK, 1 April 1998–31 March 2008, and patients on the active transplant list.

complex because organs are a scarce resource and not every individual who needs an organ will receive one.

Many of the ethical issues that require consideration in decisions to offer transplantation to one patient in preference to another are shared in common, irrespective of the specific organ or tissue to be transplanted. Factors that must be taken into account in organ allocation include:

1. Selection of the sickest patient: an offer of an organ to the patient most likely to die without it might appear the most reasonable basis for organ allocation. However, this method may also select the poorest outcome. This is not necessarily the 'best use' of a limited resource.

2. Selection of the patient most likely to benefit based on medical or other criteria: if the major emphasis in organ allocation is placed on guaranteeing that the greatest number of transplanted organs are accepted and survive for the longest time, a preference should be for the best possible tissue match in the patient with the best outlook. Whilst this approach appears acceptable in isolation, it conflicts with a number of other criteria. This would disadvantage any potential recipient with advanced disease and result in an impaired chance of success. The best way of applying this criterion is, having identified patients with similar priority for allocation on other grounds, further choice might favour that case most likely to be successful.

3. Selection of the patient on the waiting list for the longest period: the length of a prior waiting period appears fair. This criterion has identifiability and defensibility. Against adopting this as the sole criteria is the fact that if a patient has survived for a long period after meeting the requirements for entry to a waiting list this might indicate that he or she was in better condition than others on that list. The question might then be whether his or her 'need' was less.

4. All patients on the waiting list should have an equal chance of selection: it has the advantage of being seen to be free of any favouritism. However, its application is impractical. The method could only have a place in rare situations where several possible recipients are judged to have equal priority on medical and other grounds (this sometimes happens in the case of kidney transplantation).

5. Selection of patients on the basis of their importance for the well-being of others: is it appropriate for a patient with a young family, dependent upon him or her for support, or an individual with the capacity to make a unique contribution to his or her community, to be accorded priority. This criterion raises questions about the manner in which selection attributes are to be quantified and of who is entitled to do so. During the early years of kidney transplantation programmes in the USA this was considered and subsequently rejected.

6. Preference or not in selection to patients who have previously had one or more transplants: patients who have already been transplanted but who have had the misfortune of a failed graft, and so received no benefit, might be seen to have a claim for priority for another try or conversely – 'have had their chance'. Here the type of organ graft is of importance. For example, recipients with failing liver or heart grafts facing imminent death may achieve priority for this reason. Renal recipients may return to dialysis following graft failure, but the basis of loss of the first graft may persist (for example, high antibody titres) and remain transplantable at a later date.

7. Capacity of the patient to pay: equal access to medical care for all, irrespective of capacity to pay, is a basic principle of the NHS.

8. What about a potential recipient's lifestyle in selection for transplant allocation? There are many who would argue that self-inflicted illnesses such as alcoholism and drug abuse, necessitating liver transplantation due to alcoholic cirrhosis or HCV cirrhosis should lessen a patient's eligibility to be allocated a donor organ. The concern revolves around the extent to which recurrence of alcoholism or HCV in the new graft may compromise a successful outcome to transplantation. Any case for exclusion from organ transplantation because of a self-inflicted illness involves non-medical 'social' judgements. Whenever the issue of possible exclusion of patients with a particular lifestyle from access to any form of treatment that remains available to others is considered, it is essential that attention be given to the development of processes that will ensure adequate representation of the views and needs of marginalised groups and this includes HIV co-infection in haemophiliac patients as well.

9. Can we exclude patients on the basis of anticipated lack of compliance: apart from recidivism leading to a recurrence of the disease that required treatment originally, grounds for exclusion might arise if there was considerable likelihood that a patient would not be prepared to participate in essential post-transplant treatment, for example the use of immunosuppressive agents. The reliability of any prediction leading to exclusion creates a substantial ethical issue in most transplant units.

In *Transplantation Ethics*, Robert Veatch outlines an interesting way of assessing need [3]. He calls it the 'over-a-lifetime perspective'. This approach takes into consideration a person's entire life when determining who is worst off. A 17-year-old and an 80-year-old both dying of liver failure are equally badly off, but this perspective allows that the person who has had 63 more years of life is better off, so the 17 year old is neediest. Veatch writes, 'from this over-a-lifetime perspective, justice requires that we target organs for these younger persons who are so poorly off that they will not make it to old age without being given special priority – the younger the age of the person, the higher the claim.' This furthers the goal of utilising organs to their maximum potential. Presently, our system of allocation gives priority to those who are the sickest or most in need of a transplant. But sometimes those who are the sickest and in the most immediate need will not receive the same benefit from the transplant as someone whose medical condition is currently more stable. They may be so sick that they have a higher chance of dying regardless of treatment. There is a moral obligation, due to the scarcity of organs, to maximise the potential longevity of donated organs and place them where they are most likely to do the most good (bring the most health) over the longest period of time.

Donors and the donor procedure

The widening gap between organ demand and supply has resulted in the relaxation of the criteria for organ donation as the clinician must weigh up the risk of transplanting the organ against dying on the waiting list. There are however, contraindications, all of which are relative (Table 25.2). It is highly unlikely however that an individual with an active extra-cranial malignancy would be considered as a donor.

It is important to note that organs used in transplantation can come from very different clinical scenarios (Table 25.3).

Death confirmed by brainstem testing

The majority of donors in the UK come from heart-beating donors. Death is defined as irreversible loss of capacity for consciousness and the irresversible loss of the capacity to breath. Before organ procurement can commence, death by brainstem testing needs to be performed according to the UK code, which involves three steps.

1. Preconditions – comatose patient with irreversible injury, on a ventilator (>6–24 hours after last intervention aimed at reversing injury), with an identified underlying cause for coma.
2. Exclusions – no drugs, alcohol, neuromuscular blocking agents or hypothermia.
3. Clinical testing – these tests (two sets of tests at least 2–3 hours apart performed by two senior medical personnel) demonstrate absent brainstem relexes and total apnoea (Table 25.4).

All the major religions of the UK support the principles of organ donation and transplantation. However, within each religion there are different schools of thought, which mean that views may differ. All the major religions accept that organ donation is an individual choice.

The donor operation

The principles are as follows:
Preparation with antibiotics and neuromuscular blockade (to prevent spinal reflexes). Exposure is achieved through a midline laparotomy and sternotomy with pericardotomy. The colon and small bowel are reflected superiorly to expose the inferior mesenteric vein (IMV) and the aortic bifurcation. Hepatic vasculature is dissected to their origin (alternative arterial vasculature is identified), portal dissection and division of the bile duct is performed. The thoracic organs are then dissected.

Table 25.2 Organ donation (relative) contraindications

- Human immunodeficiency virus (HIV)/active hepatitis B infection
- Extra-cranial malignancy (current) or cranial
- Glioblastoma/medulloblastoma
- Severe systemic sepsis
- Disease of unknown aetiology

Table 25.3 Donor categories

Category	Description	
Non-heart beating donors (Maastricht classification)		
I	Brought in dead	Uncontrolled
II	Unsuccessful resuscitation	Uncontrolled
III	Awaiting cardiac arrest	Controlled
IV	Cardiac arrest after brain-stem death	Controlled
V	Cardiac arrest in a hospital inpatient	Uncontrolled
Heart beating donors (brain stem dead)	Usually patients in intensive care units having sustained irreversible brain damage (e.g. intracranial haemorrhage, cerebrovascular accident or head injury)	
Live donors	Increasingly common in kidney and liver donation	

Table 25.4 Brainstem death tests

- Absent brainstem relexes
- No pupillary response to light
- Absent corneal reflexes
- Absent vestibulo-ocular reflex
- No motor response to adequate stimuli in cranial nerve distribution
- No gag reflex to bronchial stimulation by suction catheter
- Apnoea testing
- No attempt to breathe despite a $P_aCO_2 > 6.5$ kPa. Hypoxia avoided by preoxygenation with 100% oxygen for 10 minutes

- Perfusion cannula is placed in the aorta, the aorta is cross-clamped and 4l of cold perfusate passed through the cannula. The inferior vena cava (IVC) is opened in the chest and the abdomen filled with ice.
- Procurement of the liver is by done by dividing the arterial supply with an aortic patch, dividing the IVC just above the renal veins, the superior vena cava (SVC) during the cardiectomy and the portal vein preserving maximum length. Procurement of the kidneys is done by dividing the ureters as long as possible (with adequate tissue around

them to preserve blood supply), preserving the renal arteries on an aortic patch and the renal veins on an IVC patch. Important steps in procurement of the pancreas (in combination with liver procurement) involve identification and division of the splenic artery, preservation of the superior mesenteric artery and the length of the portal vein. After removal of the liver the duodenum is stapled at the pylorus and 4th part, and remaining attachments to the small bowel and transverse colon are divided. Following pericardotomy and mobilisation of the great vessels, the SVC is ligated and divided, the aorta cross-clamped and the heart perfused with a cardioplegic agent via an anterior aortic puncture. After cardiac arrest the heart is emptied via incisions in the IVC and left pulmonary vein. The heart is excised by dividing all the remaining attachments. The procurement of the lungs follows as for the heart, except a perfusion cannula is placed in the pulmonary artery, and the left heart is vented via the tip of the atrial appendage as opposed to the pulmonary vein. Following manual venting the trachea is stapled and divided above to keep the lungs inflated during transport.

- Completion of the procurement involves removing a portion of spleen and mesenteric lymph nodes (tissue typing and cross-matching), iliac vessels (conduits) and removal of blood and neat abdominal closure.

Operative technique
Liver transplantation
The operative technique can be classified based on the position of the graft in the receipient (orthotopic if graft is placed in the usual position and heterotropic if placed elsewhere in the body), whether all or part of the graft is transplanted (whole graft or partial graft transplantation) and whether the native liver (or part of it) is retained (auxiliary graft). Partial grafts can be a split liver, when the liver is divided for implantation into two recipients, or a reduced-size graft, when only one part is retained to be transplanted.

Living donor transplantation and rarely domino transplantations are other techniques used.

Standard liver transplantation technique
In this method recipient hepatectomy is performed en bloc with the retrohepatic cava. Subsequently the whole graft is implanted by end-to-end anastomosis of the supra and infra hepatic inferior vena cavae to the graft's vena cava. Then the donor portal vein is anastmosed end-to-end with the recipient's portal vein, following which the graft is revascularised. The arterial anastamosis is performed between the graft artery and the recipient hepatic artery. If the recipient hepatic artery is not suitable then the graft artery can be anastamosed directly to the recipient's aorta or by using an arterial conduit. Lastly biliary anastamosis is performed using a duct-to-duct technique or a Roux-en-Y biliary reconstruction. T-Tubes are not routinely used.

The operative technique has evolved with time and more and more surgeons perform liver transplantation using some, if not all, of the following modifications.

Veno-venous bypass
Cross clamping of the vena cava, which is a requirement for the classical method, often results in haemodynamic instability and congestion of splanchnic circulation. Diverting the

blood from the portal vein and inferior vena cava to either the jugular or axillary vein on one side (veno-venous bypass) overcomes this problem.

Preservation of vena cava

In this technique the recipient's retrohepatic inferior vena cava is preserved during initial hepatectomy by dissecting the liver off the vena cava. This maintains the blood flow in the cava thus avoiding the need for systemic venous bypass. In addition a transient porto-caval shunt may also be constructed to maintain splanchnic flow.

With the recipient cava intact the caval anastamosis can be performed with direct end-to-end anastamosis of the donor cava to the unified stump of the recipient's hepatic veins or alternatively performing a lateral cavo-cavostomy on the anterior wall of the recipient vena cava.

Kidney transplantation

The kidney transplant operation has been standardised over the last few decades. Unlike liver transplantation, the transplanted kidney is placed in a heterotropic extraperitoneal location, usually in the iliac fossa. A curvilinear incision in a lower quadrant of the abdomen (Gibson's incision) is made, with division of the muscles of the abdominal wall and dissection of the preperitoneal space to expose the iliac vessels and the bladder. The renal vein and artery are anastamosed to the recipient iliac vein and artery, respectively. Then an ureteroneocystostomy is created, with or without placement of a ureteric stent. If a stent is used it is important to remove this in a few weeks to prevent complications of a non-removed stent (e.g. haematuria, renal stones, infection).

The kidney may be placed on either side, depending on history of previous transplantation, surgeon preference and the side of the donor kidney.

Pancreas transplantation

The pancreas may be transplanted simultaneously with a kidney (SPK), sometimes following a kidney transplant (PAK – pancreas after kidney) or as a pancreas alone (PTA).

The back table preparation of the pancreas is a crucial part of the procedure and this can usually take 2 hours. Following careful ligation of all peri-pancreatic tissue to prevent bleeding at re-perfusion, an iliac Y graft from the donor is anastamosed to the superior mesenteric artery (SMA) and the splenic artery of the pancreas graft. The Y graft construction avoids the need for two separate arterial anastamoses betwen the donor and the recipient to vascularise the pancreas graft. Futher important preparation of the graft involves merticulous attention to controlling the route of the small bowel mesentary, as well as preparing the portal vein.

In SPK transplantation, the pancreas is implanted first due to the lower ischaemia tolerence of the pancreas. The pancreas is usually placed in an intraperitoneal position, although extraperitoneal placement can also be done. The graft portal vein is commonly anastamosed to the recipient lower inferior vena cava. Alternatively the venous drainage can be put into the portal circulation (graft superior mesenteric vein), giving the theoretical benefit of avoiding hyperinsulinaemia, which has been linked to atherogenesis. The Y graft is anastamosed to the lower aorta or the common iliac artery (CIA). The management of exocrine secretion is still a matter of considerable debate. The donor duodenum can be anastamosed to a Roux-en-Y loop of recipient small bowel (enteric drainage) or alternatively this can be anastamosed to the recipient urinary bladder (bladder drainage).

Postoperative complications

Organ transplantation is susceptible to all the recognised complications of any major surgical procedure (e.g. bleeding, infection, hernia). There are, however, issues that can arise that are specific to organ transplanation. There are complications that are common to all transplants and some specific to individual organs. The manifestation of each complication can differ according to the organ involved. Complications are classified into early and late.

Liver

Early

1. Primary nonfunction – this can manifest as haemodynamic instability, hypoglycaemia, elevated transaminases, coagulopathy, minimal bile output, encephalopathy, systemic acidosis and renal failure. This is not compatible with life and most patients require re-grafting (incidence: 1–3%). More commonly one sees a less dramatic version of this scenario called initial poor function or delayed graft function. This is often related to graft ischaemia and will improve.
2. Vascular thrombosis – arterial thrombosis can be early or late. This is more common in the paediatric population and can manifest as rapid or slow deterioration of graft function or as necrosis of bile ducts (incidence: adult liver transplant 2–4%; paediatric liver transplant 8–10%).
3. Bile leak – occurs usually due to ischaemia of the donor duct or rarely an operative technical problem (incidence: 20%).
4. Infection – this remains the most significant complication in liver transplantation and is responsible for most of the early mortality from bacterial infections with resistant gram-positive bacteria dominating in the first month. Multi-resistant bacterial and fungal infections become a more prominent and life-threatening issue if infection persists.
5. Acute rejection – with the advent of the newer and more potent immunosuppressive drugs this has become less of an issue in transplantation in general. It may present with fever, abdominal pain and elevated liver enzymes. The diagnosis is confirmed by a liver biopsy and most episodes are responsive to augmentation of immunosuppression with high dose corticosteroids.

Late

1. Arterial stenosis – presentation is with slow deterioration of graft function.
2. Infection – late infections are usually due to opportunistic pathogens such as cytomegalovirus, candida, aspergillosis, cryptococcus, legionella.
3. Chronic rejection – this is seen months or years after transplantation with poor synthetic liver function and hyperbilirubinemia.
4. Biliary stricture – patients present with obstructive jaundice, usually due to an ischaemic stricture.
5. Recurrent disease – recurrence of viral hepatitis is likely within a short time in infected patients but this may be mild and in many cases will not result in graft loss.
6. Cancer – recurrence if the patient was transplanted for HCC (outcome for small tumours: 75% 5-year survival). De Novo tumours such as skin cancers, lymphomas and others may occur in up to 3% of transplant recipients. This is most often secondary to immunosuppression.

7. Others – diabetes, hyperlipidaemia, hypertension and metabolic bone disease – these are related to the immnosuppression agents.

Kidney

Early

1. Acute tubular necrosis (ATN) and delayed graft function – some degree of ATN occurs in 5–30% of all heart-beating cadaveric donor transplantations. Delayed graft function may be associated with a reduction in the 5-year graft survival by up to 10% in some studies.
2. Primary non-function – the kidney never functions.
3. Arterial thrombosis – causes early postoperative oliguria or anuria. Immediate re-exploration is the only chance for salvaging such a graft.
4. Venous thrombosis – can result from technical error or kinking or compression of the renal vein.
5. Acute rejection – incidence varies but with newer immunosuppression and pre-emptive treatment most centres report acute rejection rates of 10–20%. Diagnosis requires biopsy and treatment usually involves steroid boluses.
6. Ureteral obstruction – could be due to blood clot in catheter, haematoma or oedema.
7. Urinary fistula – this occurs due to disruption of the ureteroneocystostomy or ureteral necrosis. Fluid biochemistry showing urea content several folds higher than that of serum is diagnostic.
8. Infection – 30–60% will suffer some type of infection during the first year. Conventional bacterial infections occur during the first month. Infections can be confused with rejection.

Late

1. Renal artery stenosis – patients present with hypertension and diminished renal function. This presentation can be confused with that of rejection. The aetiology of renal artery stenosis is frequently technical. Most instances can be managed with percutaneous transluminal angioplasty.
2. Ureteral obstruction – late presentation could be due to ureteral stenosis.
3. Lymphocele – manifests weeks or months postoperatively with swelling of the wound, oedema of the scrotum or labia and lower extremity and urinary obstruction from pressure on the collecting system or ureter. The treatment of choice is fenestration of the cyst into the peritoneal cavity and external drainage should be avoided as this puts the kidney at risk of infection.
4. Infection – the period between 30 and 180 days postoperative is the usual time for opportunistic infections as this coincides with the period of maximal immunosuppression. Viral infections are more important (e.g. cytomegalovirus). Other pathogens include aspergillosis, blastomycosis, nocardiosis, toxoplasmosis, cryptococcosis, candida and *Pneumocystis carinii*.
5. Hypergylcaemia – this is generally attributed to corticosteroid administration and previously normoglycaemic patients may become diabetic.
6. Hyperparathyroidism – patients could suffer from tertiary hyperparathyroidism with significant hypercalcaemia and elevated parathyroid hormone levels despite a functioning graft. This is treated by total parathyroidectomy.

7. Cancers – in renal transplant recipients an incidence of 6% is reported for de novo malignant neoplasms. This is related to the duration and degree of immunosuppression rather than to any particular agent. More prevalent tumours are skin cancers (squamous cell carcinomas), lymphomas, renal cancers, Kaposi's sarcoma, carcinoma of the vulva and uterine cervix.
8. Post-transplant lymphoproliferative disease (PTLD) – term used to cover the spectrum of disease from benign hyperplasia to malignant lymphomas. Epstein–Barr virus is implicated as the most important factor in PTLD.
9. Chronic allograft nephropathy – this complication is characterised by a progressive decline in kidney function, which is not attributable to a specific cause. Chronic changes to the kidney allograft are mediated by both immune and non-immune factors.
10. Recurrent disease – Glomerulonephritides (eg, mesangiocapillary glomerulonephritis type 1, IgA nephropathy) are most likely to recur; however, loss of the kidney generally occurs late, and, thus, these diseases are not contraindications to transplantation. Similarly, patients with diabetes mellitus have poorer outcomes following transplantation than do patients without diabetes; nearly all patients demonstrate histological evidence of diabetic nephropathy within 4 years. Hence the treatment of choice for diabetics with renal failure is combined kidney and pancreas transplantation.

Pancreas
Complications and issues specific to pancreas transplantation are discussed below.

Early
1. Vascular thrombosis – this is the most common non-immunological cause of graft loss.
2. Allograft pancreatitis – this occurs in 10–20% of all pancreas graft recipients. In its most severe form it can result in graft necrosis and arterial thrombosis. This entity is difficult to detect and can be confused with rejection and pancreatic fistula.
3. Pancreatic fistula – this is more common in enteric-drained than in bladder-drained grafts.
4. Rejection – hyperglycaemia is a late indicator of rejection as islet damage results by the time such physiological evidence results. Rejection of a kidney and pancreas transplanted simultaneously from the same donor often occurs at the same time. In such patients careful monitoring of serum creatinine level is a sensitive indicator of rejection.

Late
1. Urological complications – haematuria, urethritis, recurrent urinary tract infections, and bicarbonate loss are common in bladder-drained recipients. This can necessitate enteric conversion if it does not respond to conservative treatments.
2. Autoimmune recurrence – the autoimmnune response to native islets can be responsible for loss of transplanted pancreatic β-cells.

Graft rejection and immunosuppression
With the exception of identical twins the organ donor and recipient are genetically different. Without medical manipulation a transplanted graft will be rejected within a number of days. Understanding the rejection process is a prerequisite to understanding the principles of immunospressive medication.

The rejection process

Organs are rejected as the recipient body recognises the graft as 'foreign'. This recognition is based on the fact that the graft major histocompatability complex (MHC) is different to that of the host cell. The role of the MHC is to present antigens for other immunological cells to screen. The antigens relevant to transplantation were first defined seriologically on leucocytes and are therefore called the human leucocyte antigens (HLAs). Minor histocompatability systems (miHs) are of limited clinical importance in solid organ transplantation. Major histocompatability class I proteins are found on most nucleated cells. They present antigens and are recognised by the T-cell receptor (TCR) on T-cells bearing the CD8 protein. CD8 T-cells cause lysis of the target (graft) cell. Major histocompatability class II proteins are found on B lymphocytes and dendritic cells (antigen-presenting cells). They present antigens and are recognised by the T-cell receptor on T-cells bearing the CD4 protein. CD4 cells are referred to as 'helper' cells and have crucial specialised functions in the generation of the immune response (and therefore graft rejection) such as cytotoxic T-cell generation, B-cell maturation.

For immunological cells to be activated however, in addition to this MHC (with antigen)–T-cell receptor (TCR) interaction, various co-stimulatory signals are needed. Many have been detected (e.g. Il-2, the CD28-B7 and CD40ligand-CD40 family), which is important when searching for immunosuppressive agents. It is noted that other cellular (natural killer cells) and humoral (antibodies) mechanisms of rejecton exist.

Immunosuppressive agents

The main immunosuppressive groups and their mode of action are documented in Table 25.5. In solid organ transplantation, many immunosuppressive protocols have been used, but broadly speaking most protocols are based on the principles outlined below a calcineurin inhibitor, an antimetabolite and a reducing dose of steroid. In selected cases protein immunosuppressives are given. The calcineurin inhibitor is sometimes exchanged for sirolimus at 3 month post-transplantation (Table 25.5).

Outcome

Outcomes have steadily improved due to better surgical techniques and more effective immunosuppressive treatments and the development of transplant specialists and teams. Transplants are now so successful in the UK that a year after surgery:

- 94% of kidneys in living donor transplants are still functioning well;
- 88% of kidneys from people who have died are still functioning well;
- 86% of liver transplants are still functioning well;
- 84% of heart transplants are still functioning well;
- 77% of lung transplants are still functioning well;
- 73% of heart/lung transplants are still functioning well.

Longer-term outcomes are similarly improving although most organs, with the exception of liver grafts, suffer from 'chronic fatigue' otherwise known as 'chronic rejection'. Most transplanted organs are still functioning at 5 and 10 years but the percentage attrition rate varies from 10% at 5 years for livers through to 25% for lungs. A recent analysis based on 3673 adult liver recipients for whom the 15-year patient survival rate was 58% (95% confidence interval

Table 25.5 Immunosuppressive agents

Immunosuppressive agent group	Examples	Mode of action	Side effects (in addition to infection)
Drugs acting on immunophillins – calcineurin inhibitor (CNI) It has been in use since 1983 and is one of the most widely used group of immunosuppressive drugs	Tacrolimus Cyclosporin	Forms a complex with immunophillins and inhibits calcineurin, which under normal circumstances induces the transcription of interleukin-2. The drug also inhibits lymphokine production and interleukin release, leading to a reduced function of effector T-cells	Nephrotoxicity Neurotoxicity Diabetes Marrow suppression
Corticosteroids	Prednisolone	Multiple immunomodulatory effects e.g. reduces interleukin (IL) production and hence activation of B- and T-cells, reduces immune cells protein transcription.	Multiple including hyperglycaemia, obesity, osteoporosis, skin fragility
Antimetabolites	Azothiaprine Mycophenolate Mofetil	Inhibits synthesis pathway of B- and T-cells.	Gastrointestinal (nausea, vomiting, diarrhoea, ulcers, gastritis) Bone marrow suppression
mTOR inhibitor (mammalian target of rapamycin)	Sirolimus	Inhibits response to IL-2 and hence blocks activation of B- and T-cells.	Hyperlipidaemia Leukopenia Thrombocytopenia Poor tissue healing
Protein immunosuppressives	Antithymocyte globulin	Contains cytotoxic/blocking antibodies (anti-CD2, 3, 4, 8, 11a, 18, 25, 44, 52, HLA classes I and II) to circulating lymphocytes	
	Anti-IL-2 (CD25) receptor Dacluzumab Basiliximab	Blocks IL-2 and the resulting activation of B and T-cells.	
	Anti-CD52 Alemtuzumab	Causes apoptosis of circulating lymphocytes, monocytes, macrophages and natural killer cells	

54–62%) suggests that adult liver transplant recipients have an average life expectancy of 22 years. The average life expectancy of the equivalent UK adult population is 30 years, and so on average 8 years of life are lost. Furthermore, female recipients lose fewer life-years than male recipients, and younger recipients lose more life-years than older recipients.

References

1. Devlin J, O'Grady J. Indications for referral and assessment in adult liver transplantation: a clinical guideline. British Society of Gastroenterology. *Gut* 1999; **45** Suppl 6: VI1–VI22.
2. Neuberger J, Gimson A, Davies etal. and Liver Advisory Group; UK Blood and Transplant. Selection of patients for liver transplantation and allocation of donated livers in the UK. *Gut* 2008; **57**: 252–7.
3. Veatch RM. Transplantation Ethics. Washington, DC: Georgetown University Press 2000.

Further reading

1. British Transplant Society. Standards for solid organ transplantation, 2003. http://www.bts.org.uk/Forms/standards%20document%20edition%202%20-%20final.pdf (accessed 1 March 2010).
2. Forsythe JLR. *Transplantation – A Companion to Specialist Surgical Practice*, 3rd edn. Philadelphia, PA: Elsevier Saunders, 2005.
3. United network for organ sharing. http://www.unos.org/ (accessed 1 March 2010).
4. *The Practice of Liver Transplantation.* Oxford: W.B. Saunders, 1995.
5. Talbot D, D'Alessandro A. *Organ Donation and Transplantation after Cardiac Death.* New York: Oxford University Press, 2009.
6. Clavier P-A, Petrowsky H, OeOlveira ML, Graf R. Strategies for safer liver surgery and partial liver transplantation. *NEJM* 2007; **356**: 1545–59.
7. Neuberger J, James O. Guidelines for selection of patients for liver transplantation in the era of donor-organ shortage. *Lancet* 1999; **354**: 206–14.
8. Hirschfield GM, Gibbs P, Griffiths WJH. Adult liver transplantation: what non-specialists need to know. *BMJ* 2009; **338**: b1670 1321–7.

Index